NARRATIVE THERAPY WITH OLDER ADULTS

NARRATIVE THERAPY WITH OLDER ADULTS

STORIES, WISDOM, RESILIENCE

Esther Oi-Wah Chow, Lauren Taylor, and Ada C. Mui

COLUMBIA UNIVERSITY PRESS   NEW YORK

COLUMBIA UNIVERSITY PRESS
Publishers Since 1893
New York   Chichester, West Sussex

Library of Congress Cataloging-in-Publication Data
Names: Chow, Esther Oi-Wah author | Taylor, Lauren (Social worker) author |
    Mui, Ada C., 1949– author
Title: Narrative therapy with older adults : stories, wisdom, resilience /
    Esther Oi-Wah Chow, Lauren Taylor, and Ada C. Mui.
Description: New York : Columbia University Press, [2025] |
    Includes bibliographical references and index.
Identifiers: LCCN 2024045442 | ISBN 9780231196062 hardback |
    ISBN 9780231196079 trade paperback | ISBN 9780231551625 ebook
Subjects: LCSH: Psychotherapy for older people | Narrative therapy
Classification: LCC RC480.54 .C46 2025 | DDC 616.89/1650846—
    dc23/eng/20250210

LCCN 2024045442

Cover design: Julia Kushnirsky
Cover images: Shutterstock

GPSR Authorized Representative: Easy Access System Europe,
Mustamäe tee 50, 10621 Tallinn, Estonia, gpsr.requests@easproject.com

CONTENTS

PREFACE

IN THIS PREFACE, we embark on a nontraditional approach, likening our book to a royal tapestry. We share the formation of our team and the start of our journey, while focusing on the central theme of educating our diverse readers—students, scholars, practitioners, older adults, and families—about the science, power, and significance of life-story narratives shaped by various cultures, societies, family, and social identities. Throughout this book, we delve into the art of storytelling, examining how individuals weave together the threads of their unique identities and experiences. By exploring the transformative impact of narrative practice, we illuminate how storytelling enables individuals to comprehend their lives, find meaning in their experiences, and navigate the complexities of their identities. Each person's story emerges as a tapestry interwoven with cultural, familial, and societal threads that shape their understanding of themselves and the world around them.

Our journey began in 2018 when Esther Chow, an esteemed gerontologist, teacher, researcher, and clinician in narrative practice, who was also a social work professor at the Department of Social and Behavioral Sciences of the City University of Hong Kong, visited Ada Mui, a distinguished professor at Columbia University School of Social Work. Both Chinese scholars, their collaboration was fueled by Esther's dream to write a book on narrative practice. Recognizing the richness that could be added to the book by examining how Eastern and Western cultures influence how older people remember, tell, and retell their life stories, Ada, serving as Esther's adviser, suggested the inclusion of another gerontologist. Lauren Taylor, an experienced psychotherapist, oral historian, and adjunct professor at Columbia University School of Social Work, was invited to join the team. With Ada at the helm, this dream team set out to craft a narrative tapestry, weaving together the threads of Chinese and American older adults' aging experiences, Eastern and Western cultures, aging research and clinical expertise, narrative theories, and practice skills, as well as the life stories of Chinese and American older adults.

Through the narrative skill *retelling*, we share the science and art of our professional and personal experiences in narrative practice, encompassing theories, research methods, measurements, and clinical encounters in both Hong Kong and New York City. This sharing allows the wonder and complexity of wisdom from the research participants and older adults and their families who have entrusted us with their personal narratives, to be contemplated, or even just enjoyed by future generations, like a shimmering royal tapestry in the finest gallery.

Our hope is that readers from all gerontological disciplines — students, scholars, and professionals — will benefit from its contents, finding their work with older people and families to be both more strategic in its effectiveness, and filled with deeper wonder and meaning. Additionally, we invite older individuals, regardless of their physical or cognitive challenges, and family members from diverse cultures to explore this book, seeing the value of life-story narratives and discovering pathways to meaning-making.

Our passion for studying and working with older adults arises from a profound sense of empathy and compassion, nurtured by our upbringing as well as by our professional social work training and practice in the field of aging. This book serves as a continuous learning project for all of us.

We extend our deepest gratitude to these cohorts of older adults and their families, and not-for-profit organizations, in our research and clinical work who have generously shared their personal narratives, life struggles, wisdom, and triumphs in the face of insurmountable challenges throughout their lives.

INTRODUCTION

1

ENGAGING OLDER ADULTS THROUGH NARRATIVE PRACTICE IN GERONTOLOGICAL SOCIAL WORK

MR. CHAN'S STORY   *Mr. Chan, a seventy-eight-year-old patient with lung cancer, was receiving hospice care. He came to the United States when he was in his thirties and lived by himself as an undocumented immigrant in New York City, working extremely hard in restaurants in order to send remittances to support his wife and five children in China. Before coming to the United States, Mr. Chan's family had left China in the 1960s and become refugees in Hong Kong during the traumatic Cultural Revolution, which was a sociopolitical movement in China. After he came to the United States, Mr. Chan was separated from his family for more than twenty years before he was granted asylum, at which point his family could migrate to New York. At the end of his life, Mr. Chan had depression. He had a deep sense of guilt and shame because he had conflictual relationships with his adult children. Mr. Chan felt that his life was a total failure and he was a "failed father" because he was not able to maintain harmonious relationships with his adult children as a result of his absence for so many years when they were growing up. Using narrative therapy, a social worker helped Mr. Chan to reflect on his "failed father" identity narrative, and to reconstruct the new preferred identity of "unsung hero." The amazing transformative journey, similar to Mr. Chan's experience from "failed father" to "unsung hero", is at the core of this book.*

GERONTOLOGICAL SOCIAL WORK AND NARRATIVE PRACTICE: DEFINITION AND APPLICATION

Narrative practice is a person-focused, democratic, bottom-up, and respectful intervention approach designed to support individuals, groups, and communities as they tackle the fraught existential question, "How has my life been meaningful?"[1] Narrative practice or intervention is based on the belief that people are the experts in their own life-story narratives. Narrative intervention uses people's life-story narratives as tools to help people define themselves through something other than their life's problems, while working from the assumption that people have strengths, insight, life skills, capacities, beliefs, values, commitments, and abilities that will help them reduce the impact of problems on their lives. In the dialectic conversation process of narrative intervention, gerontological social workers empower older adults to tell their life stories, reconnect to their core values, organize their thoughts, uncover opportunities for growth and development, find meaning and purpose, and revitalize preferred identities to reduce the negative impact of life challenges. This form of therapy was developed in the 1980s by Michael White and David Epston.[2] Narrative intervention can stand on its own, or it can be integrated into care plans for older adults across a variety of different care settings, ranging from community-based and home care to hospitals, nursing homes, and hospice care.[3] Mr. Chan is one example of those whom gerontological social workers serve by providing narrative therapy and an array of other intervention services to meet his biopsychosocial and spiritual needs and to provide support to his family. In addition to narrative intervention, Mr. Chan and his family also received case management, family therapy, mutual help groups, grief counseling, and end-of-care services.

Narrative intervention has been used to support people of all ages with different problems in different cultures.[4] This form of counseling is especially helpful for diverse client populations affected by life trauma who experience a problem-saturated identity, including immigrants; minorities; gender groups; racial, multiethnic, interracial, and biracial groups; and interreligious individuals, couples, groups, and communities.[5] In the context of providing services to older populations, narrative intervention encourages older adults to tell, retell, reflect, reauthor, and understand their life stories and to learn how societal and cultural discourses affect their life-story narratives and how they interpret the problems they have faced and overcome.

Mr. Chan's depression may have been due to multiple levels of personal and social trauma associated with being an undocumented immigrant, asylee, low-wage earner, non-native-English speaker, absent father, failed father, and dying patient. For Mr. Chan, his most salient problem-saturated social identity was "failed father." In Chinese culture, the father's role as a guide and discipliner is one of the most important values. In his life-story narrative, Mr. Chan expressed that he had been negatively affected by his problem-saturated "failed father" identity, but no other social identities. Narrative work focuses on people's ability to reconceptualize and externalize their life problem and reflect on the impact of the dominant discourses on their perception of the problem. Dominant discourses include the ideas, values, norms, and expectations that define social and family roles, gender identity, and race or ethnic identity. We are all part of multiple cultures and subcultures that influence our perception of success, failure, conformity, deviance, thoughts, feelings, and behaviors. Older people may experience mental health problems and challenges when these influences on personal identify formation conflict with the dominant societal discourses and expectations.[6] By creating space and providing support for older adults, social workers can empower them to use their self-knowledge, life experiences, and abilities to reflect on and reinterpret life's challenges, change their perception of them, and take action to change and deal with them.

Narrative practice can have powerful, transformative effects. Mr. Chan's ability to change his problem-saturated "failed father" identity narrative to a reconstructed positive identify of "unsung hero" provided healing and gave him an sense of positive meaning in his life. The new identity honored his lifetime contribution to his family, especially during the time when they were separated. The new identity gave him comfort and peace about his purpose in living before he died. When reflecting on his life, Mr. Chan was able to connect the dots of his lifetime positively as a provider for his family, and for the first time, he was able to feel proud of himself for the role he played in his children's accomplishments and express that pride to them. This reflects a new sense of shared pride between him and his children, acknowledging both their achievements and his contributions. Two of his adult children earned doctoral degrees and three earned master's degrees in the United States after they reunited with Mr. Chan.

Gerontological social workers use a foundation of strengths-based and empowerment approaches when providing all services, including narrative intervention, to older adults; several strengths-based knowledge bases (chapter 3) that underpin these approaches are supported by empirical evidence (chapter 2) from strengths-based narrative interventions and will be explored in part I. Social workers who provide narrative intervention (chapter 4) to help transform older adults' beliefs should be as curious as a journalist and ask poignant questions respectfully. It is essential for social workers to work collaboratively with older adults, as a sort of coauthor in the older adult's life-story narrative conceptualization, formulation, and intervention processes.[7] Several different terms are used among professionals to describe narrative practices, and these differences are also reflected in this book. The terms *narrative* or *life story* are commonly used among social workers serving individual older clients in clinical settings. The term *narrative theory* is preferred over *life story* because narrative practice is more inclusive and, as it grows in use, it has become more nuanced, with many social workers providing different levels of interventions by revisiting their life stories with older people in both group and community settings. Parts II and III are a how-to, providing detailed discussions on transformative narrative practice with older people as individuals, families, groups, and collectives.

In this book, we share the knowledge, methodology, applications, and outcomes of narrative practice with Chinese older adults in Hong Kong and American older adults in New York City. We identify the distinctiveness and the commonalities between two different cultures—Eastern (relational-based) and Western (individual-based)—in terms of practice skills, efficacy, and effectiveness of narrative interventions for the unfolding wisdom of older adults. Specifically, one of the authors, Lauren Taylor from the United States, will share her narrative practice with older Americans in New York City in part II. The lead author, Esther Oi-Wah Chow, from Hong Kong, will share from her practice research on narrative work with older adults in a Hong Kong Chinese cultural context in part III. We hope that the research, knowledge, and skills that we share will shed light on how Eastern and Western dominant discourses influence older adults' life-story narratives, as well as the processes by which narrative interventions can best be provided to diverse older people in individual, group, and community settings. At the end of the book, we will summarize the salient lessons and practice wisdom learned from both Eastern and Western cultures. Life-story narratives of older individuals (all with disguised names) reflecting on different life stages will be shared throughout this book to illuminate the incredible beauty, the power, and the efficacy of narrative intervention with aging populations across cultures. To provide conceptual frameworks regarding how older persons from different cultures formulate and author their life-story narratives, in this introductory chapter, we will provide an overview of the ways that cognitive, psychological, social, and cultural factors could influence the formation, construction, and reconstruction of life-story narratives.

CULTURE'S EFFECT ON OLDER PERSONS' AUTOBIOGRAPHICAL MEMORY AND LIFE-STORY NARRATIVES

Culture has a strong effect on how a person both initially experiences the world and remembers the world.[8] Research suggests that the older adult life-story narrative is also affected by autobiographical memory.[9] Autobiographical memory is a complex set of memories—single, recurring, and extended events integrated into a coherent story of self that is created and evaluated through the sociocultural lens of the person who tells the life story.[10] These memories contain information that helps shape and define who we are. When we recall personal experiences by constructing a life-story narrative, we tell the memories of the sense of self, identity, social relationships, culture, and socialization processes. Cultures affect how older people experience and perceive the world as well as how they remember their lived experience during the life course.[11] Based on social cultural developmental theory,[12] people's memories of their autobiographical past were, and are, shaped by culture in terms of family and social norms and values, language and ways of communication, family and social expectations, and the individual's role in the family and society. This theory defines autobiographical memory as a function of various sociocultural factors that interact with basic memory systems, such as the acquisition of language, goal setting, family and social relationships, and psychological understanding of family and societal expectations.[13] Autobiographical memory emerges gradually and is influenced by ongoing cognitive development and social interaction throughout the lifespan. Cognitively speaking, autobiographical memory guides life-story narrative construction, content choice and selection, and presentation with themes and meaning; and it helps to define the sense of self and identity in time, the social expectation, and relationship network within a culture.[14] Research in this area has concluded that people coming from Eastern cultural backgrounds tend to have fewer and more generalized collective memories, whereas people coming from Western cultural backgrounds tend to have clearer, cohesive, highly specific memories.[15] This finding is interesting and intriguing.

Psychological research has shown that a strong correlation exists between individualistic and collectivistic cultures on the retrieval and the content of autobiographical memories.[16] According to empirical evidence, these cultural orientations influence people's memories starting from their formation in early childhood and continuing its influence into adulthood.[17]

In autobiographical memories, connections between self and the past are told and reminisced. In the narrative intervention process, life-story narratives are told based on memories. To use a metaphor, a narrative practice that will also be discussed in this book, our memories and sense of life meaning are in an ongoing, evolving dance. Social workers are needed to help in this dynamic of memory and meaning; social workers should not challenge the accuracy and content of the life-story narratives and need to respect older persons' narratives and their interpretation of life stories. Social workers also need to help coauthor those narratives that are problem saturated and that may cause a person to sit outside the dance and disengage in life; eventually, they need to guide them to reauthor their narrative and enjoy the dance again.

WESTERN INDIVIDUALISTIC AND EASTERN COLLECTIVISTIC CULTURES AND LIFE-STORY NARRATIVES

Culture is a complex variable. Some research in this area has conceptualized culture in terms of individualism or collectivism and its impact on autobiographical memory.[18] In narrative intervention, older people who are encouraged to tell and retell their life-story narratives are retrieving and expressing their autobiographical memories. The effect of the linguistic and cultural environment on autobiographical memories among older adults in Eastern (e.g., Chinese) and Western (e.g., American) cultures have also been examined.[19] How do social scientists study cultures? Research has used the concepts of individualism, group-based identity, and collectivism at the individual level as proxy measures of Western and Eastern cultures and participants' expression of self, identity, cultural traits, feelings of happiness, shame, guilt, personal success, and failure.[20] Findings suggest that people in Western individualistic cultures focus more on individual rights, assertiveness, creativity, self-enhancement, personal enjoyment, achievement, and the emotions of the protagonists; whereas people in Eastern relational and collectivistic cultures put greater emphasis on collective duties, humility, self-sacrifice, self-effacement, group identity and glory, social conformity, and compliance with moral and social standards, and place less emphasis on the emotions of the protagonists.[21] This trend continues into adulthood and late adulthood.

Research examining how individualism or collectivism affects people's description of the self and self-concepts has identified consistent findings.[22]

In individualistic cultures, the self is characterized as an independent and autonomous being. On the contrary, in collectivistic cultures, the self is regarded as only a part of the group and is interdependent. In individualistic cultures, people are more likely to focus on personal success and distinguish themselves from others; in collectivistic cultures, people are socialized to put the need and mission of the group, such as family, community, or political party, before their personal preference and to conform to family and social norms. With respect to the impact of culture on self-evaluation, the tendency to promote the "self" differs across cultures.[23] People in individualistic cultures report higher levels of self-enhancement than people in collectivistic cultures; conversely, the need for family enhancement (or even work enhancement) is more prevalent in Asian cultures than in Western individualistic cultures. Studies have also indicated that people in collectivistic cultures are more likely to express a modesty bias or other enhancement than people from individualistic cultures.[24] In Asian cultures, modest self-presentation is considered a virtue and strength.[25]

Studies on families and intergenerational characteristics have shown that individualistic cultures value autonomy, personal success, self-reliance, independence, and ambition. Collectivistic cultures value family cohesion, solidarity, conformity, cooperation, and personal sacrifice.[26] In other words, people from different cultures are different in their perception and description of self, family and social obligations, and world views as well as self-views.

From a life-course perspective, a few more research studies that have compared Eastern and Western cultures and autobiographical memories are worth adding to one's knowledge base when reading this book. Research showing how the sociolinguistic environment in which children grow up shapes their autobiographical memories.[27] Results have shown that American children's memories are focused on specific events, details, emotional expression, and lengthy individual experiences. For example, one child was described by positive traits and was viewed as being the protagonist in the narrative. In contrast, Chinese children's memories were found to be general, skeletal, less emotional, and more neutral in their expression and were focused on routine events, collective activities, social interactions, and relations with others. These patterns are seen because Western cultures promote autonomy and emphasize the individual's qualities, and children in these cultures are encouraged to assert and express themselves. Eastern cultures, however, promote cohesiveness and emphasize the group, and children in these cultures are discouraged from talking about themselves and instead to focus more on the family, society, and others around them.[28] These cultural influences on memory persist into adulthood and late adulthood, as seen in the life narratives shared in this book.

Another body of research found that American college students' memories were discrete, focused on specific events, and the individual's feelings, whereas Chinese college students' memories were more general, about routine activities, focusing on family and groups. Americans also stressed personal preferences and autonomy in lengthier narratives than the ones reported by the Chinese.[29] We do not make a value judgment in terms of inferiority or superiority of either Eastern or Western cultures. Our discussion provides evidence based on social science literature and stresses the importance of cultural competence and cultural humility in narrative practice. We also suggest that social workers be aware of and pay attention to individual variations, because research findings are merely statistical guides representing the group being studied.

Using this cultural lens, we hope our audience will increase their understanding of the cultural orientation of the older adults in Hong Kong, an example of Eastern (collectivistic) culture) as well as in New York City, an example of Western (individualistic) culture. At this point, the question is how Chinese and American older adults make meaning of their culturally shaped life-story narratives. These research findings are educational. As social work educators, we have learned to appreciate the diversity of learning and expression styles among our students. Social workers and social work educators need to be culturally competent and respect the diversity of cultural expressions in feelings and thoughts. We hope our readers will also be open and respectful while looking into and working with older adults from different cultures.

As part of this introduction, we will also provide a brief discussion on global and American population aging, Hong Kong Chinese aging, and important conceptual frameworks when working with older people.

POPULATION AGING AND ETHNIC DIVERSITY: A GLOBAL PERSPECTIVE

In the U.S. context, the sixty-five and older population is projected to nearly double from fifty-two million in 2018 to ninety-five million by 2060 (16 percent to 23 percent of the total U.S. population). The older U.S. population is becoming more racially and ethnically diverse.[30] Globally, by the year 2050, most Eastern and Western countries will have populations in which more than 20 percent of the people are over the age of sixty-five years, and there will be more people over the age of sixty than under the age of fifteen years.[31] Statistically, population aging is happening much faster in Asia than in most European and U.S. societies.[32] For example, the aging populations in Hong Kong, Macau, Singapore, and mainland China will increase by 243 percent from 2005 to 2050, as compared with the world's average of 113 percent.[32] By 2051, China's aging population is expected to peak at 438 million, which, in all likelihood, will outnumber the entire U.S. and European populations.[31] Because of cultural similarities, our research and knowledge on narrative intervention with Hong Kong Chinese older adults may shed light on the critical mass of older Chinese living in mainland China as well as older Chinese immigrants around the globe.

In the U.S. context, the diverse Asian American older adult population makes up one of the fastest-growing ethnic groups. The population of Asian American older adults increased by 76 percent during the 1990–2000 decade, and it has been projected to grow by 246 percent from 2000 to 2025. This growth is comparable with the 9.2 percent (in 2000) and 73 percent (in 2025) growth rates among the older white population.[33] Despite the rapid increase in the Asian American aging population, empirically based research with this population has been limited. At least thirty different Asian subgroups have been identified in the United States, including Asian Indian, Bangladeshi, Cambodian, Chinese, Filipino, Hmong, Indonesian, Japanese, Korean, Laotian, Malaysian, Pakistani, Sri Lankan, Taiwanese, Thai, and Vietnamese.[34]

Among all the nationalities within Asian American groups, the Chinese ethnic group was the largest group (25.4 percent). Note that there is diversity within diversity among the Chinese American populations as well.[35] Chinese American older adults represent several nationalities, including the majority from mainland China, Hong Kong, and Taiwan who speak Mandarin, Cantonese, Taiwanese, Taishanese, Fujianese, and many other languages. There are also ethnic Chinese older adults who came from southeast Asian countries, including Cambodia, Indonesia, Laos, Singapore, and Vietnam. Narrative intervention is one way to explore subcultural experiences and values and ethnic identity, and it also contributes to older adults' ability to cultivate deeper meaning in life by closely examining their lived experiences.

HONG KONG CHINESE AGING POPULATION: HISTORICAL AND CULTURAL BACKGROUNDS

Hong Kong had a population of just over seven million, with a density of approximately 6,300 people per square kilometer. According to the 2021 Hong Kong Census and Statistics information, about 12.17 percent of the population in Hong Kong were between birth and fourteen years old, 68.22 percent were between 15 and 64, and 19.6 percent were 65 years of age or older. The percentage of elderly people age sixty-five and above in the total population will gradually increase from 20.8 percent in mid-2022 to 25.3 percent in 2028, and then to 35.1 percent in 2069. Since 2010, Hong Kong boasts one of the longest life expectancies in the world, and it has been ranked number one worldwide for the longevity of its residents.

Aging is a meaning-making process, and older people set both their earlier and later life goals by internalizing the values and norms of their cultures. Aging and human development are a complex totality of personal and social experiences throughout the life course.[36] Cross-cultural evidence suggests that Chinese older people value the importance of interpersonal relatedness and interdependence more than their North American counter-parts.[37] Chinese older people value family and social connectedness more than self-esteem measures, and North American older adults scored higher in self-esteem measures than social relationship measures.[38]

Most Chinese in Asian regions and around the globe continue to be influenced by these Confucian values that have been passed down for centuries. The findings seem to be consistent with dominant Chinese cultural values that flow from Confucianism and Daoism. Main concepts of these Eastern philosophies are similar and include altruism and humility, righteousness, loyalty, knowledge, filial piety, submission, and obedience to authority. Confucianism, based on the teachings of Confucius (from 551 to 479 BC), is mainly a holistic moral code for human relationships with an emphasis on the importance of rites, and it has a long history in Chinese culture. Daoism is a religious philosophy that emphasizes living in har-mony with Tao, which is the principle of nature. Confucianism emphasizes that the family is the most important social institution of a society and that family members should show absolute loyalty and solidarity to their family and older parents. Adult children are expected to take care of their parents regardless of difficulties or circumstances. The most important social value is to achieve harmony and collective good in terms of interpersonal relatedness and interdependence.[39]

Statistically, more than 50 percent of older Chinese in Hong Kong were refugees from mainland China; therefore, they are more likely to have experienced accumulated trauma as a result of historical unrest in China over the past seven decades.[38] Chinese older people in mainland China born in the 1930s spent their early childhood years under Japanese military occupation and spent their adolescent years in the civil war between the Nationalists and the Communists, which followed the defeat of Japan in World War II. A significant number of Chinese fled to Taiwan or Hong Kong, and others stayed behind to witness Mao Zedong proclaim the establishment of the People's Republic of China in 1949. People of this generation who remained in mainland China spent their young adulthood under various land reforms and Mao's economic program known as the Great Leap Forward, which was an attempt to transform China from an agricultural economy to an industrial communist society.[40] This resulted in a famine that killed twenty million to forty million people. During their thirties and forties, this cohort experienced the Cultural Revolution as well as the destruction of the "Four Olds" (i.e., customs, culture, habits, and ideas) by the Red Guards, a group largely composed of youth carrying out Communist policies.

As this historical background illustrates, Chinese older people living in China or in Hong Kong have lived through many traumatic events, and it is important to understand how these events have been remembered and have shaped their life-story narratives. Research on long-term psychological effects of trauma has been limited to studies with Holocaust survivors. These studies suggest that when older people experienced life challenges and losses in later life, prior trauma may resurface.[41] Delayed onset, reemergence, or exacerbation of symptoms and behaviors associated with posttraumatic stress may appear during the aging process. Different sociohistorical periods provide different opportunity structures, migration, and social roles for individuals with different personal characteristics that shape their autobiographical memories. These opportunities and roles, in turn, determine the particular life events that people experience and the adaptive resources with which they respond to these life events. In part I, we will provide well-documented scientific knowledge of narrative practice by reviewing related research literature. Before we do that, however, we would like to highlight important conceptual and theoretical approaches that apply to working with older populations regardless of cultures.

GERONTOLOGICAL SOCIAL WORK AND NARRATIVE PRACTICE: GLOBAL AGING PERSPECTIVES

ACTIVE AGING FRAMEWORK

The World Health Organization (WHO) advocates for "Active Aging" as the policy and program framework for older populations in all countries. WHO defines active aging as "the process of optimizing opportunities for health, participation and security in order to enhance quality of life as people age."[42] Population aging raises many important questions for policymakers and program planners to help societies adapt with aging populations and remain socioeconomically viable. To achieve this, global aging policies and programs need to be more supportive than ever of older people for them to remain healthy, active, autonomous, and socially engaged as they age. According to the WHO definition, health refers to the physical, psychological, and social well-being of individuals and societies. Thus, in an active aging framework, policies and programs that promote health, mental health, and meaningful social engagements are important factors associated with older people's dignified quality of life. Active aging applies to both individuals and societies to allow older people to realize their potential within society for physical, social, and psychological well-being throughout the life course.

The active aging approach is based on the recognition of the human rights of older people and is based on the United Nations principles of independence, participation, dignity, care, and self-fulfillment. This approach shifts the focus of strategic planning away from a "needs-based" approach to a "rights-based" approach that recognizes the rights of individuals within the productive framework of their societies to equality of opportunity and treatment. The active aging approach also recognizes and encourages older adults' right to be involved in the political process and other civic affairs in the community. Older adults also have the right to learn new health-protecting skills and services, such as narrative intervention, to tackle life challenges and regain or maintain well-being.

LIFE-COURSE PERSPECTIVE

The life-course perspective focuses on understanding the divergent views of human development and recognizes that the aging process is the accumulation of life events and changes experienced.[43] An older person's life is not a snapshot at a particular point in time, rather it is the culmination of a person's time course as shaped by historical, political, cultural, social, and family contexts, as well as by individual development factors and personal choices. Early life experiences and decisions affect opportunities later in life. Chinese older adults in Hong Kong who came from mainland China may have gone through World War I, World War II, famine, the Cultural Revolution in China, and migration stress when they stole away to Hong Kong. Therefore, cultural adaptation, cumulative historical trauma, coronavirus pandemic, and resilience may become part of their life-story narratives. The life-course perspective places older people into a larger historical context, with the focus not on a linear path but on the sum total.[44] Mr. Chan's life-story narrative is a perfect illustration for our need to understand an older person and his family life experience as the sum total (from mainland China to Hong Kong to the United States).

An older person's gender, ethnicity, race, socioeconomic status, educational attainment, and other personal factors may limit or streamline his or her opportunities early in life, depending on one's perspective. This narrowing of options can turn into limitations that may lead to future disparities.[45] Conversely, this streamlining can also foster greater resilience. The life of this author is one example: having gone through extreme poverty when she grew up in Hong Kong, she was able to persist and by the grace of God, and became a professor. This author could write a life-story narrative titled "From Poverty to Professorship."

From a life-course perspective, this active adaptation and coping with losses and life challenges is viewed as a long-term personal growth process. The life-story narrative has enormous emotional power to help an older person heal and grow, as they gain profound meaning from their narratives, furthering their insights and strengths in the process, and inspiring others to do likewise and flourish. Research conducted in Korea, China, India, and the United States has found that the intricacies of culture (language, cultural norms, family values or expectations, gender roles, birth order, faith practices) have significant implications for the ways older people conceptualize their life stories.[46] As we discussed earlier, such studies also have found that encoding and retrieval of autobiographical memory is linguistically marked.[47]

STRENGTHS-BASED AND EMPOWERMENT APPROACHES

Gerontological social work advocates for a strengths-based approach to serve our older adult populations. Working with older people demands a holistic approach because the belief that older people have the capacity to continue to learn and to grow is foundational for social workers. In the context of narrative intervention, social workers need to challenge themselves to focus on older persons' strengths, abilities, values, beliefs, and potential rather than on their problems and needs.[48] It can be tempting for a social worker to look at an older person as a similar group and first think a good thought, "What are their problems and what services do they need to solve the problems?" The better thought, or even guiding principle, should be, "Who is this person in relation to others, how can the person's talents contribute to society, and what services will help this person contribute?"

Gerontological social workers recognize older persons' strengths and aspirations, and narrative intervention with older people focuses on capacity as they view and continue constructing their life stories in the context of social and life challenges. Narrative intervention with older adults exercises both older persons' and social workers' commitment to empowerment and self-determination. In narrative practice, social workers will support older people to further develop their self-esteem and self-confidence and will activate older adults' internal and external resources to deal with their life challenges.[49] Mr. Chan was able to transform his identity narrative as the "failed father" into the "unsung hero," empowering both him and his family. Meaning-making processes can provide older people and their family with a sense of perspective and gratitude.

From a strengths- and meaning-based perspective, social workers understand that older people have the ability and capacity to continue to grow and develop during the aging process. Resilience among older adults has been defined as their capacity to endure difficulties and to recover as well as thrive in the face of disruptive life challenges.[50] The concept of resiliency refers to how individuals can achieve positive outcomes following a stressful event by developing positive adaptations. This process is supported by protective factors that help mitigate the negative effects of stress.[51] Protective factors found in older individuals include previous life experience, personality, optimism, coping skills, spirituality, and self-rated health.[52] Family and community resources that serve as protective factors for older adults include social support from family, friends, and neighbors; availability of community services; religious affiliation; and cultural values and influences. These strengths and resources enable older people and their families to respond successfully to crises and persistent challenges and to recover and grow from those experiences.

In the context of gerontological social work, social workers who provide narrative intervention to older adults should empower them to construct their life-story narrative and validate their lifetime struggles and learning experiences as their rich life assets. In Mr. Chan's life-story narrative, the social worker had knowledge of his Asian cultural modesty and acknowledged his long-term goals and lifetime contributions to his family even though the children grew up poor without his presence. Mr. Chan eventually discovered meaning and learning in growing up poor, learning that poverty can be a meaningful psychological asset for his adult children. He then was able to identify the strengths of his adult children who worked hard for their graduate studies, never taking good fortune for granted, and are grateful to have had the opportunity to be immigrants in the United States. His children also realized that this was only possible because of their father's sacrifice. Because of narrative intervention, Mr. Chan's end of life was richer—he often had a cheerful disposition having revealed to himself his dignity as a good father.

How can we, as narrative practitioners in a global community, practically help future practitioners develop the use of narrative practice as an intervention? How can this practice flourish? In the next several chapters, we will explore in detail the foundations and construct of narrative practice and examine its importance and effectiveness as a therapeutic intervention. We will begin with a review of the literature on its global impact to date and its importance in social work and psychotherapy knowledge development.

NOTES

1. Diane R. Gehart, *Mastering Competencies in Family Therapy: A Practical Approach to Theory and Clinical Case Documentation* (Boston: Cengage Learning, 2017); and Alice Morgan, *What Is Narrative Therapy? An Easy-to-Read Introduction* (Adelaide, SA: Dulwich Centre, 2000).
2. Gehart, *Mastering Competencies in Family Therapy*; and Morgan, *What Is Narrative Therapy?*
3. Pei-Shan Yang and Ada C. Mui, *Foundations of Gerontological Social Work Practice in Taiwan* (Taipei: YehYeh Book Gallery, 2022).
4. Gehart, *Mastering Competencies in Family Therapy*.
5. Gehart, *Mastering Competencies in Family Therapy*; Yang and Mui, *Foundations of Gerontological Social Work*.
6. Gehart, *Mastering Competencies in Family Therapy*.
7. Gehart, *Mastering Competencies in Family Therapy*; and Yang and Mui, *Foundations of Gerontological Social Work*.

8. Sylvia Xiaohua Chen et al., "The Added Value of World Views Over Self-Views: Predicting Modest Behaviour in Eastern and Western Cultures," *British Journal of Social Psychology* 56, no. 4 (2017): 723–49, https://doi.org/10.1111/bjso.12196; Katherine Nelson and Robyn Fivush, "The Emergence of Autobiographical Memory: A Social Cultural Developmental Theory," *Psychological Review* 111, no. 2 (2004): 486–511, https://doi.org/10.1037/0033-295X.111.2.486; and Qi Wang, "The Emergence of Cultural Self-Constructs: Autobiographical Memory and Self-Description in European American and Chinese Children," *Developmental Psychology* 40, no. 1 (2004): 3–15, https://psycnet.apa.org/doi/10.1037/0012-1649.40.1.3.

9. Kate C. McLean and Marc A. Fournier, "The Content and Processes of Autobiographical Reasoning in Narrative Identity," *Journal of Research in Personality* 42, no. 3 (2008): 527–45, https://doi.org/10.1016/j.jrp.2007.08.003.

10. Chen et al., "Added Value of World Views"; and Robyn Fivush, Jordan A. Booker, and Matthew E. Graci, "Ongoing Narrative Meaning-Making Within Events and Across the Life Span," *Imagination, Cognition and Personality* 37, no. 2 (2017): 127–52, https://doi.org/10.1177/0276236617733824.

11. Chen et al., "Added Value of World Views."

12. Nelson and Fivush, "Emergence of Autobiographical Memory."

13. Janhavi S. Desai, "Intergenerational Conflict Within Asian American Families: The Role of Acculturation, Ethnic Identity, Individualism, and Collectivism," *Dissertation Abstracts International* 67 (2006): 7369, https://www.worldcat.org/title/intergenerational-conflict-within-asian-american-families-the-role-of-acculturation-ethnic-identity-individualism-and-collectivism/oclc/437348983.

14. Jessica Jungsook Han, Michelle D. Leichtman, and Qi Wang, "Autobiographical Memory in Korean, Chinese, and American Children," *Developmental Psychology* 34, no. 4 (1998): 701, https://doi.org/10.1037/0012-1649.34.4.701.

15. Mary K. Mullen and Soonhyung Yi, "The Cultural Context of Talk About the Past: Implications for the Development of Autobiographical Memory," *Cognitive Development* 10, no. 3 (1995): 407–19, https://doi.org/10.1016/0885-2014(95)90004-7; and Nelson and Fivush, "Emergence of Autobiographical Memory."

16. Desai, "Intergenerational Conflict"; McLean and Fournier, "Content and Processes of Autobiographical Reasoning"; and Nelson and Fivush, "Emergence of Autobiographical Memory."

17. Desai, "Intergenerational Conflict"; McLean and Fournier, "Content and Processes of Autobiographical Reasoning"; and Gemma Dolorosa Skillman, "Intergenerational Conflict Within the Family Context: A Comparative Analysis of Collectivism and Individualism Within Vietnamese, Filipino, and Caucasian Families" (PhD diss., Syracuse University, ProQuest Dissertations Publishing, 1999).

18. McLean and Fournier, "Content and Processes of Autobiographical Reasoning."

19. Nelson and Fivush, "Emergence of Autobiographical Memory"; Qi Wang, "Culture Effects on Adults' Earliest Childhood Recollection and Self-Description: Implications for the Relation Between Memory and the Self," *Journal of Personality and Social Psychology* 81, no. 2 (2001): 220–33, https://doi.org/10.1037/0022-3514.81.2.220; and Qi Wang, Michelle D. Leichtman, and Katharine I. Davies, "Sharing Memories and Telling Stories: American and Chinese Mothers and their 3-Year-Olds," *Memory* 8, no. 3 (2000): 159–77, https://doi.org/10.1080/096582100387588.

20. Bernardo J. Carducci, "Expressions of the Self in Individualistic vs. Collective Cultures: A Cross-Cultural-Perspective Teaching Module," *Psychology Learning and Teaching* 11, no. 3 (2012): 413–17, https://doi.org/10.2304%2Fplat.2012.11.3.413; Desai "Intergenerational Conflict"; Ying-yi Hong et al., "Cultural Identity and Dynamic Construction of the Self: Collective Duties and Individual Rights in Chinese and American Cultures," special issue, *Social Cognition* 19, no. 3 (2001): 251–68, https://doi.org/10.1521/soco.19.3.251.21473; and McLean and Fournier, "Content and Processes of Autobiographical Reasoning."

21. Nelson and Fivush, "Emergence of Autobiographical Memory"; and Wang, "Emergence of Cultural Self-Constructs."

22. Iulia O. Basu-Zharku, "Effects of Collectivistic and Individualistic Cultures on Imagination Inflation in Eastern and Western Cultures," *Inquiries Journal* 3, no. 2 (2011), http://www.inquiriesjournal.com/articles/1679/effects-of-collectivistic-and-individualistic-cultures-on-imagination-inflation-in-eastern-and-western-cultures; Hong et al., "Cultural Identity and Dynamic Construction"; and Jenny Kurman, "Self-Enhancement: Is It Restricted to Individualistic Cultures?," *Personality and Social Psychology Bulletin* 27, no. 12 (2001): 1705–16, https://doi.org/10.1177%2F01461672012712013.

23. Kurman, "Self-Enhancement"; and Harry C. Triandis, "The Self and Social Behavior in Differing Cultural Contexts," *Psychological Review* 96, no. 3 (1989): 506–20, https://doi.org/10.1037/0033-295X.96.3.506.

24. Hazel R. Markus and Shinobu Kitayama, "Culture and the Self: Implications for Cognition, Emotion, and Motivation," *Psychological Review* 98, no. 2 (1991): 224–53, https://doi.org/10.1037/0033-295X.98.2.224.

25. Toshio Yamagishi et al., "Modesty in Self-Presentation: A Comparison Between the USA and Japan," *Asian Journal of Social Psychology* 15, no. 1 (2012): 60–68, https://doi.org/10.1111/j.1467-839X.2011.01362.x.

26. Desai, "Intergenerational Conflict"; and Skillman, "Intergenerational Conflict Within the Family Context."

27. Han et al., "Autobiographical Memory."

28. Han et al., "Autobiographical Memory."

29. Carducci, "Expressions of the Self"; and Helene H. Fung, "Aging in Culture," *Gerontologist* 53, no. 3 (2013): 369–77, https://doi.org/10.1093/geront/gnt024.

30. U.S. Census Bureau, "American Counts: Stories Behind the Numbers," April 14, 2023, https://www.census.gov/library/stories.

31. Nancy Morrow-Howell and Ada C. Mui, "Productive Engagement of Older Adults: International Research, Practice, and Policy Introduction," *Ageing International* 38, no. 1 (2013): 1–3, https://doi.org/10.1007/s12126-012-9175-y.

32. Ada C. Mui, Terry Lum, and Iris Chi, *Gerontological Social Work: Theory and Practice*, 2nd ed. (Shanghai: Truth and Wisdom, 2017).

33. Morrow-Howell and Mui, "Productive Engagement of Older Adults"; and Mui et al., *Gerontological Social Work*.

34. Ada C. Mui and Suk-Young Kang, "Acculturation Stress and Depression Among Asian Immigrant Elders," *Social Work* 51, no. 3 (2006): 243–55, https://doi.org/10.1093/sw/51.3.243.

35. Mui et al., *Gerontological Social Work*.

36. Yang and Mui, *Foundations of Gerontological Social Work*.

37. Fung, "Aging in Culture."

38. Ada C. Mui and Tazuko Shibusawa, *Asian American Elders in the Twenty-First Century: Key Indicators of Well-Being* (New York: Columbia University Press, 2008).

39. Yang and Mui, *Foundations of Gerontological Social Work*.

40. Mui and Shibusawa, *Asian American Elders*.

41. Yang and Mui, *Foundations of Gerontological Social Work*.

42. World Health Organization, "Active Ageing: A Policy Framework," World Health Organization, April 2002, https://apps.who.int/iris/handle/10665/67215.

43. Yang and Mui, *Foundations of Gerontological Social Work*.

44. Mui et al., *Gerontological Social Work*.

45. Nancy R. Hooyman and H. Asuman Kiyak, *Social Gerontology: A Multidisciplinary Perspective* (Boston: Pearson Education, 2018).

46. Mui et al., *Gerontological Social Work*.

47. Carducci, "Expressions of the Self."

48. Yang and Mui, *Foundations of Gerontological Social Work*.

49. Hooyman and Kiyak, *Social Gerontology*.

50. Yang and Mui, *Foundations of Gerontological Social Work*.

51. Hooyman and Kiyak, *Social Gerontology*.

52. Mui et al., *Gerontological Social Work*.

2

VALIDATING THE POWER OF NARRATIVE PRACTICE

Exploring Efficacy and Knowledge Development

NARRATIVE THERAPY (NT) has become increasingly important in the field of psychotherapy practice. NT embodies intentionally listening to people who are living with challenging life situations, helping them to identify their values and associated skills. Its practice emphasizes personal experiences and elaborates on the meaning of those experiences.[1] In this chapter, we will investigate the validity of narrative practice's power and efficacy, examining the accumulated knowledge base of narrative practice through a review of its extensive use within psychotherapy practice.

Narrative practice focuses on a person's expressions or memories of their life events[2] and was developed by Michael White and David Epston during the 1970s and 1980s.[3] Such expressions provide a chance for people to reconstruct their life stories and make sense of their lives. Nevertheless, older adults, as they advance in age, may experience different health situations, which may create restrictive and problematic narratives when their personal identities conflict with dominant societal discourses and expectations.[4] Therefore, narrative therapists work collaboratively with their patients to rediscover an alternative story by helping them deconstruct, coconstruct, and reconstruct their life story from a strength- and meaning-based perspective.

Narrative gerontology has provided a new approach to responding to the stories of older people.[5] With the growing interest in the exploration of life narratives in clinical practices, it is crucial to delineate the backbone of the narrative, which include autobiographical information, life review, and reminiscence. Autobiography, which has cultural aspects as discussed in chapter 1, refers to a person's written introspective report of their life, while reminiscence is a recall of pleasurable memories.[6] Life review is a critical analysis of one's life history. This type of review helps the person to resolve past conflicts and achieve ego integrity by examining their developmental stages.[7] Narrative therapists use conversational skills to work with people and collaboratively reauthor their life stories and to coconstruct their preferred identities, thus enabling them to grow from self-selected life events and plan for the future. NT is a respectful approach in that it views problems as separate from the individual and appreciates that everyone has valuable skills that can help them deal with the challenges in their lives.[8]

Although NT has been validated as a clinical practice, ongoing evaluation is important to adapt this practice for different cultures and populations. Practice evaluation uses systematic methods to examine the effects of the intervention—that is, whether or not the therapist's practice has met the goals she has set with the individuals or groups.[9]

This chapter examines and evaluates evidence from previous global research on employing NT in working with older adults. After conducting systematic searches, we classified the available literature into three categories based on the following methods of inquiry: qualitative ways of knowing, quantitative ways of knowing, and a mixed-method approach that integrates both ways of knowing. Working definitions of these methods are given in the following paragraphs.

In therapeutic research, the quantitative approach allows the researchers to study the progress made during and after therapy to assess whether it was effective for the particular groups of people.[10]

NT has risen in prominence since the 1980s, but only limited studies have documented the effects of its practice. In this chapter, we review studies examining the effectiveness of NT over the past 25 years, looking at three levels of practice from both Western and Eastern societies (including Australia, Hong Kong, and the United States): (1) one-on-one casework; (2) groups involving more than two participants; and (3) collective work bringing together groups and communities who have collectively suffered from a lack of opportunities to voice their strengths, promote social realization (the process through which individuals or groups achieve their potential and goals within a societal context), and reduce partiality in various circumstances.[11]

QUALITATIVE WAYS OF KNOWING

A qualitative way of knowing encompasses interpretive knowledge, intuition, and subjective understanding.[12] The qualitative approach prioritizes in-depth understanding of individuals' interpretations of events and the meaning people give to the world around them. It also emphasizes the value derived from researcher-participant interactions. A qualitative approach investigates the behaviors, perceptions, goals, thoughts, and feelings of the patient as well as the relationship between the therapist and the person consulting them.[13]

For studies that adopt a qualitative methodology, investigators might use interviews, focus groups, and case studies to present their findings.[14] Because each case is unique, qualitative approaches allow us to assess an intervention's flexibility. These approaches also provide in-depth knowledge of the process of narrative intervention, which may help determine whether or not NT is effective in assisting individuals and couples.

EVALUATING CASE STUDIES

With the belief that every person is the expert in their own life, narrative therapists urge individuals to examine and rediscover their values, beliefs, knowledge, and skills to identify alternative ways to overcome challenging life situations.[15] Over the years, people from different backgrounds have benefited from NT, flourishing through difficult situations as well as making role transitions throughout their life course. Table 2.1 shows some of the different demographics and challenges for which NT has been a helpful intervention specifically for older adults.

By using the qualitative method, individual case studies have revealed three interconnected themes: (1) reconstructing meaning in life, (2) improving adaptability, and (3) reconfiguring peer and family support.

INDIVIDUAL CASE STUDIES

RECONSTRUCTING MEANING IN LIFE The first theme that emerged from the literature review was loss of meaning, which was the most prevalent reason for individuals to seek out narrative therapists to collaborate on creating a new narrative, often as a result of traumas and sudden changes in life. For Elizabeth, an eighty-year-old widow, the life challenge of increasing frailty in her old age had left her physically unable to do the activities that had previously given her life purpose after her husband died. The narrative therapeutic process enabled her to construct a new life story that recognized her past accomplishments in life, encouraged her to reconnect with the beloved memories of her husband, and enabled her to

TABLE 2.1 Individual case studies: Qualitative method

AUTHOR	SAMPLE	LIFE SITUATIONS	OUTCOMES OF NT
Kropf and Tandy, 1998 (United States)	Older American woman, eighty-year-old widow	• Sense of loss (from death of her husband) • Depression from decrease in physical functioning • Fear of being dependent	• New sense of self • Alternative narrative of survivorship created • Sense of continued persistence as new meaning in life
Stern, 2011 (Australia)	Two Australian centenarians	• Living in an Australian nursing home	• Focused on older people's own life skills and knowledge • Found meaning in older people's current lifestyles • Created new and updated descriptions of life
Chow, 2013, (Hong Kong)	Older Chinese couple • Husband: seventy-year-old stroke survivor; • Wife: fifty years old	• Coping with stroke as a couple • Wife adapting to role as caregiver to her husband	• Husband: Recognized wife's contributions in his rehabilitation • Wife: Reflected on the financial support the husband has provided to the family • Couple relationships: Rejuvenated the relationships and cherished their time together • Rediscovered personal strengths and reconstructed life purpose
Stern and Serrure, 2014 (Australia)	Eleven Australians, ages eighty-six to ninety-five and one in his early seventies	• Living in a nursing home in Australia	• Realized older adults can create a continuum in their lives • Learned that older adults are experts in the stresses of their own lives • Created a meaningful life through navigation
Muruthi, McCoy, Chou and Farnham, 2018 (United States)	Older American couple • Husband: seventy-four years old; • Wife: seventy-two years old	• Sexual dissatisfaction after moving to the retirement community	• Wife: Recognized her interpersonal scripts were causing her to think her husband was not attracted to her • Husband: Realized that the wife still desired him • Deconstructed the socially dominant sexual discourse that "older adults are asexual"

AUTHOR	SAMPLE	LIFE SITUATIONS	OUTCOMES OF NT
Driscoll and Hughes, 2021 (United States)	Older Caucasian American couple in their early seventies	• Sexual dissatisfaction	• Husband: Dismissed held beliefs about sexual myths • Wife: Deconstructed the socially dominant sexual script, which enabled her to find a way to feel "sexy" • Achieved sexual empowerment and liberation for older woman
Stahnke and Cooley, 2022 (United States)	Older Austrian-American man, ninety-six years old	• Holocaust Survivor (ongoing PTSD in later life)	• Externalized depression and the traumatic experiences • Reconstructed the meaning of "death" and reduced his fear of death • Repaired the relationships with spouse
Stern and Serrure, 2022 (Australia)	Individual interviews with twelve older adults from their early seventies to ninety-five years old	• Living in a care home in Australia	• Explored their experiences living in a care home • Reconnected the older adults with their past dreams and memories • Created a support system for the older adults • Facilitated meaning-making about personal lives • Rediscovered the knowledge and skills of older adults

Sources: Nancy P. Kropf and Cindy Tandy, "Narrative Therapy with Older Clients: The Use of a Meaning-Making Approach," *Clinical Gerontologist* 18, no. 4 (1998): 3–16, https://doi.org/10.1300/J018v18n04_02; Dafna Stern, "Narrative Therapy at Any Age," *International Journal of Narrative Therapy and Community Work* 1 (2011): 57–64; Esther Oi-Wah Chow, "Responding to Lives After Stroke: Stroke Survivors and Caregivers Going on Narrative Journeys," *International Journal of Narrative Therapy and Community Work* 4 (2013): 1; Dafna Stern and Caroline Serrure, "Making a Meaning-Full Life at Montefiore," *International Journal of Narrative Therapy and Community Work* 3 (2014): 21–30; Bertranna Muruthi et al., "Sexual Scripts and Narrative Therapy with Older Couples," *American Journal of Family Therapy* 46, no. 1 (2018): 81–95, https://doi.org/10.1080/01926187.2018.1428129; Janette J. Driscoll and Anthony A. Hughes, "Sexuality of Aging Adults: A Case Study Using Narrative Therapy," *Contemporary Family Therapy* 44 (2021): 373–80, https://doi.org/10.1007/s10591-021-09589-3; and Brittany Stahnke and Morgan E. Cooley, "End-of-Life Case Study: The Use of Narrative Therapy on a Holocaust Survivor with Lifelong Depression," *Journal of Contemporary Psychotherapy* 52 (2022): 191–98, https://doi.org/https://doi.org/10.1007/s10879-022-09532-z.

take initiative to prepare for her future abilities instead of focusing on her frailties.[16] In Stahnke and Cooley's study,[17] NT assisted Frank, a ninety-six-year-old Austrian-American man who lived through the Holocaust, during which time his father and sister died in a concentration camp, to reconstruct the meaning of life and death. During the therapy, Frank was able to rewrite his life story and share his wisdom with younger people.

He reported after this reduced his fear and enhanced his acceptance of death. This narrative practice enabled him to look back on his experiences and find integrity and peace in his life journey.

IMPROVING ADAPTABILITY: RECOLLECTING THE STRENGTHS DEVELOPED OVER TIME As seen in table 2.1, most people who consult narrative therapists have experienced life situations with multilayered concerns, such as dysfunctional behavioral patterns, loss of loved ones, being bullied, relational and sexual challenges, impending death, and identity rooted in dominant versus minority social structures, which can undermine social identities and personal agency. This situation requires the therapist to work with people to recollect self-knowledge, skills, values, and beliefs to cocreate a preferred identity that builds self-esteem. Among the noted situation, sexual dissatisfaction is one of the challenges that is common among Western older couples. One example of this is Susan, who in her early seventies was introduced to NT through Driscoll and Hughes's study,[18] after years of dissatisfaction with her sexual relationship with her husband. After the NT, she was able to live beyond the socially constructed "sexual script" in her role as a woman to express her sexual needs more freely. She and her husband became more considerate of each other's needs and both parties in the relationship were empowered through the therapeutic process. Similarly, in Muruthi and colleagues' study,[19] a couple in their seventies was able to successfully resolve their sexual dissatisfaction and mutual misunderstanding through the narrative conversations they had after moving to a retirement community. After engaging in narrative dialogues that helped to deconstruct the socially dominant sexual discourse that "older adults are asexual," the partners gradually were able to build a new kind of sensual and sexual bond during this life transition.

RECONFIGURING PEER AND FAMILY SUPPORT: RECONNECTING RELATIONAL ASPECTS OF SELF Peer and family support can play a significant role in a person's ability to reconstruct a narrative as they strive to give meaning to the significant people in their lives. Terminal illness and chronic pain is believed to be a familiar life topic among older adults. In the East, it is often complicated by the weight of family obligations and cultural relationships. Chow illustrated that the poststroke life narrative of Harry,[20] a seventy-year-old male stroke survivor, was that of a patient who must continue his life while adjusting to new mental and physical constraints. While overcoming this obstacle on one's own might be difficult, Harry was accompanied by his wife, Lucy, on his quest to write a new narrative for the couple. As a result, through dialogue with the therapist, the couple was able to reconstruct their purpose in life, individually and mutually, and come to the conclusion that the stroke had brought the best out of their relationship and that the illness was not defining him as a person. Additionally, having gone through this process together, the couple also grew closer, cherishing their relationship and time together. Harry realized that having his spouse there made him more than a stroke survivor, and he recognized that his role as Lucy's partner was more important than any impairment from his stroke. The presence of a loved one can help a person realize that they are an important entity in someone else's narrative, which can help them reconstruct their own narrative.

STUDIES EVALUATING GROUP PRACTICE

Early research in the twentieth century established the effectiveness of NT by conducting in-depth interviews with different target groups, such as university students and families.[21] In modern research, group NT has focused primarily on problem-oriented cases, including negative connotations and stigmatized groups, such as abusive partners, offenders, stepmothers, and homeless people.[22] Being able to narrate one's story is an essential step toward developing an alternative narrative in NT. In group practice, members act as a sympathetic audience to individuals who are narrating their stories, and members will also provide their own accounts of similar situations.[23] The recurring experience of expressing one's story to a sympathetic audience, or of being the audience for another's narrative, can validate a person's commitment to change in these situations. The participants help one another move beyond stuck narratives to more fruitful alternatives.

The study of group NT literature has shown that group settings can be adapted to a variety of demographics, which can be generalized into the following two main categories: (1) stigmatized, and (2) terminally ill.

STIGMATIZED A predominant demographic of modern NT research in group work includes those who are heavily stigmatized or carry a negative connotation, including criminal offenders, stepmothers, and people experiencing homelessness.[24] According to a group of researchers,[25] group identification can act as a buffer against the mental health consequences of

TABLE 2.2 Group- and community-based intervention research narrative therapy: Qualitative method

AUTHOR	SAMPLE	STUDY PROCEDURE	LIFE SITUATIONS/STIGMA	OUTCOMES OF NT
Jones, 2004 (United States)	Groups of stepmothers	• The location and frequency of meeting is decided by group members • One group meets every two weeks for two hours (has been meeting for three years)	• Taboo leads patients to view themselves as "useless" and "worthless" • "Evil" stepmother stereotype • Hostility from young adult stepchildren • Spouses who are unable or willing to acknowledge the situation • Caregiving without authority	• Provided an environment to disparage dominate cultural story • Provided mutual empathy • Allowed participants to share and reconstruct their stories • Allowed participants with similar experience to provide suggestions
Sliep, 2005 (South Africa)	Eastern African refugees	• Narrative theater approach to working with communities affected by trauma, conflict, and war	• Wars and the consequences of trauma, such as drinking and substance use	• Developed alternative life stories that integrated "responsibilities" and "courage"
Gardner and Poole, 2009 (Canada)[1]	Older Canadians (ages fifty-five to seventy), seven male and five female (n = 12)	• Eight-week narrative therapy sessions • Ethnographic design • Participant observation • Extensive field notes • In-depth interviewing methods	• Substance abuse • Mental health issues • Isolation • Lack of purpose	• 66% of the participants believed that story therapy had a very positive impact on their substance misuse • 33% of the participants had stopped taking substances during the study • 33% of the participants felt that narrative therapy was "helpful" for both mental health and addictions • Participants recognized the value of mutual support • Participants believed that their accumulated wisdom was helpful in helping them to "figure out life" and resist substance addiction

Rood and Bobbi, 2009 (United States)[2]	Americans, ages sixty-six to ninety-three in community nursing homes; three of the participants had dementia	• Meet with four to six seniors each week for one hour to talk about different topics • The use of remembering conversations • The use of letters, documents, and certificates • The use of archiving "solution knowledges" and sharing these knowledges between people • Ways of linking people's lives to other lives	• Dementia • Hearing loss and nerve damage affecting motor skills • Pain	• The review of life provides intergenerational continuity, integrating members, and listeners into a network of shared meaning
Trudinger, 2009 (Australia)[3]	Eighty-one elderly people; 110 care home staff living in care homes for the elderly	• Using group documents to allow respondents to recall old residents who have passed away ("Joan") • Rereading the document to the interviewees • Re-recording the collective document as a eulogy	Interviewees all shared memories of "Joan" (a respected resident)	• Provided a shared memory of someone • Used appropriate ways to talk about life's losses and what they mean • Allowed management to do something that provides a meaningful context for people to contribute
Adshead, 2011 (United Kingdom)	Psychiatric hospital in the United Kingdom: seven male legal offenders convicted of manslaughter	• Three female therapists led the weekly therapy group at the beginning • The long-running group used television and movie metaphors to start a deeper discourse	• "Offenders" stigma • Difficulty reflecting and expressing the crime	• Provided an environment for reflection • Gave the offenders a voice to tell their story

(continued)

TABLE 2.2 (Continued)

AUTHOR	SAMPLE	STUDY PROCEDURE	LIFE SITUATIONS/STIGMA	OUTCOMES OF NT
Hung, 2011 (Hong Kong)[4]	Adult Chinese women, six rape victims invited to six sessions, three hours per sessions	• Bring rape victims together to create a sense of connectedness • Tree-of-Life metaphor and constructs alternative storylines	• Sexual violence (rape) • Taboo of rape (dominate discourse): • Discriminated • Sense of loneliness	• Regained self-confidence and embraced the newfound hope as follows: • Forgetting about the past, facing the future with courage • Learned importance of serving justice to the perpetrator • Regained confidence and being happy with oneself
Wood, 2012 (Australia)[5]	Children, young people, and their family	• Recipe-of-Life metaphor	• Homelessness	• Rediscovered self-knowledge • Used the ingredients in the recipe as guidance on how to act at the school, work collaboratively, and go through hard times
Fredman, 2014 (United Kingdom)	Older people and their families and community practitioners	• Invite community practitioners as witnesses	• Diseases • Psychological problems	• Inviting external witnesses can help address power imbalances • External witnessing practices can be instrumental in bringing shared values, principles, and commitments to members and clients
Butera-Prinzi, 2014 (Australia)	• Australian families (N = 4) • Primary focus was the Anderson family	• Family discussions • Sibling group discussions • Parental group discussions • Tree-of-Life metaphor to contextualize life after acquired brain injury (ABI)	• Family member with ABI • Family coping with life after ABI	• Decreased sense of isolation by meeting other families in the same situation • Highlighted the positive things that came from the hardships • The participants accepted the complexity of their new life
Clark, 2014 (United States)	American female substance-abusing adults	• Using the Letter of Letting Go and the Narrative Novel	• Struggling to get over substance addiction	• Narrative Novel and Letter of Letting Go to help in recovery • Participants were able to comprehend the impact of drug use on their loved ones • Realized the impact of drug use on their sense of identity.

Study	Population	Method	Challenges	Outcomes
Lit, 2015 (Hong Kong)	Terminally ill Chinese cancer patients (including older adults)	• Six-week group sessions • Individual pregroup interviews • The groups used a "double listening" technique during therapy sessions • Create a "spontaneous communitas"	• Chinese cultural limitations in talking about their situation openly • Taboo leads patients to view themselves as "useless" and "worthless"	• Introduced the concept that people are "multistoried" using the metaphor of mosaic pictures • Bolster their meaning of life • Safe space was provided to them to discuss their death and cancer • Opportunity to share their legacy and leave things for their loved ones
Chow, 2015 (Hong Kong)	Older Chinese adults recovering from stroke	• The therapist utilized six steps to introduce Train of Life to the participants	• Debilitation of stroke • Social stigma of stroke in Chinese culture (dominant discourse) • Sense of isolation • Sense of personal failure • Feeling trapped	• Visualized the strengths of stroke survivors by using Train-of-Life metaphor • Regain meaning of life • Facilitate the public's understanding about stroke patients through outsider witness and a theater performance
Tan, 2017 (Singapore)	Singaporean women ages thirty-two to fifty-six (N = 4)	• Recipe-for-Life metaphor	• Experienced domestic violence from their male partner or adult sons	• Being able to externalize the dominant social discourse about domestic violence by using the metaphor of "uninvited ingredients" in the recipe, such as bacteria • Participants were empowered by alternative stories where their values in caring for their children were recognized • Rediscovered and recognized personal values
Chow, 2020 (Hong Kong)	Chinese older adults (N = 144)	• Older adults went through twenty-four four-session groups • Tree-of-Life metaphor was implemented	• Tackle stress-related aging issues and identities	• Using the Tree of Life to rediscover their wisdom, five themes were identified: • Insight about their abilities, intentions, and problem-solving capabilities • Sense of purpose and commitment to their preferred identities • Realization of personal values and beliefs • Reconnecting sense of agency and hope • Cherishing life as a journey to celebrate their wealth of wisdom for a common good
Chow and Fok, 2020 (Hong Kong)	Chinese older adults (N = 30)	• Six two-hour NT sessions • Each session had a different theme • Recipe-of-Life metaphor was implemented	• Person living with chronic pain	• Three themes were identified: • Rediscovery of personal qualities and capabilities • Validation of preferred identity • Fusion of spiritual seasoning of life

(continued)

TABLE 2.2 (Continued)

AUTHOR	SAMPLE	STUDY PROCEDURE	LIFE SITUATIONS/STIGMA	OUTCOMES OF NT
Rajaei et al., 2020 (United States)	U.S. heterosexual couples (N = 8)	• Each couple attended twenty-six sessions for a year • The couples went to counseling for one hour once a week for the first four months • Sessions were held every other week for the next two months • Couples attended once a month for the last six months	• One partner had been diagnosed with stage 1 or 2 cancer • The strain of cancer on the relationship • The strain of cancer on the partner	• Three themes emerged: • Increased vulnerability • Increased mindfulness • Improved communication
Grant, 2022 (Awabakal, Australia)	Adult Australian women	• The therapist employed the double listening technique	• Sexual violence (rape) • Sense of shame • Sense of guilt • Sense of hopelessness	• Facilitated mutual support among women who had similar experiences • Made voice of the women be heard by other social workers and counselors

Sources: Anne C. Jones, "Transforming the Story: Narrative Applications to a Stepmother Support Group," _Families in Society_ 85, no. 1 (2004): 129–38; Yvonne Sliep, "A Narrative Theatre Approach to Working with Communities Affected by Trauma, Conflict and War," _International Journal of Narrative Therapy and Community Work_ 2005, no. 2 (2005): 47–52; Paula J. Gardner and Jennifer M. Poole, "One Story at a Time: Narrative Therapy, Older Adults, and Addictions," _Journal of Applied Gerontology_ 28, no. 5 (2009): 600–620, https://doi.org/10.1177/0733464808330822; Bobbi Rood, "A Time to Talk: Re-Membering Conversations with Elders," _International Journal of Narrative Therapy and Community Work_ 1 (2009): 18–28; Mark Trudinger, "Remembering Joan: Re-Membering Practices as Eulogies and Memorials," _International Journal of Narrative Therapy and Community Work_ 1 (2009): 29–38; Gwen Adshead, "The Life Sentence: Using a Narrative Approach in Group Psychotherapy with Offenders," _Group Analysis_ 44, no. 2 (2011): 175–95; S. L. Hung, "Collective Narrative Practice with Rape Victims in the Chinese Society of Hong Kong"; Natale Rudland Wood, "Recipes for Life," _International Journal of Narrative Therapy and Community Work_ 2 (2012): 14–31; Glenda Fredman, "Weaving Net-Works of Hope with Families, Practitioners and Communities: Inspiration from Systemic and Narrative Approaches," _International Journal of Narrative Therapy and Community Work_ 1 (2014): 34–44; Franca Butera-Prinzi, Nella Charles, and Karen Story, "Narrative Family Therapy and Group Work for Families Living with Acquired Brain Injury," _Australian and New Zealand Journal of Family Therapy_ 35, no. 1 (2014): 81–99, https://doi.org/10.1002/anzf.1046; Ashley A. Clark, "Narrative Therapy Integration Within Substance Abuse Groups," _Journal of Creativity in Mental Health_ 9, no. 4 (2014): 511–22, https://doi.org/10.1080/15401 383.2014.914457; Siu Wai Lit, "Dialectics and Transformations in Liminality: The Use of Narrative Therapy Groups with Terminal Cancer Patients in Hong Kong," _China Journal of Social Work_ 8, no. 2 (2015): 122–35, https://doi.org/10.1080/17525098.2015.1039171; Esther Oi-Wah Chow, "Narrative Therapy an Evaluated Intervention to Improve Stroke Survivors' Social and Emotional Adaptation," _Clinical Rehabilitation_ 29, no. 4 (2015): 315–26; Meizi Tan, "Recipes for Life: A Collective Narrative Methodology for Responding to Gender Violence," _International Journal of Narrative Therapy and Community Work_ 2 (2017): 1–12; Esther Oi-Wah Chow, "Rediscovery of Older Adults' Life Wisdom: Application of Narrative Therapy Using a Tree-of-Life Metaphor," _Innovation in Aging_ 4, Suppl. 1 (2020): 835, https://doi.org/10.1093/geroni/igaa057.3059; Esther Oi-Wah Chow and Doris Yuen Hung Fok, "Recipe of Life: A Relational Narrative Approach in Therapy with Persons Living with Chronic Pain," _Research on Social Work Practice_ 30, no. 3 (2020): 320–29, https:// doi.org/10.1177/1049731519870867; Afarin Rajaei et al., "Striving to Thrive: A Qualitative Study on Fostering a Relational Perspective Through Narrative Therapy in Couples Facing Cancer," _American Journal of Family Therapy_ 49, no. 4 (2021): 392–408, https://doi.org/10.1080/01926187.2020.1820402; Grant Lesley, "Bringing Together Women Like You and Me: Collective Narrative Practice with Women and Trauma," _International Journal of Narrative Therapy and Community Work_ 1 (2022): 1–8.

stigmatization. Group NT provides a person with a judgment-free environment in which they can discuss their concerns among people with similar experiences. Furthermore, group NT has been effective in reducing certain symptoms of mental illness, thereby aiding in the patients' rehabilitation and their families' wellness.

TERMINALLY ILL In addition to stigmatized groups, increasing research has studied the impact of NT on those suffering from terminal illnesses,[26] possibly delaying mortality.[27] Studies have shown that NT plays an important role in reducing symptoms of depression by improving mindfulness among patients with cancer, which allows them to acknowledge their "new normal life," accept their emotions; and create an alternative narrative of meaning for their painful and difficult times.[28] According to the NT studies referenced previously involving patients with cancer, loneliness was their main complaint. NT improved couples' communication and enabled them to initiate discussion of difficult topics and cocreate a shared struggle, which eventually reduced loneliness. This contributed to a reduction in the anxiety associated with cancer. Similar results were found with people who were suffering from other types of illnesses, such as those with acquired brain injury (ABI). According to Butera-Prinzi and colleagues (2014),[29] the Tree-of-Life metaphoric framework has been used in NT to highlight the positive things that resulted from these hardships as a family unit. As a result, the family members reflected that they were now more capable of getting along with the member of the family (the dad) who had an ABI and navigating through problems together.

STUDIES EVALUATING COLLECTIVE PRACTICE AND USE OF METAPHORIC FRAMEWORKS FOR THERAPY Group-based NT invites people to tell their stories in ways that they prefer and invites others who are experiencing the same thing to share their elucidation of the situation.[30] For those who are struggling with the intricacies of a more problem-saturated narrative, metaphor as a communication device for NT has been developed to help them probe complex storylines at a deeper level. Metaphor is also used to build cohesion among several groups of people facing similar difficulties. Just as with general NT use, the added use of these metaphors has allowed therapists to cocreate a safe distance from and perspective of the negative life scripts held by participants suffering from terminal illnesses, trauma, cancers, stigma, and ongoing rehabilitation for noncommunicable diseases.[31] There are three primary metaphoric frameworks used by therapists to help individuals to narrate their stories; Tree of Life (ToL),[32] Train of Life,[33] and Recipe of Life.[34] These metaphoric frameworks create a safe environment for participants to talk about their life issues, especially when it carries stigma and taboo; for example, women who had experienced rape were able to develop an alternative narrative from that of a victim to that of a survivor.[35] Ultimately, as they regained self-confidence, they were able to contribute to the lives of other victims by sharing their experiences either verbally or through collective documents. The collective narrative practices that were done in adult and older adult groups are listed in table 2.3, and detailed processing on the use of these three metaphoric frameworks will be discussed in chapters 11 through 13.

STRENGTHS AND LIMITATIONS OF THE QUALITATIVE APPROACH

Studies on the qualitative approach have been useful in documenting responses and validating narrative strategies that improve the conditions of a person. Qualitative research, however, cannot be used to study the effectiveness of the therapeutic processes, unlike quantitative studies that endeavor to study effectiveness. As such, qualitative research is judged on the subjective interpretations in the interviews.

QUANTITATIVE WAYS OF KNOWING

A quantitative way of knowing includes positivistic, scientific, and observable characteristics to develop an objective worldview.[36] Using numerical terms, the researcher examines the influence of a set of factors (independent variables) on a certain outcome (the dependent variable).[37] In quantitative NT studies, researchers will often adopt an evidence-based approach using methods, such as randomized clinical trials (RCTs).[38] This sort of research may be assessed by examining whether the intervention group improved more than the control group compared with a baseline.

EVALUATING GROUP AND COLLECTIVE PRACTICE

The use of evidence-based research has added to the credibility of NT. Although past studies have used other forms of evidence-based research, such as a quasi-experimental design,[39] RCT designs are considered to be the gold standard for evidence-based research because they reduce the chance for researcher bias and measure the cause-and-effect relationship of an intervention and its results.[40] The RCT design randomly assigns participants to either an intervention group or a control group. Pre–post tests are given to compare the effectiveness of the therapy with results before and after the therapeutic interventions. In the recent decade, RCT has been employed by researchers to study the effectiveness of NT in helping people with mental health concerns. Table 2.3 shows studies that have employed RCT designs in their NT studies.

Eight RCTs were included in this review with 896 participants, 439 of whom were assigned to the NT treatment groups and 445 to the control groups. Each study included four to ten sessions, which were held either weekly or biweekly. Additionally, the treatment sessions' lengths varied for each trial, spanning from thirty minutes to two hours. Furthermore, as seen in table 2.3, the primary target for the RCT studies was to utilize NT in helping people overcome mental health hurdles. In all of the RCT studies, the treatment group consistently showed improvements in the posttest of their outcome variables. Nevertheless, the most commonly tested mental health diagnosis was depression, which was found in five of the eight RCTs. To test depressive symptoms, different scales were employed, including the following: Geriatric Depression Scale Short Form (GDS-SF),[41] Patient Health Questionnaire-9 (PHQ-9),[42] Center for Epidemiologic Studies—Depression Scale (CES-D),[43] and Beck Depression Inventory (BDI-II).[44] In each of these studies, the treatment groups showed greater improvement in their depressive symptoms compared with the control group. Additionally, the use of different types of scales validated the significance of NT in helping people reduce symptoms of depression.

Table 2.3 also includes studies conducted in Hong Kong that showcase different variations of the RCT design, including studies for stroke survivors, chronic pain survivors, and caregivers of people with schizophrenia.[45] In these studies, the undertaken procedural measures were vital to the results, which showcased the effectiveness of NT. In the study on life wisdom, a single-blind waitlist RCT approach was used, the study on stroke survivors used a double-blind RCT approach, and the study of chronic pain survivors used a waitlist RCT approach. A double-blind RCT is a scientific method that does not disclose the research topic to the participants, nor is the group assignment disclosed to the NT intervention group or psycho-education intervention group.[46] For the single-blind RCT method, the researchers are aware of the group assignments, while participants remain unaware of their assigned group. These approaches are useful because they reduce

TABLE 2.3 Literature review of randomized control trials in group-based narrative therapy: Quantitative method

AUTHOR AND COUNTRY	VARIABLES	FINDINGS

Korte et al., 2011 (The Netherlands)	• Depression
	• Anxiety
	• Positive mental health
	• Quality of life
		• Intervention group had lower depressive symptoms and a positive effect on the following:
		  • Anxiety
		  • Positive mental health
		  • Quality of life

Chow, 2018 (Hong Kong) (Stroke survivors)	• Stroke knowledge
	• Mastery
	• Hope
	• Meaning in life
	• Life satisfaction
	• Depression
		• Intervention group reported lower depressive symptoms, and improvement in the following:
		  • Mastery
		  • Hope
		  • Meaning in life
		  • Life satisfaction
		  • A better understanding of stroke

Chow, 2018 (Hong Kong) (Chronic pain survivors)	• Depression
	• Mastery
	• Hope
	• Meaning in life
	• Life satisfaction
		• Intervention group reported lower depressive symptoms, and improvement in the following:
		  • Mastery
		  • Hope
		  • Meaning in life
		  • Life satisfaction

Moreira et al., 2020 (Portugal) (IPV victims)	• PTSD • CPTSD • Depression	• The intervention reduced depressive and PTSD symptoms • Increased CPTSD symptoms postintervention
Shakeri et al., 2020 (Iran) (People with amphetamine addiction)	• Depression • Quality of life • Anxiety	• The intervention reduced the levels of depression and anxiety • The quality of life remained unaffected
Chow and Fung, 2022 (Hong Kong) (Chinese older adults)	• Life wisdom	• Intervention group showed improvement in their perceived wisdom
Sun et al., 2021 (China) (Oral cancer patients)	• Stigma • Self-esteem • Social support	• The intervention reduced stigma and improved self-esteem • There was no significant difference found in social support

AUTHOR AND COUNTRY	VARIABLES	FINDINGS
Zhou et al., 2020 (Hong Kong)	• Family relationship • Caregiver experience • Inner resource • Hope • Mental health	• The collective narrative therapy group was effective in improving the following: • Family relationships • Caregiving experience • Inner resources • Hope • Mental health of the caregivers

Sources: J. Korte et al., "Life Review Therapy for Older Adults with Moderate Depressive Symptomatology: A Pragmatic Randomized Controlled Trial," *Psychological Medicine* 42, no. 6 (2012): 1163–73, https://doi.org/10.1017/S0033291711002042; Esther Oi-Wah Chow, "Narrative Group Intervention to Reconstruct Meaning of Life Among Stroke Survivors: A Randomized Clinical Trial Study," *Neuropsychiatry* 8, no. 4 (2018): 1216–26, https://doi.org/10.4172/Neuropsychiatry.1000450; Esther Oi-Wah Chow, "Narrative Group Interventions to Rediscover Life Wisdom Among Hong Kong Chinese Older Adults: A Waitlist RCT Study," *Innovation in Aging* 2, Suppl. 1 (2018): 992, https://doi.org/10.1093/geroni/igy031.3666; André Moreira, Ana Cristina Moreira, and José Carlos Rocha, "Randomized Controlled Trial: Cognitive-Narrative Therapy for IPV Victims," *Journal of Interpersonal Violence* 37, no. 5–6 (2022): NP2998–NP3014, https://doi.org/10.1177/0886260520943719; Jalal Shakeri et al., "Effectiveness of Group Narrative Therapy on Depression, Quality of Life, and Anxiety in People with Amphetamine Addiction: A Randomized Clinical Trial," *Iranian Journal of Medical Sciences* 45, no. 2 (2020): 91–99, https://doi.org/10.30476/ijms.2019.45829; Esther Oi-Wah Chow and Sai-Fu Fung, "Narrative Group Intervention to Rediscover Life Wisdom Among Hong Kong Chinese Older Adults: A Single-Blind Randomized Waitlist-Controlled Trial," *Innovation in Aging* 5, no. 3 (2021): igab027, https://doi.org/10.1093/geroni/igab027; Lying Sun et al., "Narrative Therapy to Relieve Stigma in Oral Cancer Patients: A Randomized Controlled Trial," *International Journal of Nursing Practice* (2021): e12926, https://doi.org/10.1111/ijn.12926; and De-Hui Ruth Zhou et al., "An Unexpected Visitor and a Sword Play: A Randomized Controlled Trial of Collective Narrative Therapy Groups for Primary Carers of People with Schizophrenia," *Journal of Mental Health* (2020): 1–12, https://doi.org/10.1080/09638237 .2020.1793123.

research bias. Moreover, complying with institutional review board (IRB) ethical standards, a waitlist control group includes participants who do not receive the experimental treatment, but who are put on a waitlist to receive the intervention after an active treatment group.

STRENGTHS AND LIMITATIONS OF QUANTITATIVE APPROACHES

Quantitative approaches add value in terms of observing the magnitude of change that therapy was able to prompt in individuals. Moreover, having empirical backing positively affects the credibility of the studies using NT. Because of the interpretive nature of NT, quantitative research alone does not account for the unique experiences of subjects in different contexts. Quantitative evidence, however, does show a positive trend in promoting well-being among a diverse range of demographics.

MIXED-METHOD RESEARCH: FUTURE DIRECTIONS

According to the mixed-method approach, researchers gather and analyze both quantitative and qualitative data in the same study.[47] An example is a collective study using a mixed-method design that proposes that cohesive, resilient communities are important to the well-being of residents.[48] One such study combined in-depth interviews and survey results from volunteers according to the perspective that healthy communities act as "social cures," which means that the social networks and social identities can promote adjustment, coping, and well-being for individuals who are dealing with a range of illnesses, injuries, trauma, and stressors.[49] By adopting a mixed-method paradigm, the study researchers uncovered the determinants of successful community identities that were essential to progressing the community health agenda. The results showed that community relationships were crucial to shaping one's sense of community belonging, providing mutual support, and promoting well-being. In addition, the results confirmed that the more groups could self-identify as "social cures," the better the health and well-being of the community.

POTENTIAL USE OF MIXED-METHOD APPROACH

Research on mixed methods is limited to date, especially applications to NT research, as a result of the discrepancy of fundamental assumptions of the quantitative and qualitative approaches. Qualitative studies are aimed at gaining a holistic understanding despite objectivity, whereas quantitative studies are aimed at identifying variables that relate to the object of study. The poststructural approach views the signifier and signified as inseparable. In this context, the mixed-methods approach could be used to infer further insight because it combines qualitative (signifier) and quantitative (signified) information in its analysis. A possible solution to ensure the objectivity of the qualitative information is to develop systematic and measurable ways for participants to report the outcome of NTs. For example, practitioners could design questionnaires with ratings of optimism about future prospects, the ability to appreciate individual strengths, and life wisdom. In this way, the signifier (statistics) may better represent the signified (quality of therapy outcome). Because of the limited NT research that adopts the mixed-method approach, further exploration is required to improve the credibility of NT research and, ultimately, to help more people in need with the use of NT.

CONCLUSION

As a relatively young form of psychotherapy, especially in the East, NT's contributions to the field are still in development. Nonetheless, thus far, NT appears to be a promising therapeutic method for practitioners working in a range of contexts, as evidenced by the literature. More emphasis is needed on individuals and groups who might be reluctant to join in a narrative conversation or to have their stories heard by others, including those with cultural barriers and stigmatized groups. The strength of NT in helping diverse and often disadvantaged groups of people comes from its intercultural sensitivity, the diversity of problems it addresses, and its ability to progressively build on strengths and resilience. In addition, NT has the flexibility to be conducted on many different dimensions from micro to macro scales of casework, group work, and collective work. Despite its strengths, NT has a long path ahead before it can become a conventional global therapeutic process. More mixed-method studies are needed that provide a holistic understanding and empirically supported evidence to reveal the potential of NT and create "social cures" among communities around the world.

Chapter 3 discusses the theories underpinning narrative practice, and chapter 4 explains in detail NT's conversational framework and skills. This framework has been consolidated from years of practical experience working from different levels of practice, including individuals, groups, and communities.

NOTES

1. Christine C. Danner et al., "Running from the Demon: Culturally Specific Group Therapy for Depressed Hmong Women in a Family Medicine Residency Clinic," *Women and Therapy* 30, no. 1–2 (2007): 151–76.
2. Donald E. Polkinghorne, "Narrative Therapy and Postmodernism," In *The Handbook of Narrative and Psychotherapy: Practice, Theory and Research*, ed. Lynne E. Angus and John McLeod (Thousand Oaks, CA: Sage, 2004).
3. Michael White, Made Wijaya, and David Epston, *Narrative Means to Therapeutic Ends* (New York: Norton, 1990).
4. H. Theron and D. Bruwer, "More About . . . Mental Health in the Community," *CME* 24, no. 8 (2008): 449–50.
5. Christopher Faircloth et al., "Disrupted Bodies: Experiencing the Newly Limited Body in Stroke," *Symbolic Interaction* 27, no. 1 (2004); Ruthellen Josselson,

"Narrative Research and the Challenge of Accumulating Knowledge," *Narrative Inquiry* 16, no. 1 (2006): 3–10; William L. Randall and Gary M. Kenyon, "Time, Story, and Wisdom: Emerging Themes in Narrative Gerontology," *Canadian Journal on Aging (La Revue canadienne du vieillissement)* 23, no. 4 (2004): 333–46; and Kate De Medeiros, *Narrative Gerontology in Research and Practice* (New York: Springer, 2013).

6. Randall and Kenyon, "Time, Story, and Wisdom."

7. De Medeiros, *Narrative Gerontology in Research and Practice.*

8. Maggie Carey and Shona Russell, *Narrative Therapy: Responding to Your Questions* (Adelaide, SA: Dulwich Centre, 2004).

9. Martin Bloom, Joel Fischer, and John G. Orme, *Evaluating Practice: Guidelines for the Accountable Professional*, 6th ed. (Boston: Pearson, 2009), 2.

10. Wolfgang Lutz and Clara E. Hill, "Quantitative and Qualitative Methods for Psychotherapy Research: Introduction to Special Section," *Psychotherapy Research* 19, no. 4–5 (2009): 369–73, https://doi.org/10.1080/10503300902948053.

11. David Denborough, "The Team of Life with Young Men from Refugee Backgrounds," *International Journal of Narrative Therapy and Community Work* 2 (2012): 44–53, https://doi.org/10.3316/informit.627063623957215.

12. Joe M. Schriver, *Human Behavior and the Social Environment: Shifting Paradigms in Essential Knowledge for Social Work Practice*, 5th ed., Connecting Core Competencies Series (Boston: Allyn and Bacon, 2011), 27.

13. Kathrin Mörtl and Omar Carlo Gioacchino Gelo, "Qualitative Methods in Psychotherapy Process Research," in *Psychotherapy Research: Foundations, Process, and Outcome*, ed. Omar C. G. Gelo, Aldred Pritz, and Bernd Rieken, 381–428 (Vienna: Springer, 2014).

14. John Ward Creswell, *Qualitative Inquiry and Research Design: Choosing Among Five Approaches*, 3rd ed. (Los Angeles: SAGE, 2013), 160.

15. Teresa Legowski and Keith Brownlee, "Working with Metaphor in Narrative Therapy," *Journal of Family Psychotherapy* 12, no. 1 (2001): 19–28, https://doi.org/10.1300/J085v12n01_02; and Athlone Christine Besley, "Foucault and the Turn to Narrative Therapy," *British Journal of Guidance and Counseling* 30, no. 2 (2002): 125–43, https://doi.org/10.1080/03069880220128010.

16. Nancy P. Kropf and Cindy Tandy, "Narrative Therapy with Older Clients: The Use of a "Meaning-Making" Approach," *Clinical Gerontologist* 18, no. 4 (1998): 3–16, https://doi.org/10.1300/J018v18n04_02.

17. Brittany Stahnke and Morgan E. Cooley, "End-of-Life Case Study: The Use of Narrative Therapy on a Holocaust Survivor with Lifelong Depression," *Journal of Contemporary Psychotherapy* 52 (2022): 191–98, https://doi.org/https://doi.org/10.1007/s10879-022-09532-z.

18. Janette J. Driscoll and Anthony A. Hughes, "Sexuality of Aging Adults: A Case Study Using Narrative Therapy," *Contemporary Family Therapy* 44 (2021): 373–80, https://doi.org/10.1007/s10591-021-09589-3.

19. Bertranna Muruthi, Megan McCoy, Jessica Chou, and Andrea Farnham, "Sexual Scripts and Narrative Therapy with Older Couples," *American Journal of Family Therapy* 46, no. 1 (2018): 81–95, https://doi.org/10.1080/01926187 .2018.1428129.

20. Esther Oi-Wah Chow, "Responding to Lives After Stroke: Stroke Survivors and Caregivers Going on Narrative Journeys," *International Journal of Narrative Therapy and Community Work* 4 (2013): 1.

21. Jean-François Lyotard, *The Postmodern Condition: A Report on Knowledge*, trans. Geoff Bennington, Brian Massumi, and Fredric Jameson, vol. 10, *Theory and History of Literature*, 12th ed. (Minneapolis: University of Minnesota Press, 1984); and Alan Carr, "Michael White's Narrative Therapy," *Contemporary Family Therapy* 20, no. 4 (1998): 485–503.

22. Gwen Adshead, "The Life Sentence: Using a Narrative Approach in Group Psychotherapy with Offenders," *Group Analysis* 44, no. 2 (2011): 175–95, https:// doi.org/10.1177/0533316411400969; Anne C. Jones, "Transforming the Story: Narrative Applications to a Stepmother Support Group," *Families in Society* 85, no. 1 (2004): 129–38, https://doi.org/10.1606/1044-3894.242; and Barbara Baumgartner and Brian Dean Williams, "Becoming an Insider: Narrative Therapy Groups Alongside People Overcoming Homelessness," *Journal of Systemic Therapies* 33, no. 4 (2014): 1–14, https://doi.org/https://doi.org/10.1521 /jsyt.2014.33.4.1.

23. Dean Ruth Grossman, "A Narrative Approach to Groups," *Clinical Social Work Journal* 26, no. 1 (1998): 23–37.

24. Adshead, "The Life Sentence"; Jones, "Transforming the Story"; and Baumgart-ner and Williams, "Becoming an Insider."

25. Tessa L. Dover, Jeffrey M. Hunger, and Brenda Major, "Health Consequences of Prejudice and Discrimination," in *The Wiley Encyclopedia of Health Psychology*, vol. 2, ed. Lee Cohen, 231–38 (Chichester, UK: Wiley, 2020).

26. Yun-He Wang et al., "Depression and Anxiety in Relation to Cancer Incidence and Mortality: A Systematic Review and Meta-analysis of Cohort Studies," *Molecular Psychiatry* 25, no. 7 (2020): 1487–99, https://doi.org/10.1038 /s41380-019-0595-x; and Claire L. Niedzwiedz et al., "Depression and Anxiety Among People Living with and Beyond Cancer: A Growing Clinical and Research Priority," *BMC Cancer* 19, no. 1 (2019): 943, https://doi.org/10.1186 /s12885-019-6181-4.

27. Guillaume Fond et al., "End of Life Breast Cancer Care in Women with Severe Mental Illnesses," *Scientific Reports* 11, no. 1 (2021): 10167, https://doi.org /10.1038/s41598-021-89726-y; Guillaume Fond et al., "Association Between Mental Health Disorders and Mortality Among Patients with COVID-19 in 7 Countries: A Systematic Review and Meta-analysis," *JAMA Psychiatry* 78, no. 11 (2021): 1208, https://doi.org/10.1001/jamapsychiatry.2021.2274; and QuanQiu Wang, Rong Xu, and Nora D. Volkow, "Increased Risk of COVID-19

Infection and Mortality in People with Mental Disorders: Analysis from Electronic Health Records in the United States," *World Psychiatry* 20, no. 1 (2021): 124–30, https://doi.org/10.1002/wps.20806.

28. Afarin Rajaei et al., "Striving to Thrive: A Qualitative Study on Fostering a Relational Perspective Through Narrative Therapy in Couples Facing Cancer," *American Journal of Family Therapy* 49, no. 4 (2021): 392–408, https://doi.org /10.1080/01926187.2020.1820402; and B. Rodríguez Vega et al., "Mindfulness-Based Narrative Therapy for Depression in Cancer Patients," *Clinical Psychological Psychotherapy* 21, no. 5 (2014): 411–19, https://doi.org/10.1002/cpp.1847.

29. Franca Butera-Prinzi, Nella Charles, and Karen Story, "Narrative Family Therapy and Group Work for Families Living with Acquired Brain Injury," *Australian and New Zealand Journal of Family Therapy* 35, no. 1, 81–99 (2014): 81–99, https://doi.org/10.1002/anzf.1046.

30. Emily Pia, "Narrative Therapy and Peacebuilding," *Journal of Intervention and Statebuilding* 7, no. 4 (2013): 476–91, https://doi.org/10.1080/17502977.2012 .727538.

31. Sara Portnoy, Isabella Girling, and Glenda Fredman, "Supporting Young People Living with Cancer to Tell Their Stories in Ways That Make Them Stronger: The Beads of Life Approach," *Clinical Child Psychology and Psychiatry* 21, no. 2 (2016): 255–67, https://doi.org/10.1177/1359104515586467; Suvi-Maria K. Saarelainen, "Life Tree Drawings as a Methodological Approach in Young Adults' Life Stories During Cancer Remission," *Narrative Works* 5, no. 1 (2015): 68–91, https://journals.lib.unb.ca/index.php/NW/article/view /23785; Butera-Prinzi, Charles, and Story, "Narrative Family Therapy and Group Work"; Suzan F. M. Jacobs, "Collective Narrative Practice with Unaccompanied Refugee Minors: 'The Tree of Life' as a Response to Hardship," *Clinical Child Psychology and Psychiatry* 23, no. 2 (2018): 279–93, https://doi .org/10.1177/1359104517744246; Esther Oi-Wah Chow, "Narrative Therapy an Evaluated Intervention to Improve Stroke Survivors' Social and Emotional Adaptation," *Clinical Rehabilitation* 29, no. 4 (2015): 315–26, https://doi.org /10.1177/0269215514544039; Nhlanhla Ncube, "The Tree of Life Project: Using Narrative Ideas in Work with Vulnerable Children in Southern Africa," *International Journal of Narrative Therapy and Community Work* 1 (2006): 3–16; Grant Lesley, "Bringing Together Women Like You and Me: Collective Narrative Practice with Women and Trauma," *International Journal of Narrative Therapy and Community Work* 1 (2022): 1–8, https://doi.org/10.3316 /informit.429037128627631, https://search.informit.org/doi/10.3316/informit .429037128627631; and Yvonne Sliep, "A Narrative Theatre Approach to Working with Communities Affected by Trauma, Conflict and War," *International Journal of Narrative Therapy and Community Work* 2005, no. 2 (2005): 47–52.

32. David Denborough, *Collective Narrative Practice* (Adelaide, SA: Dulwich Centre, 2008).

33. Chow, "Narrative Therapy."

34. Natale Rudland Wood, "Recipes for Life," *International Journal of Narrative Therapy and Community Work* 2 (2012): 34–43; Meizi Tan, "Recipes for Life: A Collective Narrative Methodology for Responding to Gender Violence," *International Journal of Narrative Therapy and Community Work* 2 (2017): 1–12; and Esther Oi-Wah Chow and Doris Yuen Hung Fok, "Recipe of Life: A Relational Narrative Approach in Therapy with Persons Living with Chronic Pain," *Research on Social Work Practice* 30, no. 3 (2020): 320–29, https://doi.org /10.1177/1049731519870867.

35. Suet Lin Hung, "Collective Narrative Practice with Rape Victims in the Chinese Society of Hong Kong," *International Journal of Narrative Therapy and Community Work* 1 (2011): 14–31, https://doi.org/10.3316/informit.870589297245238.

36. Schriver, *Human Behavior and the Social Environment*, 20.

37. M. Lakshman et al., "Quantitative vs. Qualitative Research Methods," *Indian Journal of Pediatrics* 67, no. 5 (2000): 369–77, https://doi.org/10.1007 /BF02820690

38. Allen Rubin and Earl R. Babbie, *Research Methods for Social Work*, 9th ed., Empowerment Series (Boston: Cengage Learning, 2017), 26.

39. Seyedhadi Yeganeh Farzand, Kianoush Zahrakar, and Farshad Mohsenzadeh, "The Effectiveness of Narrative Therapy on Reducing the Fear of Intimacy in Couples," *Practice in Clinical Psychology* (2019): 117–24, https:// doi.org/10.32598/jpcp.7.2.117.

40. Eduardo Hariton and Joseph J. Locascio, "Randomised Controlled Trials— The Gold Standard for Effectiveness Research: Study Design: Randomised Controlled Trials," *BJOG: An International Journal of Obstetrics and Gynaecology* 125, no. 13 (2018): 1716, https://doi.org/10.1111/1471-0528.15199; and Lars Bondemark and Sabine Ruf, "Randomized Controlled Trial: The Gold Standard or an Unobtainable Fallacy?," *European Journal of Orthodontics* 37, no. 5 (2015): 457–61, https://doi.org/10.1093/ejo/cjv046.

41. Emerson L. Lesher and Jeffrey S. Berryhill, "Validation of the Geriatric Depression Scale-Short Form Among Inpatients," *Journal of Clinical Psychology* 50, no. 2 (1994): 256–60.

42. Jaivir S. Rathore et al., "Validation of the Patient Health Questionnaire-9 (PHQ-9) for Depression Screening in Adults with Epilepsy," *Epilepsy and Behavior* 37 (2014): 215–20.

43. L. S. Radloff, "Center for Epidemiologic Studies Depression Scale (CES-D)" (2012).

44. Aaron T. Beck, Robert A. Steer, and Gregory Brown, "Beck Depression Inventory–II," *Psychological Assessment* (1996).

45. Esther Oi-Wah Chow, "Narrative Group Intervention to Reconstruct Meaning of Life Among Stroke Survivors: A Randomized Clinical Trial Study," *Neuropsychiatry* 8, no. 4 (2018): 1216–26, https://doi.org/10.4172/Neuropsychiatry.1000450; Esther Oi-Wah Chow, "Narrative Group Interventions to Rediscover Life Wisdom Among Hong Kong Chinese Older Adults: A Waitlist RCT Study," *Innovation in Aging* 2, no. Suppl. 1 (2018): 992–92, https://doi.org/10.1093/geroni/igy031.3666; Esther Oi-Wah Chow and Sai-Fu Fung, "Narrative Group Intervention to Rediscover Life Wisdom Among Hong Kong Chinese Older Adults: A Single-Blind Randomized Waitlist-Controlled Trial," *Innovation in Aging* 5, no. 3 (2021): igab27; and De-Hui Ruth Zhou et al., "An Unexpected Visitor and a Sword Play: A Randomized Controlled Trial of Collective Narrative Therapy Groups for Primary Carers of People with Schizophrenia," *Journal of Mental Health* (2020): 1–12, https://doi.org/10.1080/09638237.2020.1793123.

46. Ted J. Kaptchuk, "The Double-Blind, Randomized, Placebo-Controlled Trial," *Journal of Clinical Epidemiology* 54, no. 6 (2001): 541–49, https://doi.org/10.1016/S0895-4356(00)00347-4.

47. Allison Shorten and Joanna Smith, "Mixed Methods Research: Expanding the Evidence Base," *Evidence-Based Nursing* 20, no. 3 (2017): 74–75, https://doi.org/10.1136/eb-2017-102699.

48. Mhairi Bowe et al., "A Social Cure in the Community: A Mixed-Method Exploration of the Role of Social Identity in the Experiences and Well-Being of Community Volunteers," *European Journal of Social Psychology* 50, no. 7 (2020): 1523–39, https://doi.org/10.1002/ejsp.2706.

49. Jolanda Jetten, Catherine Haslam, and Alexander S. Haslam, introduction to *The Social Cure: Identity, Health and Well-Being*, ed. Jolanda Jetten, Catherine Haslam, and Alexander, S. Haslam (London: Psychology Press, 2011), https://doi.org/10.4324/9780203813195.

3

NURTURING ROOTS

The Theoretical Foundations of Narrative Practice

MANY YEARS AGO, as social work students, we wanted to help transform people's lives for the better and sought out different theories along our journeys as the basis for our continued passion to support others. Four theories in particular (i.e., humanism, structuralism, poststructuralism, and social constructionism, which are explored in this chapter) awaken in us the knowledge that people have a lot of power to transform their lives individually and collectively. We discovered that our role could be to guide them on their journeys, much like a first mate to the captain navigating a ship. We developed this metaphor as a tool to help others identify their framework for life: imagining one's life as a vast starry sky, with each star symbolizing a life event or an experience. With all the stars coming together, the starry sky is composed of diverse episodes of one's whole life. How do we understand the complexity of our lives when we look at them? It is amazing to see which stars (life events) a person identifies when unfolding their life story to connect those life-challenging or perplexing events and to learn how the person infuses meaning to each of those events.

People need support in creating their frameworks, to make sense of the negotiation process that emerges from those challenges, and to determine how that person validates their self-worth, values, beliefs, and identities over a lifespan. Narrative therapy (NT) provides the means for us to understand, recollect, and interpret our life experiences. Connecting different sparkling moments provides the possibility to narrate the respective storylines of rich and diverse life experiences that are expressed, told, and remembered, even as other events are forgotten, ignored, and denied. Among a myriad of life experiences, however, what are the factors that trigger an individual to connect specific dots of particular experiences when presenting a particular storyline? Does this happen in response to interrogation? Or does it come from one's self-understanding of a particular theme?

UNDERSTANDING LIFE-STORY DEVELOPMENT

Throughout our lifespan, we are exposed to diverse life events, either good and uplifting moments or bad and trying times. We try to make sense of our lives and experiences by attributing meaning to them through our lived experience, which emerges within and is inevitably influenced by immediate social and cultural discourses. We gradually acquire and display the beliefs, values, and practices of our family, groups, organizations, and community that are part of the cultural traditions as we grow up. As spiritual development accompanies crucial life transitions and challenges, such as facing a critical life decision, dealing with a dilemma, recovering from an illness, confronting physical disabilities, or facing impending death and the loss of loved ones, one may begin to question and discard or refine some of their commonly held beliefs and practices. During these moments in life, a person may feel that her identity is entrapped in a difficult life-situation and may adopt a problematic label. A person makes sense of their behavior and life through personal beliefs, social norms, and feedback from others. In this narrative, dominant social standards, norms, and expectations regulate the person's access to experience in the form of authority. Thus, problems arise from the frustration of a person's failure to meet social standards and social expectations. In other words, when a person's experience contradicts society's dominant narrative, there is a high chance that the person is being denied by the dominant narrative and being internalized as a problematic person. As a result, they may develop a problematic identity. Several theories oppose this negativistic view.

FOUNDATIONAL THEORIES FOR USING NARRATIVE THERAPY: HUMANISM, STRUCTURALISM, POSTSTRUCTURALISM, AND SOCIAL CONSTRUCTIONISM

According to humanism, everyone has an intrinsic drive to grow and improve into a better version of themselves. Everyone wants to achieve self-realization, emphasizing that individuals have self-awareness and are capable identifying their own problems through self-reflection and feedback, which leads to self-actualization. This theory's most popular representatives are Abraham Maslow and Carl Rogers. Maslow proposed the hierarchy of needs theory, which classifies the basic needs of human beings. He advocated a

focus on human "self-needs and self-actualization," clarified the motivation of human behavior as a subject, and made it clear that human needs
and instincts differed from those of animals. He also argues that human
development is based on the continuous satisfaction of different levels of
need, with the distinct characteristic of human nature being "continuous
growth."[1] Rogers's view of human nature is based on the ideas of "self-concept,"
"self-actualization," and "self-direction." His theory advocates an optimistic
view of human nature that is "human centered."[2] He believes that the main
characteristic of a human being is to maximize their potential in becoming
a self, and he advocates focusing on one's abilities and potential, believing
in oneself, and developing one's motivation and self-confidence.

In short, humanistic theory holds the highest respect for human nature as
good. Yet, across the lifespan, when and where do we acquire and develop
our moral values? Is it when we are born into diverse societies and cultures,
with different perspectives on our beliefs about human nature? Who are the
socializing agents that construct social and cultural values and impart them
on the people? And what is the impact of such constructs on the individual and human growth and development on respective personal and social
identities? And what is the impact of these constructs on the identities of
the most vulnerable, those who have become disadvantaged and are being
marginalized? This question provides a critical point of entry to learning
how social and human service professionals perceive people, emphasizing
the need for the therapist to share that these beliefs and attitudes for humans
are positive, advocating empathy and sympathy to form a good helping relationship with the people who consult social and human care workers and
services providers.

Structuralism assumes that the meaning of life is essentially the same for
all people and reflects their values. It views social roles as the core elements
and believes that these defined elements determine the only truth of life.[3]
According to this view, all people's life meaning and existence are virtually
static. Moreover, structuralism ignores the manifestation of human subjectivity, dismisses distinct characteristics, and falls somewhat into fatalism.[4]
Poststructuralism, in contrast, emphasizes individual uniqueness, including
the specific details and particular facts of a person's life story.[5] It promotes
multiple perspectives on storytelling and emphasizes that the life of each
individual in society has value, especially inner knowledge. It believes that
each person has the power to construct and interpret life's meaning, particularly through action and storytelling. The difference with poststructuralism
does not simply refer to a different view of life's meaning but rather it also

incorporates some ideas from philosophical hermeneutics. Gregory Bateson argues that one cannot know the objective world and that all "knowing" of the objective world is given meaning through one's own interpretation, not as a methodology but as a way of making meaning.[6] For example, in the case of an unhappy family, traditional therapy would suggest that the family's dysfunction has led to tensions between members and their individual behavior. When NT is used in a poststructural context, however, it focuses on the meaning that family members give to events that determine the direction of their relational behavior. Instead of focusing on the causes of events, it focuses on what conditions enable the "problem" to survive, how these conditions affect people's lives, and how they perceive such conditions.

Poststructuralism is a philosophical and theoretical movement that emerged in the 1960s and 1970s, primarily in France. Its chief concern is with the ways in which a person's sense of life meaning is produced and maintained through a society's language, discourse, and power relations. Poststructuralists argue that language is not simply a neutral tool for expressing ideas, but rather that it is itself a site of struggle and contestation, with different cultural subgroups vying for control over how a group's life significance is constructed and communicated. Key figures in poststructuralism include Michel Foucault, Jacques Derrida, and Gilles Deleuze.

Social constructionism, in contrast, is a more specific approach within the social sciences that emerged in the 1970s and 1980s. It is concerned with the ways in which a culture's social phenomena—such as gender, race, and sexuality—are not simply natural or biologically determined, but instead are constructed through social processes and institutions. Social constructionists argue that these categories are not fixed or stable. Instead, they are constantly being created and recreated through social interactions and practices. Key figures in social constructionism include Ian Hacking, Peter Berger, and Thomas Luckmann.

Although poststructuralism and social constructionism share similarities— for example, both reject the idea of an objective reality that exists independently of a culture's language and social context—they differ in their theoretical roots and specific approaches. Poststructuralism is more concerned with the ways in which life meaning is produced and maintained through language and power relations, whereas social constructionism is more focused on the ways in which social phenomena and life meaning are constructed through social processes and institutions.

The "self-identity" perspective among poststructuralism has particularly profound implications for NT. For example, older people who have experienced a chronic illness, such as stroke, diabetes, or dementia may be overly concerned with aspects of the dominant social status as a patient who is chronically ill, with culture's unjust values of themselves as no longer useful to society, while ignoring the fact that they still have other significant identities, such as being good parents who care for their families. In NT, the therapist is not concerned with how the elder person "lacks value" in life, but rather discusses what it means to have had a stroke, how one sees oneself with a stroke, and how one sees themselves in the eyes of their family, even if they can no longer care for them. Through this dialogue, older adults can depersonalize a stroke—moving them away from the idea that they are worthless after the stroke and shifting their identity to a more global view. The beauty of NT infused with the helpfulness of these three theories is that it allows people to see the "problem" as separate from their identities. NT enables them to acknowledge and use their strengths, values, beliefs, and abilities to reauthor their life-story narratives with meaning, wholeness, and goodness.

HOW NT ADAPTS TO JUDGMENTS ABOUT HUMAN NATURE UNDER HUMANISM AND POSTSTRUCTURALISM

From humanism to poststructuralism, there has been a major epistemological shift from "essence" to "structure" and from "independence" to "self-value." This shift has greatly affected the orientation of NT and the therapeutic relationship. First, traditional psychotherapy has focused on the individual, on the individual's upbringing and life circumstances, and on the development of the individual's personality, thinking, and attitudes, with little regard for the influence of others on the individual. Therefore, Gergen has called traditional psychology "the psychology of the absence of others."[7] Conversely, NT focuses more on the person's interpersonal relationships and how they interact with dominant discourses in everyday life. The emphasis is on using one's own story and one's own strength to gradually escape the negative effects of unfair social values. The aim of the "problem externalization" technique is not only to separate the person from the problem but also to make the person aware of the fact that they have been placed in a social framework to the point of being immobilized. As a result, the person is able to see clearly how their interaction with the problem has fueled it and extended its the influence and control over them. In addition, narrative therapists often ask people to invite significant others in their life to act as witnesses to the changes they have learned from these experiences. NT assumes that an individual's problems are not the result of a disruption or malfunction in the internal structure of the individual's nature but instead are constructed by maladjustments with the sociocultural environment. Incompatibility with the dominant social culture creates the problem. NT, therefore, focuses on the "relationship" and the "constructive process" of the problem as a therapeutic concern.

Second, NT no longer places the therapist as an expert above the person, but rather the person is viewed as the expert in solving their problems. Because knowledge, including certain psychological knowledge, is no longer an objectively true reflection of the person's psychological phenomena, the therapist is no longer qualified to present her- or himself as an expert. On the contrary, because the person's so-called psychological problems result from the construction of daily life, no one knows more about their life and the construction of those problems than that person. Therefore, they are rightly entitled to play the role of an expert in solving their problems. Whatever the person says, the narrative therapist gives sincere acceptance and approval because the narrative therapist believes that what the person is saying is what he or she believes to be a fact of life, a life experience, and a feeling that has had a significant impact on her or him. What the narrative therapist can do is accept and accompany the person throughout the process. The relationship between therapist and person is no longer that of expert and ordinary person (i.e., active intervention and passive acceptance), and therapy is no longer a set procedure in which the "knower" conveys "knowledge" to the "unknowing." Instead, both the therapist and person coconstruct the therapeutic process through consultation and collaboration as therapy participants.

ADAPTING NARRATIVE THERAPY TO THE CHARACTERISTICS OF PEOPLE IN THE EASTERN CONTEXT

The value base of NT remains essentially rooted in the Western philosophy of individualism. The therapist's practice of NT emphasizes the individuals' ability and potential to change and develop themselves, with full respect for individual values. This implicit Western value-ethical principle is a key component of resolving problems. This implied Western value-ethical principle, however, does conflict with and have some inconsistencies with Eastern collectivist and paternalistic values and therefore it needs to be further localized. In collectivist cultures, the family strongly influences the individual, so the family and community largely govern the self-expression and self-actualization of the person. People who are from Eastern cultures may be uncomfortable with detailed and individual-focused narrative models of therapy as well as with revealing events to strangers that may damage self-esteem or cause them to lose face.

The relational orientation of NT is well suited to people of Eastern culture who largely have a relational view of themselves. The story that the person tells inevitably includes specific situations, significant people, and relationships between people. In family therapy, Michael White has stated that problems in the life of one family member can affect other family members. In most cases, the individual's problems are linked to poor interactions with other family members.[8] NT, therefore, incorporates the family, the school, the workplace, and even institutions of power and cultural traditions in the field of study. The individual is not an entity until herself, but a being that exists as a result of being in relationships with others. In this respect, the Eastern view of the self coincides with the postmodern view of the self as a relationship-centered self.[9] The practice of NT provides flexibility in the definition of the individual or the problem, making it possible for the person and therapist to revise, recall, and re-recall a story from different perspectives.[10] Formally, these relational recreative dialogues are where change is seen to occur in NT.[11] The task of NT should be to avoid, rather than produce, the "authority of experience." Instead, the story needs to be interpreted by the person with the intent of producing alternative narratives, if the person finds the story's outcome to be desirable.

People often seek help for problems or difficulties because they feel trapped, stuck, or overwhelmed by their problems. The therapist cannot assume that they have an analysis of their situation, that they are not trapped in an unhelpful dominant narrative, or that they can move beyond existing, often unhelpful, ways of coping. The therapist and person will interpret and make sense of the experience through therapeutic dialogue. In NT, the therapist and the person externalize problems together, reclaiming important pieces of the person's life. Externalizing the problem creates an appropriate space for the person to see the negative narratives they have developed of the "problem" as a result of unjust social values. It is also possible to see that these "problems" are formed because of the constant interactions between people—that is, the existence of relationships that expose the person to unjust social values. Next, the positive narrative of the person is reinforced through the witnessing of the outside witness, whose validation and support help affirm the individual's experiences and perspective. The therapist simply plays the role of the audience in this session, which is intended to avoid the influence of the therapist's perceived authority over the person, free from the representation that the person is the expert or authority on their experience. Finally, through a series of processes in the narrative dialogue, a person rediscovers the ability to face life's challenges and their relationship with competence is strengthened.

CONCLUSION

Because NT arising from a Euro-American cultural context is culturally different from other societies, it is difficult to effectively respond to the needs of other communities from different cultural backgrounds by relying unilaterally on Euro-American culture-based concepts and assumptions in therapy. To better develop localized NT to accommodate people from different cultural backgrounds, therapists should pay more attention to respective spiritual and political narratives to give more legitimacy and recognition to indigenous use of language expressions. In addition, local knowledge and cultural traditions are embedded in the methods and techniques of NT. Therapists must pay attention to the local relevance of the techniques and theories used in practice and tap into the traditional therapeutic approaches embedded in local knowledge.

How the therapist integrates the spirit and strategies of Western NT with the dominant narrative interpretation in this context is the main issue that should be considered in localizing NT. Furthermore, the importance of art and writing has emerged as people think about NT, and art and writing therapies are widely used in NT. Art and writing can be used as an adjunct to verbal expression to complement the limitations of verbal expression and provide a diverse medium for personal expression and reflection. At the same time, similar physical expressions act as a referent to explore the person's deeper emotions and meanings, enhance the person's insight, and facilitate change in the person.

With the influx of immigrants in Europe and the United States, therapists have been exploring more culturally relevant interventions in working with different immigrant groups. The therapeutic approaches, techniques, and theoretical models used by therapists need to be adapted to serve different immigrant groups and ethnic minority groups in a culturally relevant way. To develop an NT model appropriate to the different groups served, especially ethnic minority groups, the therapist should first understand the local culture, knowledge, the way people think, and their cognitive patterns. Therapists should be interested in identifying and questioning their own cultural biases so that they can try to make the dialogue culturally appropriate for a wider range of people. Narrative therapists should be curious about each person's locality and learn how each person has been influenced by their culture's dominant story and learn to value each person's distinct story. Culture shapes our ontology, epistemology, worldview, and value presuppositions. In addition, language and culture are inextricably linked to the style of the communication process. Therefore, developing an NT practice requires the therapist to understand the forms and processes of communication in the community and to prevent the therapist's own culturally laden perspective from dominating the language and communication patterns of the community. These NT forms, processes, and conversational skills will be laid out as essential tools in the next chapter.

In short, the therapist needs to be aware of how the problems that plague the person are formed, understanding why many possible outlets for the person's life are excluded from consciousness. By discovering the dimensions of the problem and the processes and mechanisms by which it has developed, the person can revisit the cultural assumptions that have been defaulted and internalized, allowing them to recognize assumptions that constitute the problem. We are all often pulled by these invisible strings, these cultural assumptions, and are controlled by them.

In addition to using these NT essential tools well, the salient attribute of a narrative therapist lies in the ability to be a safe presence, intentionally listening and reflecting, and thereby lessening a person's defenses so that they will be willing and able to tell their story truthfully and rewrite their life. The roles of faithful listener, confidant, companion on the spiritual journey, and coach of one's personal practice are inherent to this ability.

NOTES

1. Abraham Harold Maslow, *Motivation and Personality* (Prabhat Prakashan, 1981).
2. R. Hegel Mather, "Dostoyevsky and Carl Rogers: Between Humanism and Spirit," *History of the Human Sciences* 21, no. 1 (2008): 33–48, https://doi.org/10.1177/0952695107086151.
3. R. G. Smith, "Structuralism/Structuralist Geography," *International Encyclopedia of Human Geography*, ed. Rob Kitchin and Nigel Thrift, 30–38 (Oxford: Elsevier, 2009).

4. Peter Caws, "What Is Structuralism?," *Partisan Review* 35, no. 1 (1968).
5. Kalle Berggren, "Sticky Masculinity: Post-Structuralism, Phenomenology and Subjectivity in Critical Studies on Men," *Men and Masculinities* 17, no. 3 (2014): 231–52.
6. Isaac E. Catt, "Gregory Bateson's 'New Science' in the Context of Communicology," *American Journal of Semiotics* 19, no. 1/4 (2016): 153–72.
7. K. J. Gergen, "Psychological Science in a Postmodern Context," *American Psychologist* 56, no. 10 (2001): 803–13, https://doi.org/10.1037//0003-066x.56.10.803.
8. Michel White, "Family Therapy and Schizophrenia: Addressing the 'In-the-Corner' Lifestyle," *Dulwich Centre Newsletter* 1 (1987): 14–21.
9. David Marsten, David Epston, and Laurie Markham, *Narrative Therapy in Wonderland: Connecting with Children's Imaginative Know-How* (New York: Norton, 2016).
10. Ruth Madigan and Moira Munro, "'House Beautiful': Style and Consumption in the Home," *Sociology* 30, no. 1 (1996): 41–57, https://doi.org/10.1177/0038038596030001004.
11. Jeffrey L. Zimmerman and Victoria C. Dickerson, *If Problems Talked: Narrative Therapy in Action* (New York: Guilford, 1996); and Frigga Haug, "Feminist Writing: Working with Women's Experience," *Feminist Review* 42, no. 1 (1992): 16–32.

4

EMPOWERING CHANGE THROUGH NARRATIVE PRACTICE

Essential Tools

THEORETICAL FOUNDATION OF THE CONVERSATIONAL SKILLS

As discussed in chapter 3, narrative therapy (NT) was inspired by social constructionism and poststructuralism, which hold that a person's mental health status and meaning in life is extensively influenced by the symbols in their surrounding society, or spheres of influence, from the micro to the macro level. In the process of social construction, an individual (regardless of their gender, age, or cultural background) needs to assign meaning to his or her personal experiences and narrate his or her own life story. People internalize the life stories they have constructed, imbuing meaning to their lives.

We need to be alert that if a person is surrounded by negative information or narrations (e.g., stroke patients are not productive but dependent) that strengthen a negative life script, the story he or she writes will be infused with oppression and blame, and eventually will lead to a problem-saturated life story. Under such a social construction, people tend to lose sight of any of their capabilities and value, instead seeing their lives only as disappointing and meaningless, with little hope or aspirations for future, which further reinforces their problem-saturated identities.

To help people out of this problem-saturated situation, NT aims to guide them to look at things from a different perspective, leading them to explore and reflect on their life experiences and capabilities, and thus to regain the power to reauthor their life stories.

NT believes that everyone is the expert in their own lives and that they have the ability to fix their own problems. To achieve this, NT will first objectify the problem-saturated life story (i.e., separate it from the person), and then deconstruct it and reconstruct the storyline with the person's long-overlooked ability, power, and faith.

TABLE 4.1 Procedures and strategies included in narrative therapy

STEPS	STRATEGIES	UNIQUE APPROACHES
1. **Deconstruct** a problem-saturated life story	**Externalizing** conversation	**Metaphor and therapeutic documentation**
2. **Coconstruct** a new life story	**Reauthoring** conversation of the life story through the process of identifying unique outcomes	
3. **Thickening and reconstruction** of a new life story	a. **Re-membering** conversation, and b. Outsider witness practice	

Operationally, NT consists of four procedures: (1) externalizing and deconstructing, (2) reauthoring and coconstructing, (3) re-membering and thickening, and (4) outsider witness and reconstruction. NT follows two approaches: (1) outsider questions and (2) therapeutic documentation (see table 4.1). The specific approaches include metaphor, therapeutic documentation (e.g., records, letter, certification, pictures), and outsider witness.

The next section of this chapter explains the procedure of each strategy with NT case examples and provides suggested questions and guidelines for practical purposes.

EXTERNALIZATION CONVERSATIONS: DECONSTRUCTING

MR. AND MRS. CHENG'S STORY   *Mr. Cheng, an eighty-three-year-old diabetes patient, had a mild stroke five months ago. Before the stroke, he had high blood pressure for many years. His wife, Mrs. Cheng has become his caregiver and is very anxious that he will have a massive stroke if he is not careful and does not take care of himself.*

Mr. Cheng has a humorous disposition, even if at times it is dark humor used to deflect his challenging emotions about stroke. He named the stroke a "plague" and he sees his family as consistently being his adviser, a role that frequently annoys him, on how to live just like when he was diagnosed with diabetes: his family members always remind, scold, and educate him on the choice of food he is eating. He has taken to calling his family (including his wife, two daughters-in-law, and others) the "black geese and white geese of Cheng's family." This Chinese expression means he sees them as always nagging him like squawking black geese at night, and white geese by day. He named the period of time when he experienced the mild stroke as the "Inevitable Station." He believes this time is unavoidable for people

Justifying the evaluation					He considered being grateful; he had five "geese" nagging after him night and day, who care for him when he needs them.		The members of the Swan family took care of him and watched over him; he has become the king of the Swan kingdom.
Evaluating effects of the problem				He felt sad as he has become a patient and a burden of his family, and they nag after him.			
Mapping the effects of the problem			After the stroke, Mr. Cheng's family often remind him what he should or should not eat; he finds this annoying.				
Naming the problem/ concern	Naming the chronic illness as "plague" and was plagued by it.						Renaming: Because he is well taken care of by the Swan family, his wife and daughter-in-law are now known as the Black and White Swans.

Figure 4.1 Externalization conversation chart: Mr. Cheng's voices.

experiencing old age; sickness and death will occur and there is no need to be nervous about such circumstances (figure 4.1).

Mrs. Cheng loves her husband dearly and was very worried about his health after his complications, especially with diabetes. She named the stroke a "bomb," and she felt that this "bomb" had taken away the warmth between her and her husband. She named the years living with the diabetes diagnosis as a "Midway Station," and because of the Cheng's family history of strokes, she felt that the stroke was an unavoidable stage in her husband's life. She realizes a stroke happens suddenly and that with the advance of health informatics, we can reduce the chances even though we cannot avoid it. She cherishes her time with her husband and wants him to live longer through healthy behaviors, which his family feels he is not doing enough to prevent a stroke as much as possible (figure 4.2).

Through NT's use of externalizing conversations with stroke, Mr. Cheng recognizes his family's incessant exhortations are motivated by their continued love and concern for him. Mr. Cheng switched his perspective and is feeling grateful that there are five "swans" in his family who love him so much that he

					She believed that her husband's condition after the stroke would worsen and that future strokes would be unavoidable. She cherished her time with her husband and was afraid to hope he could live happily by distancing his identity from "The Bomb."
Justifying the evaluation					
Evaluating the effects of the problem				Knowing that "The Bomb" had entered their family's identity, she tried her best to reduce the chances of a future stroke. Still, her desire to minimize adverse health outcomes led to controlling behaviors for her husband's diet and health that he did not like, negatively affecting their married relationship.	
Mapping the effects of the problem			She was very worried about her husband's health condition and significant potential worsening after his stroke.		
Naming the problem	Mrs. Cheng named the stroke "The Bomb," because it adversely changed everything for her and the spousal relationship instantly.				

Figure 4.2 Externalization conversation chart: Mrs. Cheng's voices.

has become the "King of the Swan Family." His new more positive perspective is exhorted by his family, and he has renewed his behaviors to stay healthy to live a long and happy life with his family, children, and grandchildren.

This example of Mr. Cheng reveals just one of the many stories of people and their families who are troubled by chronic illnesses. In Mr. Cheng's case, he was first diagnosed with diabetes, and then recently suffered a stroke. Mr. Cheng perceives he has been trapped into the identity of a "patient": he is facing reduced physical functioning and relies on others to care for him.

On top of these difficult life situations and real health problems, he has adopted negative labels like "deficient," "useless," "burdensome," and a "failure," which reflect a detrimental impact on his self-esteem and overall well-being.

Externalization conversations in NT holds the belief and follow a working principle of a *"problem is a problem, and the person is not the problem."* The externalization conversation helps to objectify the problem to counteract the social construction of societal power, culture, and institutions. Through externalization conversations, the narrative practitioner aims to deconstruct and dissociate the person from their problem-saturated identity, moving away from feelings of useless and being a burden to helping the person expand his or her thinking. In this space, the practitioner can help the person evaluate and debate the impact of the problem. This creates an opening for the person to gradually reduce the impact of this problem-saturated identity by restoring one's positive values, beliefs, commitment, and purpose of life, leading ultimately to vindication and an embedded intentional understanding of self.[1]

When practicing externalization conversations, attention needs to be paid to the relationships between use of language and narrative practice. The language used reflects the worldview, beliefs, and personal values of the person in question. During therapy, the practitioner needs to affirm and use the person's language and expressions to complement the externalized conversations and identification of the problem. In doing so, this process respects the person's personal agency and aligns with the person's lived experience, helping them to engage in the conversation process.

The following four substeps are involved in externalization conversation: (1) naming the problem or concern, (2) mapping the effects of the problem or concern, (3) evaluating the effects of the problem, and (4) justifying the evaluation. Figures 4.1 and 4.2 show how the procedure of externalization conversation is applied to the example of Mr. Cheng and his wife, respectively. To apply the theory into practice, some practice guidelines and suggested questions for an externalization conversation are given in table 4.2.

Applying the procedure to Mr. Cheng's example, the practitioner first asked Mr. Cheng to name *the problem*, and he named his stroke problem a "plague." In the next step of *mapping out the effects of his problem,* Mr. Cheng raised the issues in relationships: the nagging by his family about his diet, and the redirection, which he found annoying. Then the practitioner asked him to *evaluate the problem* — that is, how has the problem affected him positively or negatively? Here, Mr. Cheng disclosed his inner feelings of being sad about becoming a patient and a burden to his

TABLE 4.2 Suggested questions for externalization conversations

NAMING THE PROBLEM OR CONCERN	THEORY IN PRACTICE:
	Invite the person to name the problem, concern, or experience he or she is describing. This will increase the person's ownership of the problem or concern, giving him or her the feeling of being in charge of the problem or concern, and making it a counterpart to the conversation by objectifying and personifying the stated problem or concern.
	If the person has difficulty in naming the problem, the worker needs to be restrained and be flexible in using conversational skills to wait for the conversation to develop. Of course, it is also possible to repeat words or phrases that the person has used (in describing the problem or concern) and then invite the person to pick a name to describe it.
	Suggested Questions:
	– When did the problem or concern (i.e., diabetes/stroke) first appear in your life? How long ago?
	– Did you have any prior knowledge about this problem or concern? How did you notice its arrival?
	– Where were you when this problem or concern occurred? What were you doing?
	– Were you alone? Or with other people? Who were they?
	– Did they happen to know about this problem or concern?
	– How would you describe this problem or concern?
	– What is this problem or concern like?
	– Do you like this problem or concern?
	– Can you give a name to this problem or concerns?
	-What would you call this problem or concerns if you had to give it a name?
	Example: Mr. Cheng
	Naming the stroke as a "plague" because he felt plagued by it.
Mapping the effects of the problem or concern	**Theory in practice:**
	The practitioner looks for the impact of the stated problem or concern (use the name given by the person to the identified problem or concern) on the person and assists them in discovering the extent to which the problem or concern has affected various relational factors. These complex areas of influence include the following:
	• Issues and environment: family, workplace, school, peer groups
	• Issues and relationships: family and self, friends
	• Issues and self-identity: personal intentions, expectations, dreams, aspirations, and values
	• Issues and future life possibilities
	Suggested Questions:
	– Can you share with us the ways in which the problem or concern (name given to the identified problem or concern) has affected your life?
	– How has this problem or concern affected your life? What kind of changes have been brought about by this problem or concern?

- How strong can the problem or concern become? Are there moments in life when the problem or concern becomes very strong? When is it at its strongest? When is it at its weakest?
- How much of an impact does this problem or concern have on your life now?
- What kinds of changes has it brought?
- Does it affect how you view yourself? And how you see life?
- What is living with this problem or concern like for you and your family?
- How has the arrival of this problem or concern affected your emotions?
- Does this problem or concern affect your relationships?

Example: Mr. Cheng

His family often reminds him of what to do or not to eat. He finds this redirection annoying.

Evaluating effects of the problem or concern	**Theory in Practice:**

Once it is clear how the problem or concern has affected the person's life, the practitioner has to ask the person to comment on that problem or concern so that the practitioner knows how the person understands the impact of this problem or concern.

According to the person, is the problem or concern a good thing or a bad thing? The complex stance the person takes on the issue can also be clearly identified by assessing the various changes.

Suggested Questions:

- Has this problem or concern affected you in a good or positive way? Bad or negative? Or a mixture?
- Is this problem or concern having a good or a bad effect on you?
- What would your family say about this?
- Can you describe the relationship between you and the problem or concern? Is it a happy relationship or a bad one? Or is it a mixed relationship?
- How would you rate your overall experience with this problem or concern?

Example: Mr. Cheng

He feels sad that he has become a patient and is a burden to his family, while also having to endure his family's nagging.

Justifying the evaluation	**Theory in Practice:**

Exploratory questions are used to help a person clarify and understand their intentions and also can help them develop a positive self-identity.

Suggested Questions:

- Why has their nagging affected you so profoundly?
- Why do you think they remind you of healthy behaviors?
- Please share with me why the arrival of this problem or concern was a good or a bad thing for you?
- Did this problem or concern get in the way of something that was important to you?

Example: Mr. Cheng

He considers that his family nagging is an act of love and care and he becomes grateful for it.

Source: Michael White, *Map of Narrative Therapy* (Adelaide, SA: Dulwich Centre, 2007).

family, while also having to endure the nagging from his family. Last, the practitioner asked Mr. Cheng to *justify the evaluation*, asking him to rethink how profound the problem was and how the outcome of their nagging was good or bad on him and his family. This is when Mr. Cheng realized that his family's nagging was an act of love and care, and he learned to became grateful for it.

REAUTHORING CONVERSATIONS: COCONSTRUCT

MR. HO'S STORY *Mr. Ho, a seventy-five-year-old stroke survivor, is married and has two children. Before his stroke, he was a driver and after recovering from his stroke he remained engaged in work and now works as a security guard. He suffered a stroke three years ago. In the middle of the night, Mr. Ho had a stroke and was taken to the hospital by family members who called an ambulance; he was hospitalized for three weeks. Mr. Ho was diagnosed with a left brain injury and as a result, the functioning of the right side of his body was affected. When he was discharged from the hospital, he felt weakness and numbness in half of his head and feet, as well as pain in the right side of his face, lack of movement in his right hand, and a constant tremble in his right foot when he stood up.*

Mr. Ho's view of the stroke:
The stroke has added inconvenience to Mr. Ho's life, and he cannot control his movements. Mr. Ho refers to the stroke as an "electric shock," which took away his freedom and made him feel like a "wreck." The "electric shock" was initially severe, causing him to lose his mobility and making it difficult to get out of bed.

The effects of the stroke:
The stroke did not break Mr. Ho's belief that he was "on his own." After more than a year of hard work, the destructive power of the "electric shock" diminished, and his mobility gradually returned to about half of what it was before the stroke. He was able to return to work. Although the type of work he does has changed, he is still committed to his personal belief that he has to be autonomous, on his own.

Important values in life:
During his recovery, reauthoring the conversation slowly reduced the force of the stroke. The narrative conversation provided a space for Mr. Ho to pause

and reexamine his personal values and outlook on life, thereby strengthening his personal characteristics and beliefs.

This unique experience and result opened up a narrative conversation. Naming his stroke as an "electric shock," Ho says, "The 'electric shock' vibrates all day long, like old glue around my hand, leaving me with no freedom." When Mr. Ho tells his story again, his personal beliefs and values are that he "doesn't want to bother/burden people, he wants to rely on himself." Mr. Ho is very strong and determined to fight against the "electric shock." He wanted to be free from the control of the "electric shock." He wants to be free again and not to be a "loser." Therefore, he studied actively and worked hard with support from physiotherapy and regular exercises.

He has a constant conversation about his dreams and hopes, beliefs and values, ideas about things, and the purpose of his actions. This approach enriches his identity, strengthens his personal beliefs and values, helps him to reduce the distress of his stroke, and strengthens his motivation to move forward. Mr. Ho renames his stroke as a "less dreadful electric shock"

Life stories with the future of stroke:
Mr. Ho wants to love life, continue to live independently and strive to live to his fullest.

NT holds that people have many rich life experiences, but that when they encounter a serious life situation (e.g., in Mr. Ho's case, a stroke), they are influenced by a dominant (e.g., medical) discourse and its constructs, which leads them to adopt a problem-saturated (e.g., patient who loses his mobility and freedom) identity. When these problems are oppressive, the person is being dominated and entrapped by them and internalizes them (e.g., putting on negative labels—feels like a "wreck"). In this negative state, the person, in any case, will likely forget other talents and abilities, and fail to present his or her life story entirely, thus neglecting the development of an alternative, healthier storyline. Ultimately, the person creates a self-fulfilling negative storyline.

Given the pressure of social and cultural discourse, a person may not be able to express their abilities, values, beliefs, and life achievements that have been dominant, and not in their original narration of their life stories. This is when reauthoring in NT begins to take place.

Reauthoring the conversation means revisiting old life events and shining moments, and rediscovering a person's abilities, beliefs, and values through a conversation of action and consciousness, thus enabling the person to reestablish their preferred identity and coconstruct a new way forward that aligns with their dreams and aspirations. At the same time, the person's life story can be reauthored and developed in a new way, and the direction of the person's life can be expanded.

The purpose of a reauthoring conversation is to inject new elements into the problem-dominated story, helping the person to reexamine, reorganize, and reconstruct their situation. By reconstructing a direction in life and weaving a new life story, therapists help the person to see things in a new light. Although the problem remains, it is no longer viewed as an obstacle, but instead it is looked at as one of many things in life. As a result, the person discovers a new ability to interact with people and face difficulties in the future with resilience.

Most of the reauthoring conversations begin after the discovery of what NT calls the *unique outcome* (figure 4.3). In constructing the conversation, the person can reexperience the old experience and weave this energy into a new story, allowing the person to rediscover and establish self-ownership of these values and beliefs that are, indeed, part of their self-identity. Hence, they identify a unique outcome that they can connect to other important life events and segments, tapping into inherent knowledge to enrich their life story and reinforce the importance of this unique outcome.

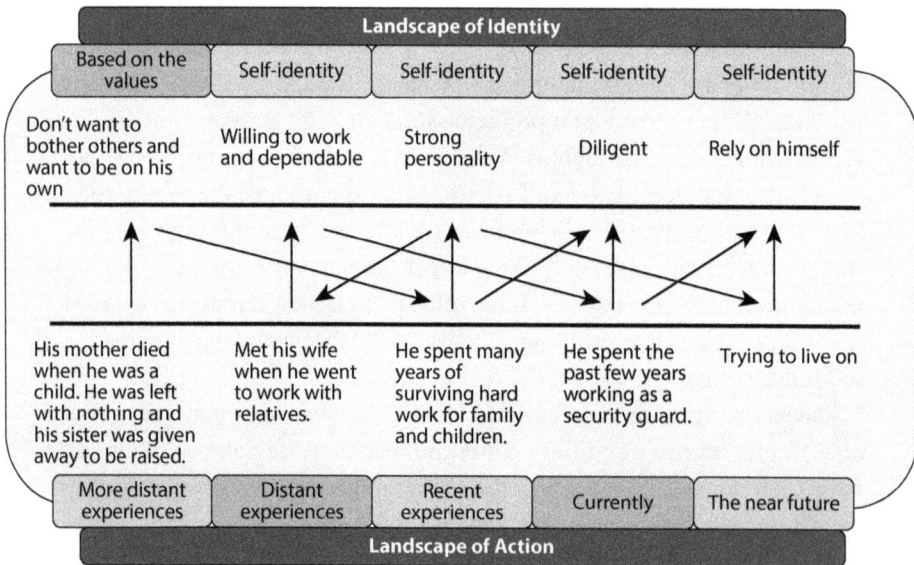

Figure 4.3 Reauthoring conversation chart: Mr. Ho's voices.

The reauthoring conversation and establishing a unique outcome is accomplished within what NT calls the *landscape of action* and *landscape of identity*. Through a step-by-step therapeutic conversation, the person moves through different times and places, such as past experiences, present situations, and hopes for the future, to enrich their commitment and contribution to the community, principles, dreams, hopes, beliefs, values, personal ideas, and purposes of behavior. Ultimately, these techniques help the person build a new self-identity, regain ownership of themselves, and move in a new direction in life.

Reauthoring conversations can be used in conjunction with additional NT techniques, such as externalization conversations, re-membering conversations, outsider witnesses, definition ceremonies, and therapeutic documentation. By enriching the person's alternative storyline, a new storyline is less likely to be pushed back or to replay problematic stories, thus building a *new self-identity* and allowing the new storyline to continue to develop for therapeutic effect.

The following five types of questions are involved in reauthoring conversations: (1) unique outcomes, (2) landscape of action, (3) landscape of identity, (4) renaming the problem, and (5) naming a new experience. To apply the theory into practice, some suggested questions for a reauthoring conversation are provided in table 4.3.

RE-MEMBERING CONVERSATIONS: THICKENING AND RECONSTRUCTION

MR. YIK'S STORY   *Mr. Yik is in his late sixties and is married with two adult children. He has recovered from a stroke. Before the stroke, he had his own business; after the stroke, he suffered from cancer, as well as a number of other chronic illnesses, and had difficulty moving around, which led him to close his business.*

Mr. Yik's view on stroke:
Because stroke is in his family history, Mr. Yik is not too surprised by it but sees it as an inevitable part of his life. He feels that a stroke is like a "wake-up call" to remind him to take care of his health. Otherwise, he would have been taken by surprise if a serious illness came along. The stroke was a "turning point" in his life; he was brought to a crossroads and was motivated to make a life decision to stop working and take care of his health.

TABLE 4.3 Suggested questions for reauthoring conversations

YYY: Identified problem/concern	
ABC: Characteristics/strengths/unique outcome	
OPQ: Naming of preferred identity	

Unique outcomes	**Suggested Questions:**
	– In your experience of "living with stroke," despite the troubles, hardships, and deficits, are there any unique parts of your life that are not troubled by YYY?
	– When was YYY least powerful?
	– Are you further away from YYY now than you were at the beginning? Or is it closer?
	– What have you done to get to the distance between YYY and where you are now?
	– What are your favorite things/skills/strengths you have done/used to keep this new distance?
	– How do you feel when you have applied these things/skills/strengths to help you? Are you happier?
	– What are the ABCs that help you to reduce the resistance/facilitate you to move forward?
	Example: Mr. Ho
	Her cherishes his life and family and his ability to be self-reliant in overcoming problems.
Landscape of action	**Suggested Questions:**
	– Please tell us how ABC has helped you when YYY was at its weakest? Or what makes you stronger?
	– Please tell us the characteristics of ABC that have kept you going despite the influence of YYY?
	– What beliefs/values in relation to ABC have helped you to get the life you want?
	– Please tell a story when you first get to know this belief/value.
	– What does this belief/value reflect about what you value?
	Example: Mr. Ho
	He went to the physiotherapy and did related rehabilitation exercises consistently, regaining half of his mobility after he had a stroke.
Landscape of identity	**Suggested Questions:**
	– In thinking about the course of action you have taken, what does this tell you about who you are and about what is important to you in life?
	– What kind of person do you feel you are through this experience? (Let the person describe his/her traits and preferred identity: OPQ.)
	– How is your life different now compared with when you had YYY?
	– How would you describe your current situation/reflect who you are as a person? (Name his/her current identity.)
	– How would you describe the situation you were in when you first had YYY/reflect who you were at the time? (Name the person he/she was when he/she confronted with YYY.)

     – Do you have the confidence to work closely with ABC in future? If so, how would you describe this situation/reflect who you would like to be OPQ? (Name a future identity.)

Example: Mr. Ho

He shared his belief in relying on himself and not bothering others, making him a reliable spouse/father to his family.

Renaming the Problem	**Suggested Questions:**
	– How do you feel about YYY (the problem) now?
	– What do you think YYY is like now? Is it the same as before?
	Example: Mr. Ho
	He renamed the stroke a "less dreadful electric shock."
Naming a new experience (in living with the problem)	**Suggested Questions:**
	– How do you now rename this new experience of life with YYY (the problem)?
	– What is this new experience?
	Example: Mr. Ho
	He loves his life and family, continuing to live independently with his wife, and striving to live to his fullest with his family.

The impact of the stroke:

Reconstructing his life after the stroke has highlighted Mr. Yik's belief that "we have to fight, there is always a way out." The stroke affected his ability to walk, and he was able to regain a little bit of it through many efforts. With the belief that "I am born to be useful," he fought his illness again. He hopes to become a fighter against his illness and to shift his life to a "fighting station."

The important values of life:

Mr. Yik's road to recovery was different from others in that he was never overwhelmed by negative emotions. He saw his stroke as a turning point in his life, one that allowed him to put aside his business to focus on his health and well-being. At the same time, he actively participates in stroke support groups to help those in need of rehabilitation, acting as a companion and walking with them through difficult times. Through this process, Mr. Yik has reinforced his belief that "we have to fight; there is always a way."

He recalls that he had developed this belief when he was five or six years old. He had fallen down a well alone, but he did not wait to be rescued. He climbed out of the well himself and escaped. In his early twenties, he got caught in a rope at the bottom of a boat while swimming, but with this belief that "there is always a way," he was able to get out of the water. As he told these stories, Mr. Yik discovered that he had inherited this belief from his father. His father had been scammed for money by friends and relatives, but he did not hold a grudge and persevered in his struggle to get through the situation.

During the re-membering conversation, Mr. Yik told his father that he was happy to have inherited all of his abilities, and his father replied that he was happy to "pass on" his spirit to someone else.

Mr. Yik said, "Many thanks, I really appreciated the teaching of my father."

Mr. Yik hopes to pass this belief on to his children, from generation to generation, and to others around the world who are recovering from stroke, to help them regain faith and to celebrate their lives. As a gift, he gave a letter to his wife to thank her for taking care of him. She is his "Guardian Angel," and he hopes that he can be the same for her.

A life story with the future of stroke:
Apart from being a stroke survivor, Mr. Yik is also a cancer patient with different chronic illnesses. He laughs that his many past experiences have turned him into an "Encyclopedia of Chronic Illnesses." In the future, he hopes to promote his belief that "there is no end to overcoming challenges" and he wants to share his experiences with other patients. In addition, he looks forward to moving toward his next life station—that is, "sharing."

A re-membering conversation is a way of thinking about other people in one's life. In re-membering conversations, relevant people or objects can be invited to participate in the conversation. Unwelcome people can be removed from the conversation to achieve the effect of self-witnessing and to be "one's own expert in life." Through this reunion with important and unimportant people at different times of life, people can connect the past "me" with the present "me," rearrange their life story, incorporate valuable experiences or remove troubling ones, and continue on the journey they want to take.

The goal of re-membering conversations is to revise the person's current self-identity and to allow them to see themselves in a new light to adapt to the ongoing development of their lives (table 4.4). In rewriting conversations, the person can find a unique outcome or establish a new self-identity; this task is then complemented by re-membering conversations, in which the new self-identity is enhanced and enriched. By examining past relationships,

TABLE 4.4 Suggested questions for re-membering conversations

Identifying the figure who contributes to person's life	Suggested Questions:
	– When did you learn/recognize these abilities/knowledge/traits/ideas?
	– Who taught you these abilities/knowledge/traits/ideas?
	– Who would be happy to know that you have these abilities/knowledge/traits/ideas?
	– Who would you most like to know that you have these abilities/knowledge/traits/ideas?
	– Who do you know who has these abilities/knowledge/traits/ideas?
	Example: Mr. Yik
	He realized that his belief that "we have to fight, there is always a way" was inherited from his father.
The person's identity through the eyes of that figure	**Suggested Questions:**
	– If the person who taught you knew what you were doing now, what do you think they would say about you? How would they praise you?
	– What would the person you miss most say if he/she knew you had these abilities/knowledge/traits/ideas?
	– If I interviewed the person who taught you, what would he/she say?
	– If the person who taught you knew you had these abilities/knowledge/traits/ideas, would they think differently of you?
	Example: Mr. Yik
	He imagined his father would say "well done" and would be happy that his spirit had been passed on.
The person's contribution to that figure's life	**Suggested Questions:**
	– If the person teaching you hears about what you are doing now, what do you think he/she will gain?
	– If you praise the person who is teaching you, does he/she appreciate your praise?
	Example: Mr. Yik
	He believes that his father would be glad and honored to be a good father.
The implications of this contribution to shape the figure's identity	**Suggested Questions:**
	– If the person teaching you knows what you are doing now, how do you suppose this affects his/her view of him/herself?
	– Do you suppose that teaching the person you are teaching knows what you are doing now and could strengthen his/her values?
	– Looking at the relationship with him/her again, do you have any new insight?
	Example: Mr. Yik
	He hopes to pass on his belief that "there is no end to overcoming challenges" and to share his experiences with other stroke and cancer patients.

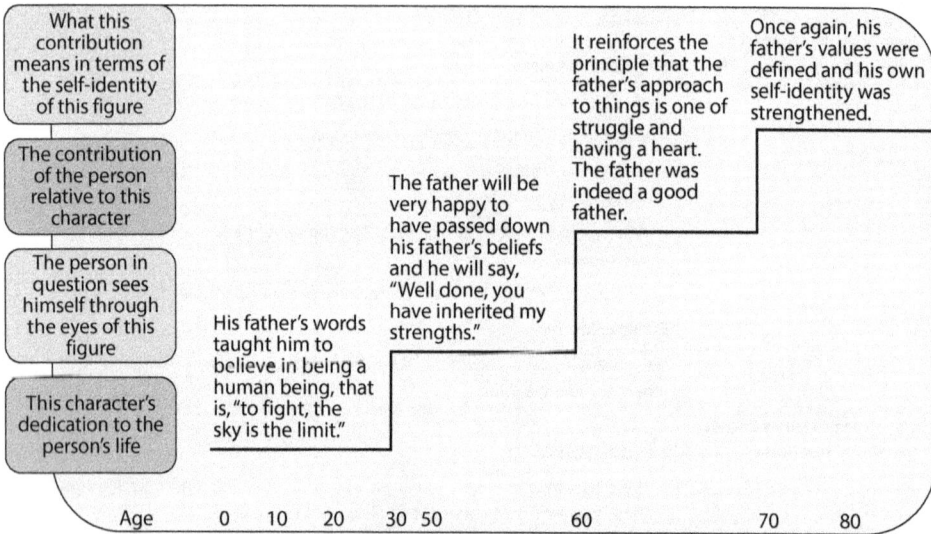

Figure 4.4 Re-membering conversation chart: Mr. Yik's voices.

reinviting important and influential people to join in the construction of the story, or by removing unpopular people, and expressing their reactions to events as an outsider witness, re-membering conversations help people develop a new direction for their future during the process. The following four substeps are involved in the re-membering conversation process: (1) identifying the figure that contributes to the person's life, (2) identifying the person through the eyes of that figure, (3) identifying contributions by the person to the figure's life, and (4) noting the implications of this contribution to the figure's identity. Figure 4.4 illustrates the procedure of a re-membering conversation through Mr. Yik's case.

OUTSIDER WITNESSES PRACTICE

MR. YIK'S STORY CONTINUED: TELLING AND RETELLING   Mr. Yik's story is a good example of the outsider witnesses practice. Following is an excerpt of Mr. Yik's sharing with other people.

The invited participant, Mr. Yik, is a recovering stroke survivor. With a family history of strokes, Mr. Yik regards his stroke as a "wake-up call" alarm bell. Although the treatment was difficult, he tried his best to manage his mood. With Mrs. Yik, his wife, by his side and assuming the lead responsibility of taking care of their family, he vowed to persevere until the very end. He is a fighter who does not fall down easily. Mr. Yik hopes that in the future, he will be a healthy person with a fighting spirit and will no longer need to be taken care of by others. He recalls three stories about his struggle: (1) At five to six years old, he fell down a well and crawled back up to safety. (2) In his teens, he was almost struck by a lightning, but eventually escaped the bad weather. (3) In his twenties, he got caught by a rope at the bottom of a boat while swimming, and struggled to get free, but eventually successfully swam by himself back to the surface. Mr. Yik found that he learned his perseverance, fight, and the strength of willpower from his father."

Three of our friends, Ms. Wong (social worker), Mr. Lee (teacher), and Miss Chow (undergraduate student) were very touched. Mr. Yik's account of his experience resonated with them as told through conversations and retold through the outsider witnesses practice. As outsider witnesses, they gave the following responses (retelling):

Mr. Yik is a fighter and has a strong life force. What touched me was the alarm bell that Mr. Yik had mentioned, which made me feel that Mr. Yik could "live with his illness." I also felt that Mr. Yik had a very optimistic personality. In the mind's painting, there is a picture of a man who does not fall down, which means that Mr. Yik is like a man who never falls down when facing a stroke. Through reflecting on Mr. Yik's story, what I have learned from him was not to give up but persevere in times of difficulty and try to live again. This is a great encouragement to me.

—MS. WONG, SOCIAL WORKER

I was very moved by Mr. Yik's story. I was impressed by Mr. Yik's spirit to fight, optimism, and perseverance. I admire Mr. Yik's strong and resilient faith and see him as a great warrior. Mr. Yik's story gives me the courage to face the difficulties I may encounter in the future, including those in the workplace.

—MR. LEE, TEACHER

I resonated with Mr. Yik's willpower, which reminded me of the struggling story of Andy Lau, a famous artist. Through years of hard work and perseverance, Mr. Lau was able to achieve great success in the fields of acting and singing. What I learned from Mr. Yik was the struggle and perseverance that would help me to face the difficulties of the present and the future, especially in my studies.

—MISS CHOW, POSTGRADUATE STUDENT

These responses from outsider witnesses were retold to Mr. Yik. Following is the retelling of Mr. Yik's response to this outsider witness practice.

Mr. Yik was very moved by these three young friends from the reflecting team, whom he did not know before. He received great encouragement from them. He saw how his life had influenced the younger generations, added value and meaning to him and them, and supported them to be self-reliant. He replied by saying he had become a "spiritual mentor" and an "Encyclopedia of Chronic Illnesses" to the young generation, including his own children and other young people.

The outsider witness is arranged after the reauthoring conversations and the people have been prepared and consented to participate. The purpose of this conversation is to allow the person to further consolidate the rediscovery of their life story by sharing their insight with an invited audience (serving in the capacity of outsider witnesses). Audience members (who may be the person's invited guests, family members, or people from outside are also welcome to participate) are invited to be listeners and are asked to share their feelings after listening to the person share his rediscovery of his life story. In Mr. Yik's case, outsider witnesses were friends of the practitioner. After listening to the person tell their recollected story, the outsider witnesses are invited to retell the conversations to the practitioner or facilitator with personal connectedness and empathy. This testimony of the person's new life story expresses how the person's experience has affected the witness's life.

After the retelling, the practitioner or facilitator may invite the person to do a retelling of the retelling and to provide feedback to the outsider witnesses, so that the person can reflect on their life and consolidate a new life story by listening to the retelling of their story. Retelling and engaging in this reconstruction process and learning that the person's traumatic experience has had a significant social impact on others enriched Mr. Yik's life with value and meaning (figure 4.5).

Table 4.5 includes suggested questions for outsider witnesses.

THERAPEUTIC DOCUMENTATION

SAMPLE WELCOME LETTER FROM AN NT FACILITATOR To acknowledge the meaningful accomplishments of the person, NT practitioners use multiple approaches applying either words or images made by the person

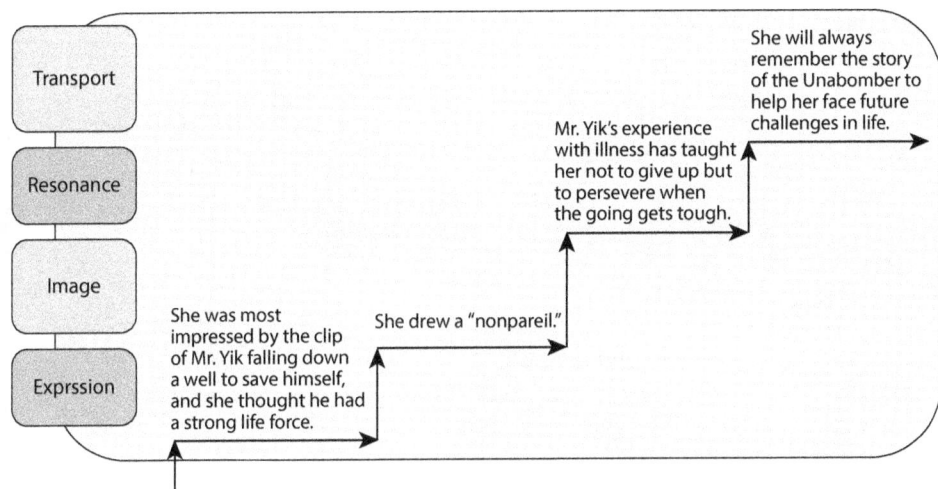

Figure 4.5 Outsider witness retelling chart: Ms. Wong's responses.

TABLE 4.5 Suggested questions for outsider witnesses

W: Social worker

OL: Outsider witness listener(s)

P: Person(s)

Expression	**Theory in Practice:** The W invites the OL to talk about the most compelling part of the P's story and asks them to identify any positive statements/phrases that caught the OL's attention. At this stage, the W pays particular attention to how the OL expresses and understands the values/characteristics/beliefs of the subject and invites the OL to retell any particularly appealing phrases in the subject's story. By listening to the OL's expressions of the most salient moments, the P can draw out different stories about themselves. **Suggested Questions:** – What phrases in their conversations do you particularly resonate with? **Example: Ms. Wong, social worker** Mr. Yik's metaphor of the alarm bell resonates with her and made her feel that he could "live with his illness."
Image	**Theory in Practice:** The W needs to pay attention to any images or pictures that are presented in the OL's mind, allowing the OL to draw images of the subject that appear in their mind and leading the OL to evaluate how these images relate to the subject's values/traits/beliefs. When the OL retells the subject's story from the perspective of an OL, the subject's position or personal identity on the issue begins to shift. **Suggested Questions:** – What do you think these clips/conversations reflect about their beliefs/values/personal values? **Example: Ms. Wong, social worker** She appreciates Mr. Yik's optimistic view of not giving up and fighting against the illness.

(continued)

TABLE 4.5 *(continued)*

Resonance	Theory in Practice:
	The OL is encouraged to express how he/she understands the stories retold in the first and second points. In doing so, the W will understand why the OL has chosen these points (phrases and images) and how the stories in particular have touched the OL; whether these resonate with the OL and how these resonances have a direct relationship with the OL and how they affect the OL's life. The aim is to allow the OL to express the ways in which his or her life experiences have resonated with others and to demonstrate that his or her narrative has some social meaning and value.
	Suggested Questions:
	– How do these clips/conversations resonate with your life experiences?
	Example: Ms. Wong, social worker
	From Mr. Yik's story, she has learned not to give up but to persevere in times of difficulty and to try to live again.
Transport	**Theory in Practice:**
	Linked to the third point of resonance, the W will ask the OL if these touching stories have influenced their own reflections on life and the lives of others.
	Suggested Questions:
	– How do you think these clips/conversations will affect your work/life in the future?
	Example: Ms. Wong, social worker
	Mr. Yik's story will be a great encouragement for her in the future when facing challenges.

Source: Michael White, "Definitional Ceremony and Outsider-Witness Responses," Michael White Workshop Notes, 2005, https://www.dulwichcentre.com.au/michael-white-workshop-notes.pdf.

through important promises, moments, scenarios, or processes that mark the reauthoring of the person's life story.

Such documentation can appear in various formats, including cards, letters, personal statements, certification of merits, manuals, pamphlets, discs, photos, drawings, and so on. The practitioner then use these materials to guide the person to express their feelings and thoughts during the therapeutic documentation. Witnesses and audiences are welcome to be present while the person shares the insights they gained from completing this therapeutic documentation. For instance, a declaration is an open treatment record in which a person is invited to write down some promises or resolutions that he or she will later read to an audience. The audience will also witness the development of the person's new life story. Consider the It All Begins with a Stroke Group as an example. The NT facilitators will write down or draw out the hopes and dreams described by the participants as encouragement for them to move in that positive direction.

DEAR MEMBERS OF THE IT ALL BEGINS WITH A STROKE GROUP

I really appreciate that you have taken the time to participate in the first gathering of the It All Begins with a Stroke Group. This gathering connects us with each other for support so that we can overcome the difficulties imposed on us by the stroke. Members will establish mutual support, rewrite our life stories about our experiences with stroke, and find the philosophy in living with the stroke.

At times, it can seem like the struggle during the recovery from the stroke outweighs the happiness from your narratives, but we are glad to see that you are persisting in the midst of these adversities. Many of you have almost been knocked to the ground, but with encouragement from yourself and your families, you have regained faith and strength to continue with physical therapies. A hosts of this group, were also have been inspired by your persistence, and we also see your ability to "never to give up" and "always have hope" shining in your attitudes. We know the importance of having mutual care among family members and quality services from organizations as a foundation for your stories.

Everything mentioned empowers us, enables us to carry on with our lives despite the obstacles put forward by the stroke, and supports us as we continue fighting for our loved ones.

We are going to have seven sessions, and I sincerely hope that I will see you face the challenges together brought about by the "bad kid"(i.e., stroke) and enrich each other's life stories.

Finally, I would like to share my appreciation to you again. Thank you very much for your participation!

Ms. Au Yeung
It All Begins with a Stroke Group

CONCLUSION

In this chapter, we demonstrated step-by-step examples for narrative practice to be used as a therapeutic tool, specifically promoting the psychosocial well-being of individual older adults with chronic illnesses. The theoretical foundation of this approach, which is based on social constructionism, was highlighted, along with the instrumental factors and conversational skills necessary to effectively implement this approach with individuals. The three main steps of NT (i.e., externalizing conversation, reauthoring, and re-membering) were discussed in detail, providing a road map for social workers and narrative therapists. By recognizing the power of narrative in shaping our lives, NT offers a valuable tool for promoting well-being and empowering individuals to rewrite their life stories.

In the next section of this book, we will look at the use of narrative practice within psychotherapy in Western culture, specifically in New York, emphasizing the powerful interplay between therapist and client.

NOTE

1. Michael White, *Map of Narrative Therapy* (Adelaide, SA: Dulwich Centre, 2007).

NARRATIVE PRACTICE WITH OLDER ADULTS IN WESTERN CULTURES

5

CRAFTING HEALING NARRATIVES

Integrating Narrative Work in Clinical Practice

Each time I tell my story, I remove one small bit of hurt from inside me.
I ease my wound.

—CAROL STAUDACHER, *A TIME TO GRIEVE*

According to John McLeod, professor emeritus of Counseling at Abertay University, "We take for granted in today's world that psychotherapy is a form of treatment for certain types of problems."[1] McLeod's work on psychotherapy and research has focused on making research more accessible through the use of narrative. He invites us to consider that unlike occupations, such as farmers, lawyers, or physicians, psychotherapy as a profession did not exist before the late nineteenth or early twentieth century. He asks us to question what made it possible for psychotherapy to become a form of treatment and posits that there are two possibilities. One places the emergence of psychotherapy within the context of "progress," based on the increase of scientific knowledge and the application of evidence-based principles. The other examines culturally sanctioned rituals that enabled people to cope with group and interpersonal tensions and emotions. McLeod holds that psychotherapy was not "invented" by scientists, but rather that it evolved from healing practices in previous historical periods: therapy is, fundamentally, about storytelling.

Jeffrey Dean Webster reminds us that it is not only through the lens of culture that we understand the meaning of our stories but also through the lens of time.[2] The past and the future share common elements that are not shared with the present. The past and the future are both infinite and enable "temporal projection." Webster points out that the duration of the present has been debated since William James described the "specious present" in 1890. The present is constantly being formed and transformed into the past. Temporal projection also allows us to anticipate events in the future. Both past and present are constructed, as memory and anticipation are innately subjective.

Our healing practices have also evolved over time. McLeod writes that the sense of personhood is different in modern society than it was in traditional societies, during which time people lived in proximity to one another.[3] The concept of "who I am" was not defined in terms of the quality of interpersonal relationships, but rather through kinship hierarchy, loyalty, and fate. The construction of the modern self has engendered new narratives, including "being in therapy." Before the modern era, religion, religious icons and leaders, and collective spiritual rituals provided help for those with psychological distress. These were the narratives that pervaded traditional societies.

In the modern era, there are many treatments for psychological distress, and within psychotherapy, various storytelling techniques are used to help those trying to make sense of suffering in their lives. A distinction had been made in the literature between the healing practices of reminiscence and life review. Robert N. Butler understood life review as a naturally occurring process that all older people experience as they attempt to make meaning of their lives and come to terms with unresolved conflicts, healing their psyches.[4] This process includes reminiscence, which Butler defined as the simple process of recalling past events, but which does not feature the deeper psychological undercurrent of a life review. While reminiscence involves the evocation of memories, life review involves a more structured and active engagement with these memories. Although considered to be a simpler process than life review, reminiscence interventions have proven to have a positive and lasting impact on depression and other mental health conditions in the elderly.[5] Research has shown that an even greater benefit is derived from the use of a life review, which allows for a reduction in negative forms of recall, while also supporting a more positive view.[6] For older clients who may not have had therapy in the past, or for whom therapy carries a certain stigma, the life narrative approach may be effective in easing them into the process. As one of my clients, new to this kind of therapy, said a few months into the treatment: "Now I get it. Therapy is like making a *shidduch* (Hebrew for a match made for the purpose of marriage) with yourself!"

Clients come to us intimately entangled with their problems, which may cause them to lose sight of themselves as beautifully whole yet complicated human beings whose narratives extend far beyond "the problem" they identify. This is not to say that we should not address their problems but rather that in helping clients uncover and appreciate their larger narratives, we assist them in discovering deeper and broader meaning of their lives. Arthur W. Frank cautions us that "typologies risk putting stories in boxes, thus allowing and even encouraging the monological stance that the boxes are more real than the stories, and the types are all that need to be known about the stories."[7] Client and therapist may collude in this process, which can impede the process of creating a new narrative based on resilience and strength. There are many ways in which to guide clients in this process, but one especially effective method is to pose the question (open another conversation?): "What would you be talking about if you weren't talking about your (fill in the blank with presenting problem; e.g., depression, anxiety, alcoholism, landlord)?"

REMEMBERING AND FORGETTING

Susan Bluck approaches remembering with a critical eye and wonders whether forgetting does not also play an equally important role in the process.[8] She poses three questions in examining this conundrum:

- What is the goal, the desired outcome of remembering-forgetting?
- Does one principle, to remember or forget, apply for both good and bad memories?
- Is it ethical to internally or externally manipulate others' memories to induce forgetting?

Bluck argues that modern psychotherapy has become too focused on self-esteem and that although self-esteem as a part of well-being is a worthy goal, it is "unlikely the original goal of the human autobiographical memory system. Memory may have evolved in part as an emotion-regulating function, but it serves many other functions, such as forging social bonds and informing future behaviors. If well-being is our goal, then should we strive to remember only the positive, and forget the negative?" Ella James et al., however, further specify this notion and believe that, in the case of traumatic memory, forgetting can improve mental health. [9]

According to William Randall, our stories are continually being "coauthored" by others, and we can become "destroyed" by these societal constraints.[10] Life narratives contain many subplots, interwoven with the narratives of others, and with the cultural themes of the larger society. As Thomas R. Cole has noted: "Growing old cannot be understood apart from its subjective experience, mediated by social condition and cultural significance."[11] How does this play out for the individual in society? It allows for both the creation of an ever-changing narrative tapestry, and the entrapping of an individual in a narrative box, so identified with the problem narrative and negative labeling that this individual cannot see a way out.

Whether events and challenges are viewed as positive, negative, or mixed, they evolve from those moments that stop us in our tracks. And, if we allow it, we can then imagine these events from a strengths-based perspective that can help us reinterpret our history. Andreea Ritivoi speaks of a "narrative view of self" and asserts that the identity of a person "emerges from the person's life story."[12] Clients often stop to reflect and process this new moment into their life story, and in doing so a new, a more comprehensive narrative ensues. The following is an example from the author's practice.

Patrick was referred to our agency by an organization that provides monetary assistance to financially needy older clients who were born in the United Kingdom. His caseworker at the organization felt Patrick needed psychological help, as Patrick was showing increasing signs of paranoia, and was convinced that his landlord and neighbors were spying on him. When I first began working with Patrick, he spoke exclusively of his landlord and did, in fact, sound paranoid. After establishing a therapeutic alliance with him (perhaps easier because I did not try to dismantle his paranoid ideation), I posed the question, "What would you be talking about if you weren't talking about your landlord?" This opened up a completely new aspect of our work together.

> Patrick was born in northern England during World War II, to a working-class family. He remembered playing in the bombed-out buildings in his neighborhood. His father was a hard-drinking man and took out his anger on the family. At sixteen, Patrick had enough of his father's violent behavior and decided to run away. He found work as a "butcher's boy" on merchant ships, which ultimately led to his career as the chief butcher on several cruise ships. Patrick traveled the world on these ships, and when he realized that I was interested in his story, he began bringing in all kinds of memorabilia of his life at sea—photos, postcards, ship records, and souvenirs. He came to New York on several occasions, and at some point decided to stay. He needed to find another line of work and ended up working as an interpreter for the Theater for the Deaf, having taught himself sign language solely because he was attracted to the concept of

this job. He brought me a newspaper article with a picture of himself, praising his work with the theater. But his work required that he be on the road much of the year, and traveling was taking a toll on him. He returned to New York and found work as a host in an exclusive restaurant club, where he remained until his retirement. Unfortunately his pension was not enough to live on, and he began to suffer financially, and he then in a period of vulnerability and misaligned hope, succumbed to a ploy that scammed him out of the $20,000 he had managed to save. Eventually his health began to deteriorate, and Patrick went into a nursing home.

Although Patrick never lost his paranoid ideation, our work over the two years he was in treatment was much richer as a result of my encouraging him to share his story. This was the first time anyone had expressed an interest in his story, and he became immersed in that experience. Although we did discuss his living situation, it was no longer the central focus of his therapy.

WRITING WITH AND FOR CLIENTS: ANOTHER WAY TO INTRODUCE NARRATIVE

Life review and reminiscence are adaptable to many creative modalities. Meredith Flood and Kenneth Phillips have studied the benefits of utilizing creativity as a therapeutic intervention with older adults. [13] Writing, in particular, lends itself to this aspect of narrative. Numerous studies have demonstrated that writing can help older adults make meaning of their lives, connect with others, and reduce depressive symptoms and negative affect. But some clients feel they cannot write, whether for psychological or physical reasons. In those cases, creativity on the part of the therapist can bridge this gap. The following two examples highlight a range of possibilities.

Clients tell me stories of suffering and happiness, trauma and resilience, stories about family and places, and often stories about their mothers. Many clients begin the stories of their mothers with the words "I had a mother who . . ." For those clients who cannot write, the idea came to me to write these stories together—the client would dictate and I would type— beginning their stories with the words "I had a mother who . . ." Although I hesitate to look at a computer screen during a session, especially as many of my clients complain that their doctors no longer look at them but rather at the computer, I was delighted to find that a number of clients were enthusiastic about my proposal and so I decided to give it a try. As much as I disliked having to take typing in school (I grew up before the advent of computers), it has become a treasured talent for narrative therapy (NT), as I am able to type rapidly and listen at the same time.

Two clients in particular have found the project therapeutic. In one case, a widow who deeply missed her husband found humor and solace in recounting tales of her mother's life. In the other, a client found a connection with his mother he had never experienced when she was alive, and he felt her love as he had never felt it before. The following is a recounting of the stories of these two individuals.

RITA'S STORY: "MY MOTHER ROLLED CIGARETTES IN EGYPT"

Rita's mother wasn't feeling well when she went to the doctor. Her abdomen was swollen and she had no energy. Fearing a dread disease, she finally went to the family doctor. Much to her surprise, the doctor informed her she was several months pregnant. Knowing that Rita's mother already had all the children she wanted, he offered to adopt the baby, as he and his wife were childless. When Rita was born, her father fell in love with her and refused to give her up, but Rita's mother never let Rita forget she was an "accident."

Rita's mother was born in Montmartre, to a Sephardic Jewish family. The family left France after World War I, and traveled to a number of countries, arriving in Egypt when Rita's mother was nine years old. Shortly after their arrival her father was run over by a horse carriage and suffered fatal injuries. His widow and children were left to fend for themselves. Their mother set the children to learning how to roll cigarettes and then sell them to passersby in the street. When Rita's mother was a young woman, she met Rita's father and they immigrated to the United States.

Rita was born in the Bronx, NY. Her mother left much of Rita's care to her older sister. Her sister married and had two young children, and Rita came to live with her. Her sister died of influenza at age twenty-two, which was a great blow to Rita.

When Rita was fifteen she met Harry. They fell in love and became inseparable, and when Rita was nineteen they married. Harry was charming but moody, and not an easy man to live with, but Rita loved him passionately. She had a number of medical problems that prevented her from having children, so Harry became the center of her universe. He worked in the record business as a recording engineer, and his work took him all over the world. Rita was always by his side. Every story she told about Harry ended with, "Everyone loved Harry."

GEORGE'S STORY

When I gingerly proposed the idea of a collaborative writing project to George, he was eager to begin. George grew up in a small, conservative town in western Canada. His father, who had been ill for most of George's young life, died when George was only four, leaving George's mother to raise George and his two siblings alone. She was outwardly a timid and conventional woman, or so George had always thought, until he began telling her story. At every subsequent session, after we discussed the practical problems of the week, George would ask: "When can we get to my mother?" This was a signal for me to turn to the computer, as George would begin his narrative.

As this process unfolded, George discovered that his mother was a much more three-dimensional figure than he had ever recognized and that she loved and cared for him in ways that he had not previously realized. George identifies as homosexual and, although he never discussed his sexual orientation with his mother, he suspects she must have known. George is an artist, and his mother supported his artistic leanings in subtle ways, although he was not aware of this when he was young.

In telling the story of his growing up years, and specifically the stories about his mother, George began to feel a closeness and a deeper love for her, although she had been dead for many years. This new-found love—both his love for his mother and his recognition of her love for him—has helped him move forward in other areas of his life. He no longer experiences the anger and depression he felt before he began this process. This is evident in the following excerpt from his story:

Much of what I have told you happened when I was very young. When I was in my teens, Mother had moved to Toronto. My sister lived there, and my brother, for a time. We went to dinner at this woman's house, a woman who had been a friend of my mother in Vancouver. Her name was Georgia, and she had been a friend of my mother in Vancouver. Her husband had died and she had remarried. She was a nice woman. This new husband of Georgia was somebody my mother did not know, and she obviously did not feel close to this man. He glommed onto the idea—this is what I surmised—that I was not masculine enough as a dining companion. The way he chose to exhibit this was to tell me during the dinner that I should join the Army, as it would "make a man out of me." What happened next was totally uncharacteristic of my mother. They served wine, and my mother had a wine glass in her hand.

My mother grabbed that glass until it broke, and she said to this man, with fury in her voice: "I didn't raise my boy to be a soldier." If you knew my mother, you would know how uncharacteristic this was of my mother. She never displayed this kind of love of support for me. My brother had been in the army, and my mother succeeded in getting him out. She wrote letters to doctors, and convinced them she needed him at home. Obviously she was steeped in what mothers of soldiers felt. I think she felt this love for me, but I have to emphasize for you, Canadian Anglo-Saxon life was so unemotional, so unaffectionate. I once remember having dinner with my brother, and referring to our home as a "loveless household." He denied it, but as her firstborn, I think she had a special feeling for him. When I said this to him, it offended him. What he said was that our mother had always referred to "Little Geordie" (I was called Geordie by my mother). But that phrase she used that night, those were her exact words, and they resonated so much to me all of my life.

A CAUTIONARY TALE: WHEN THE STORY OVERSHADOWS AN UNDERLYING PROBLEM

Although some people can adapt therapeutic tools to narrating their life stories with minimal guidance, others can get lost in continually retelling their own dramatic stories and require keen intervention from the therapist. As a therapist, I can become so fascinated by some clients' narratives that even I may be distracted from underlying problems. I have educated students that there are times when "seduction" by the story may mask important information for the treatment; leaving critical elements of the client's life unattended from healthy therapeutic intervention. As a new therapist, I was assigned a client who had had nineteen therapists before me. My supervisor warned me that I would be number twenty, but the client's narrative was so compelling that I did not see it coming. One day during a session, the client left in the middle without any explanation, never to return. Looking back after many subsequent years of experience, I can now understand that the stories this client told me about her profound disconnection from her daughter should have served as a red flag, but instead I was drawn into her narrative about her loves and adventures.

The following is an illustration of an instance in which I allowed myself not only to be enticed by the story but also, because of the cultural dynamic involved in this case, almost missed an underlying diagnostic problem.

HARRIET'S STORY

Harriet, an African-American woman in her mid-sixties, had been in treatment with a colleague of mine for about two months. Both Harriet and her therapist had come to realize they were not well matched. Harriet called our clinic director and requested another therapist. I was asked to step in because the clinic director felt that my relational/cultural perspective might be more conducive to Harriet's needs. My colleague, a Caucasian woman of the same generation as the client, described Harriet as an angry woman. And she found herself angry at what she described as Harriet's attempts to "control" the sessions. She thought Harriet was "too goal oriented," and could see that her own psychodynamic approach was ineffectual.

Harriet is a tall, heavyset woman of coffee-colored complexion. She wears casual clothes, and often sports a colorful striped scarf made of African woven cloth. She keeps her sunglasses on at all times to protect the health of her eyes, which has been endangered by Type II diabetes, and occasionally takes off her black cap to reveal a shaven head. In a word, she looks imposing.

Harriet had been married to a successful actor when she was young. Their jet-set lifestyle suited her well at the time, but his recreational use of alcohol and cocaine became problematic, and she decided to leave her husband and pursue a career as a writer. She earned a master's degree from a prestigious university, published several books, and taught college-level writing courses. However, her career went downhill because of her struggle with depression, and she could no longer work. She had been in treatment for years before coming to our clinic, with an African-American Marxist feminist therapist, who had focused on the social and historical roots of Harriet's distress.

As we sat down for our first session, I decided at once to put something out on the table. I asked Harriet how she felt about having a white therapist. Harriet laughed and, with a wave of her hand, said: "Oh, I got over that a long time ago." I felt we were off to a good start. Harriet told me in a subsequent session that I had earned "brownie points" with her friends when she told them I had asked her that question.

Harriet showed me a chart she had made for herself which she called "Renaissance." This chart depicted six boxes, each detailing a personal goal. Harriet's goals included improved health, return to work, home improvement, and social network. She decided that tending to her health was the most important place to start. Harriet's experience with the healthcare system as a Medicaid patient had been unpleasant. She felt her position as an older, less

*affluent woman of color was at the root. I gave her a couple of recommenda-
tions for medical clinics where she might get more help.*

*Under the rubric of improved health Harriet had written "exercise." Harriet
had been taking classes at a downtown yoga center, but stopped when the trip
became too difficult. At my suggestion, she decided to try a class closer to home.
She chose a free program for seniors run by a Jewish organization. Harriet tried
a class, but came to her session complaining about the other members. She
described the scene. In a more animated voice than she usually used with me,
she said: "Those white bitches. They think they are at the coffee shop. They don't
stop talking. Yoga's supposed to be about keeping' quiet and setting' up your
personal space." She went on to tell me about how the woman next to her kept
interrupting the teacher to tell him about her brother-in-law. Harriet laughed
and so did I. Harriet used to be a performance artist, and I told her I thought
this scene would make a wonderful one-woman show. She was flattered.*

*She also used to take dance classes. I take dance classes. I saw this as a
point of connection. When I told her of my interest in dance it did, indeed,
become a point of connection. We compared notes, and I promised to bring
her a brochure for the extension division of a major dance studio. I suggested
she inquire about lower rates for senior citizens. Harriet showed me a flyer
she and a friend had created proposing a dance program for older people in
underserved communities. They were trying to get it funded. I felt a twinge of
envy, because I had recently been talking to people about a similar idea. My
client had jumped my gun on this, and I wanted to be part of it. This was a
clinical red flag for me.*

*As I began to analyze my work with Harriet I realized that in my eagerness
to build rapport with her I had been trying to erase my own whiteness. I fed
her resources to keep her connected, and she received this information as a
gift. As long as I kept giving her "gifts," I felt she would be happy. I wanted
her to be happy. I wanted to impress her with my knowledge of racial/cultural
mythology (e.g., the myth of the strong Black woman; Romero, 2000). But we
had not yet really talked about feelings. I had not asked her what had gotten
in the way of her realizing her goals. I was stuck in the engagement phase. I
really liked Harriet. She was interesting, and entertaining. I looked forward
to my sessions with her, and I was afraid of losing her. I felt as though I were
treading a fine line, with race relations hanging in the balance, but I had
missed an important piece of her treatment in failing to address other factors
contributing to her depression. Harriet had left her former therapist because
her depression was not getting better, and, although I was enjoying her stories,
I was not making much headway either.*

I spoke to Harriet about her willingness to have a psychiatric evaluation. She agreed and was given a diagnosis of bipolar disorder. Today she is taking medication to help with her mood swings. She finds the medication helpful in enabling her to participate more fully in her psychotherapy.

STORYTELLING: THEN AND NOW

Stories can cry out: these things happen; I embody what happened.

—ARTHUR W. FRANK, *LETTING STORIES BREATHE*

If, as McLeod reminds us, therapy is a form of storytelling, and a way of making connections between then and now, then we consider the shifting meaning and manner of telling stories from past to present.[14] As discussed previously, in earlier times, storytelling was primarily a communal, participatory activity, with themes embedded in a collective experience.[15] Heroes and myths shared moral and religious underpinnings, understood by the community. The modern story, in contrast, especially as it is told in the therapeutic setting, encourages the deconstruction of earlier narratives. As McLeod has written, the internet has also changed the face of storytelling, and given us seemingly vast and limitless possibilities for choices and solutions.[16] We must keep this pluralism in mind when working with older adults, as many may be embedded, either culturally or by virtue of the times in which they grew up, in a form of storytelling that is different from our own.

One aspect of narrative therapeutic work is very challenging for me: the death of a beloved client. Handling death is rarely discussed in our modern, death-avoidant society, even in the therapeutic relationship. What happens to the narrative when the client dies? We therapists are the keepers of so many confidential tales and, although we may preserve them in progress notes, treatment plans, and assessments, we are bound to confidentiality by virtue of the profession. But as cocreators of the therapeutic narrative, it is honoring to our clients that their stories affect our lives as people and therapists. Do we not also need to find healthy ways to honor our clients' stories, both in life and in death?

One client with whom I had a powerful connection, a man named Joe, died a few years ago. He and I had worked together on the writing of his story, including his recovery from depression. I was devastated when his wife called to tell me that he had died suddenly. His widow gave me permission to share a poem he wrote. To me, it is an invaluable autobiographical narrative legacy and a tribute to the stories he shared with me. Most of all, it captures the joy he experienced, after emerging from many years under the dark cloud of depression.

RECIPE FOR LIVING

*Simply place one foot in front of the other and
lean slightly forward; do not walk into walls or
closed doors. Smile a "good morning" yourself
in the bathroom mirror and if your image doesn't
return that smile, simply yawn and go back to bed.
Move about in ways that attract and excite you for
there is no one correct path to seek out; turn
toward light unless you prefer the darkness.
Open your mouth and let sound freely spew forth
like waves of the ocean. Trust that your heart-
inspired brain will furnish the words you wish to
say. If you are bored, keep searching until you
find whatever excites you. Forget about what you
read in newspapers and view on television, well,
maybe, not completely; but keep an open mind . . .
Be receptive, yet don't waste your time living
vicariously. Don't spend a lot of time trying to
solve your daily newspaper's crossword puzzle
because life, itself, is a puzzle; so sort out the
clues to your happiness and seek the solutions.
Do not attempt to monitor, criticize or evaluate
yourself in the living moment. Never expect to
find happiness in some escapist's realm, like a
bourbon bottle. Instead sing out all the music
contained in your heart without restricting your
voice. New ingredients can be mixed in at any
time and discarded, likewise. Living is cooking
continually and being consumed at the same time -
figure that out. It's meant to be shared
with loved ones; but there are no obligations.
SAVOR LIFE!*

—JOE GIMPEL (1938–2019)

This chapter has explored the intricate interplay between client and therapist in NT with older adults. As the field of NT evolves, recognition is increasing of the significance of the storied relationship as a powerful agent of change. The therapeutic relationship becomes a vibrant tapestry, in which the lived experience, wisdom, and resilience of the client are interwoven with the empathic responsiveness and attuned presence of the therapist. Within this dynamic, intersubjectivity is a vital lens through which to understand and engage with clients, fostering connection, empathy, and collaborative exploration. By examining the role of intersubjectivity in NT, we further our ability to develop interventions to help older adults coconstruct authentic life narratives, giving renewed purpose and meaning to the lives they have lived.

NOTES

1. John McLeod, "Psychotherapy, Culture, and Storytelling: How They Fit Together," in *Narrative and Psychotherapy* (London: SAGE, 1997), 1–27.
2. Jeffrey Dean Webster, "Is It Time to Reminisce About the Future?," *International Journal of Reminiscence and Life Review* 1, no. 1 (2013): 51–54, http://143.95.253.101/~radfordojs/index.php/IJRLR.
3. McLeod, "Psychotherapy, Culture, and Storytelling," 1–27.
4. Robert N. Butler, "The Life Review: An Interpretation of Reminiscence in the Aged," *Psychiatry* 26, no. 1 (1963): 65–76, https://doi.org/10.1080/00332747.1963.11023339.
5. Gerben J. Westerhof, Ernst Bohlmeijer, and Jeffrey Dean Webster, "Reminiscence and Mental Health: A Review of Recent Progress in Theory, Research, and Interventions," *Ageing and Society* 30, no. 4 (2010): 697–721, https://doi.org/10.1017/S0144686X09990328.
6. Sanne M. A. Lamers et al., "The Efficacy of Life-Review as Online-Guided Self-Help for Adults: A Randomized Trial," *Journals of Gerontology Series B: Psychological Sciences and Social Sciences* 70, no. 1 (2015): 24–34, https://doi.org/10.1093/geronb/gbu030.
7. Arthur W. Frank, *Letting Stories Breathe: A Socio-Narratology* (Chicago: University of Chicago Press, 2010).
8. Susan Bluck, "Remember and Review of Forget and Let Go? Views from a Functional Approach to Autobiographical Memory," *International Journal of Reminiscence and Life Review* 4, no. 1 (2017): 3–7, http://143.95.253.101/~radfordojs/index.php/IJRLR.
9. Ella L. James et al., "The Trauma Film Paradigm as an Experimental Psychopathology Model of Psychological Trauma: Intrusive Memories and Beyond,"

Clinical Psychology Review 47 (2016): 106–42, https://doi.org/10.1016/j.cpr .2016.04.010.

10. William Randall, "Storied Worlds: Acquiring a Narrative Perspective on Aging, Identity and Everyday Life," in *Narrative Gerontology: Theory, Research, and Practice*, ed. Gary M. Kenyon, Philip G. Clark, and Brian De Vries (New York: Springer, 2001).

11. Thomas R. Cole, *The Journey of Life: A Cultural History of Aging in America* (New York: Cambridge University Press, 1992).

12. Andreea Deciu Ritivoi, *Yesterday's Self: Nostalgia and the Immigrant Identity* (Lanham, MD: Rowman and Littlefield, 2002).

13. Meredith Flood and Kenneth D. Philips, "Creativity in Older Adults: A Plethora of Possibilities," *Issues in Mental Health Nursing* 28, no. 24 (2007): 389–411, https://doi.org/10.1080/01612840701252956.

14. McLeod, "Psychotherapy, Culture, and Storytelling," 1–27.

15. Lauren Taylor, "Sharing a Narrative Meal," in *Narrative in Social Work Practice*, ed. Ann Burack-Weiss, Lynn Sara Lawrence, and Lynne Bamat Mijangos (New York: Columbia University Press, 2017).

16. McLeod, "Psychotherapy, Culture, and Storytelling," 1–27.

6

HARMONIZING VOICES

Embracing Narrative Intersubjectivity

> *Being intensely engaged in a relationship with another person is one of the greatest joys of being human. It is, perhaps, the most vital manifestation of consciousness.*
>
> — CHRISTIAN DEQUINCY, "INTERSUBJECTIVITY:
EXPLORING CONSCIOUSNESS FROM A SECOND PERSON PERSPECTIVE"

INDIVIDUAL THERAPY

THE TRANSFERENCE VERSUS COUNTERTRANSFERENCE DEBATE

Intersubjectivity is an interactive, relational process, whereby the therapeutic work takes place in the meeting space between therapist and client. Cassandra L. Bransford posits that U.S. social work has been divided between two models of practice: a paternalistic approach and an empowerment model.[1] In the paternalistic model, the therapist is the expert who knows what is in the client's best interest, whereas in the empowerment model, the client is viewed as "possessing inherent strengths, resources, and knowledge, which the social worker, by dint of her or his authorized role, may be in a position to help foster." Bransford argues that the dichotomy between these two models is artificial and that an intersubjective approach allows for a greater understanding of both clients' strengths and vulnerabilities.[2] Cathy Seibold believes this shift is the most significant change to have occurred in psychoanalytic theory in the past three decades.[3]

Historically, the literature on intersubjectivity is focused on psychoanalytic theories of transference and countertransference. The concept of transference, in which the patient transfers to the therapist unconscious feelings and desires from childhood, and countertransference, the redirection of the therapist's feelings toward the patient (often considered an emotional entanglement with the patient), were first mentioned by Sigmund Freud in the early 1900s.[4] Alberto Stefana, in his historical examination of countertransference, presents the struggle experienced by Freud in facing his own countertransference.[5] The following excerpt is from a letter Freud wrote to Jung:

> Such experiences, though painful, are necessary and hard to avoid. Without them we cannot really know life and what we are dealing with. I myself have never been taken in quite so badly, but I have come very close to it a number of times and had a narrow escape . . . But no lasting harm is done. They help us to develop the thick skin we need and to dominate "countertransference" which is after all a permanent problem for us; they teach us to displace our own effects to best advantage. They are a "blessing in disguise" (quoted phrase is in English in original).

Freud's view was designed to create neutrality in the therapeutic relationship, but even Freud knew this was not possible. As he wrote in 1937, "anonymity to the degree that it exists is at best an ideal fiction." Idell Natterson believed that countertransference is too closely entwined with its original meaning of "unconscious pathological response of the psychoanalyst to the analysand."[6] She argued for the development of a new terminology that would address the way in which the therapist's subjective experience "comes into play throughout the course of treatment." Del Lowenthal questions the validity of countertransference by asking: "Why is it if transference is when the patient/client 'wrongly' projects onto the therapist someone from their past, the same isn't true for the psychological therapist's countertransference, which seems an increasingly popular modus operandi for psychological therapists? Also, to what extent can the client read the therapist's unconscious?"[7] We need not discount the usefulness of countertransference but, rather, regard it as a tool to enhance our connection to the client's world. As Christin J. Fort has written: "Understanding the dynamic world of one's own experience, as well as its potential impact on the client, creates room for deeper reflection, more holistic conceptualization, and careful acknowledgement of one's own perspective."[8]

Moving beyond the confines of transference and countertransference, Jean Baker Miller, a psychiatrist and a founder of the Stone Center for

Research on Women, developed the reciprocal *relational-cultural model* of psychotherapy in response to traditional unidirectional models of therapeutic authority.[9] The goal of the relational-cultural model is to foster mutually growth-enhancing relationships, in which both parties feel they play an important role. Miller believed that isolation is one of the most damaging human experiences and that the therapist must foster connection with a client, even at the expense of the therapist's neutrality. Miller refers to this as "therapist authenticity," but she makes a distinction between relational responsiveness and reactivity: "Reactivity is impulsive, entirely spontaneous, and based only on the internal experience of one person. . . . Relational response involves a consideration of context and concern about the possible impact of our actions and words on the other person and the relationship."[10]

WITHIN NARRATIVE THERAPY AND ORAL HISTORY

Interestingly, the emergent recognition of intersubjectivity in oral history parallels a similar phenomenon in psychotherapy, as discussed in chapter 5. Intersubjectivity is at the core of both the oral history interview and the psychotherapeutic relationship. As Penny Summerfield has written: "The process of the production of memory stories is always dialogic or inter-subjective in the sense that it is the predictor of a relationship between a narrator and a recipient subject, an audience."[11]

Glen O. Gabbard states that the therapeutic relationship or alliance is "the single most potent predictor of psychotherapy outcome regardless of modality" and appears, as well, to be the single most robustly evidence-based finding in psychotherapy research.[12] How do clinicians recognize when the client's construction of a narrative may be a diversion from therapeutic dialogue? Here, understanding our own reactions can be invaluable, and intersubjectivity shapes the outcome. Maureen Walker describes this process as "empathic attunement to emergent experience and openness to movement through mutual influence."[13]

How can intersubjectivity be used to a therapeutic end within a narrative approach? The following case examples illustrate a range of ways in which I have used narrative intersubjectively. In the majority of cases, narrative intersubjectivity helped the client come to a deeper understanding of the emotional issues at hand. Nevertheless, in some instances, sharing one's story with a client can make the client feel uncomfortable. In this chapter, I present examples of both types of outcomes.

The first case example, titled the "The 'Ooh-Ooh' Syndrome," converges with the "eureka" (or "aha" or "sparkling") moment discussed by Esther Chow in chapter 12. Both examples illustrate moments of powerful connection that can be used to enrich the therapeutic work. The ooh-ooh syndrome occurs when the therapist identifies with something going on in a client's life—for example, something that resonates with a similar issue the therapist may be experiencing outside of the treatment room. The therapist may feel like saying, "Ooh-ooh, if you knew what was going on in my life!" The therapist may share this personal experience in the interest of deepening the connection with the client but must be careful to ensure that the therapist's issue does not become the client's concern or supersede the therapeutic needs of the client. In contrast, a "eureka" moment is a poignant moment when a person senses a deepened individual insight into one's experiences.

CASE EXAMPLES

THE "OOH-OOH" SYNDROME   I am by nature a storyteller. My kindergarten report says, "Lauren enters the classroom every day with her cheerful 'You know what?' and proceeds to launch into a story." I come by it honestly. As my daughter says, "In our family, we narrate our lives." My grandmother was the keeper of the family stories, and I spent many hours listening to the tales of Junior Munker, who "was up to no good," or red-haired Alex (my grandfather's brother) who joined the Foreign Legion and saved his battalion from starvation by fashioning bread from tumbleweed.

For someone who loves narrative as much as I do, it is often difficult not to reply with a parallel story about my own life. I must carefully weigh my narrative tendencies to make sure this is in the service of the client. My social work students are always curious about therapeutic boundaries. How much of ourselves should we share with our clients? Cathy Seibold believes that intersubjectivity "provides a way to understand the meaning a patient may consciously and unconsciously give to disclosures, particularly personal disclosures, by the therapist."[14] If this meaning is addressed in the therapy, it can lead to a deepening of the therapeutic relationship and a means of opening channels of communication that may previously have been blocked by the inherent structure of the therapist-client dyad. I underscore, however, the importance of caution in self-disclosure. There have been instances in my practice during which I revealed personal information, thinking it would be helpful to the client, but the client felt as though I were undervaluing, or even usurping, her narrative with my own.

A therapist friend of mine coined the phrase "the ooh-ooh syndrome," to describe those moments when a client says something that really hits home, and you, the therapist, want to reply: "Ooh-ooh, if you knew what was going on in my life!" Many times in my years as a clinician and, more recently as an oral historian, I have experienced these "ooh-ooh" moments. The question then arises as to whether or not to share one's own personal material.

JACK'S STORY: POINTS OF CONNECTION *Jack, a seventy-four-year-old man, requested treatment after his partner of thirteen years abandoned him for a much younger lover. Jack's previous partner, with whom he had been living for twenty-six years, died of a brain tumor after a long illness. Jack had lived alone for a period of time before he met G, although he had had other relationships and has many friends. G represented for Jack the ideal of classical beauty. Jack describes his lover as having been the "quintessential WASP," beautifully groomed and dressed, but emotionally remote. To Jack, G was perfect in every way, but in retrospect, he sees the relationship in a different light. Among other things, G drank too much.*

In our very first session, Jack said to me: "I don't want you to be fooled by my charm. I want you to help me get underneath the mask." Jack had had a successful career as a performer, and he was used to putting on a mask. There are many aspects of Jack's romantic life that are consistent with my own. I don't share intimate details of my relationships with Jack in the way that he does with me, but the overall picture of our experiences is strikingly similar. Yet, at times when I interject with something of my own experiences, Jack will say: "There you go firing a rocket at me again and making me face what's really going on in my life."

In the beginning Jack was perplexed, as his former therapist had had a more traditional approach. We discussed my rationale for sharing parts of my story, and over time he came to see that there was often a message in my story that helped him clarify his own. There is a feeling of shared vulnerability in this therapeutic experience, and had I not taken the chance of sharing my experience, we might never have felt this deep bond. It does not always work this way, and sometimes it even works in the opposite way: learning to stay with painful material presented by a client or interviewee is a critical part of the work, and at times, the desire to share one's own story can be a way to distance oneself from the client's pain, instead of a way to draw closer. As an interviewer, one must assess each individual and each particular situation before venturing to tell one's own story. At moments, however, doing so can create a profound human connection. This client described it by saying that when we share our stories, we "become more human."

TIMOTHY'S STORY: DEEPENING THE CONNECTION   Sometimes a deep connection with a client comes as a surprise. This is what happened with Timothy. Although it was unspoken, I sensed we had been searching for this connection from the beginning of our work together. His question caught me off guard, but he had obviously been thinking about it since our previous session. I hadn't realized until that moment that the therapy touched him so deeply.

Timothy describes himself as having been "drop-dead gorgeous" when he was young. He is not self-aggrandizing when he says this, as he is still strikingly handsome. Even with his thick glasses and long white canes, tap-tapping as he feels his way into the treatment room, he has the regal bearing of the statue of David.

   Timothy was transferred to me after a colleague left the agency. By the time I first met him, he had worked through a lot his childhood trauma, and was ready to move on to other issues in his life. He shared with me the horrible abuse he had suffered at the hands of his father, but felt he had explored this enough in his previous treatment. What concerned him now was the present. Nine years ago, at the age of fifty-nine, Timothy suffered a massive stroke, which left him virtually blind and partially paralyzed. He has regained some of his functioning, although not his vision, but he has pain all over from muscle contractions. He considers himself lucky that he didn't lose his hearing, as music plays a critical role in his recovery.

My conversations with Timothy had seemed superficial at times, and I couldn't find the key to help him open up. We shared a love of music, and this played a role in our attempt to connect with one another, but it wasn't enough. I don't remember having asked him the question in a previous session, but he brought it to my attention with the following question: "Last week you asked me how I see my life. May I ask you how you see yours?" The question both surprised and challenged me. I had not thought that the treatment was affecting this client outside of the sessions; but his question showed me otherwise. The challenge was in how much of myself to reveal in a therapeutic relationship that had, until then, been rather formal and distant.

I began by saying that I consider myself to have had a privileged life. I decided to be as open as possible with the client, while making sure I did not reveal personal information that was not in the service of the treatment. Although I did not see parallels in my life story and my client's, he found points of identification that were important to him. As I spoke, his demeanor softened, and when the session ended and I stood up to say goodbye, I felt as though a wall had come down between us. For a brief moment we stood facing one another in silence, and it was clear to me that we were both feeling the connection. Then we said goodbye. In a subsequent session, I asked Timothy about his reaction to my answer. He said: "Knowing more about you helps me, because I also feel it helps you understand more about me."

Kenneth Pargament et al. call these therapeutic encounters "sacred moments."[15] In their research, they found that the greater the number of sacred moments in the therapy, the greater the sense of well-being in the outcome, for both client and therapist. In another publication on the therapeutic use of narrative, I refer to this as "sharing a narrative meal." Bransford concludes: "Ultimately, social workers may provide far better modeling for their clients if they openly acknowledge the vulnerabilities and possibilities inherent in all of our lives."[16] What better way to do this than through narrative?

MARY'S STORY: SACRED MOMENTS   Being a listener is another way of sharing oneself with a client. Stories are cocreations and, for some clients whose voices have never truly been heard, listening and bearing witness as a therapist is a significant part of the therapeutic relationship. Regardless of differences or similarities, "sacred moments" can occur in any therapeutic encounter. The following story of Mary, a client with whom I worked only briefly, touched me deeply. Even though I did not share details of my personal narrative with Mary, sharing my presence with her as a listener was a significant factor in the narrative intersubjectivity of my interaction with this client.

I had been told by my supervisor that Mary might be a "problem client." Seventy-four-years old, she had been hospitalized multiple times for depression and had made two serious suicide attempts in her life, the first when she was in her teens. I was to be on alert, as she was considered a high-risk client. Before I met her, I had read her profile on the intake sheet and was feeling some trepidation about my ability to connect with her.

How would I describe her in an initial psychosocial evaluation? I wrote: "Mary is a seventy-four-year-old African American woman, neatly groomed and appropriately dressed, wearing a flower-print cotton dress and color-ful straw hat. She is small in stature, and uses a walker. Her demeanor is friendly but somewhat guarded. She has a long history of depression."

Mary had been "in the system" for so many years that she knew well how to tell the story of her depression. "I had no one to talk to when things went wrong, so I would talk with the doctor and then I would go to the hospital and it felt like a community there." Mary's chief complaint was loneliness. She had been taking an antidepressant for twenty years and wanted to get off it. She felt as though there might be a better way for her to cope.

When I asked Mary to tell me her story, she opened up. Here is her story, in my words:

Mary was born in Georgia, the oldest of ten children. She has no recollection of her father, but when he left, she became her mother's scapegoat. "Mary do this, Mary do that. Where's Mary? Why ain't you doin' what you're supposed to do?" Mary had no one to comfort her, so she sought refuge in the arms of men. When Mary became pregnant at 15, her mother and the mother of the baby's father got together and decided that their children should get married. Mary had no choice. Her husband abused her, and when two more pregnan-cies followed in short order, Mary felt overwhelmed and took an overdose of sleeping pills. She was in a coma for two days and woke up in the hospital. Her husband was nowhere to be found.

Mary showed me the scars on her arms and legs from the time she cut herself. She was going with a man who invited many visitors into their home and she thought he was ignoring her. She went into the bathroom and cut herself with a razor down to the bone. She needed multiple stitches, and the scars are also a reminder today of the abuse she suffered.

Mary got involved in one abusive relationship after another. As she described her experience she told me that as soon as a man told her she was beautiful, she was trapped and became his victim. She smiled, flashing a gold tooth, and stroked her arm to show me how a man could win her over. Eventu-ally she fought back, but her abuser died of a heart attack after she beat him, and Mary ended up in jail for second-degree murder. Her lawyer brokered a plea bargain, and instead of twenty-five to life she was sentenced to five years.

Prison life was cruel. "I got beat up a lot by the other prisoners." Mary spent a lot of her time in "the lock," because she refused to put up with the abuse she suffered at the hands of the prison guards. "Sir, I finished washing the floor. Can I go now?" "You ain't goin' nowhere. Wash that floor again." "Who do you think you are taking two pieces of bread? Put one back immediately."

Mary refused to bend. But when she wasn't in "the lock," she found solace in the prison library, and she began to write the story of her life. Sadly, she didn't save what she wrote, but the writing she did in prison led her to reflect on her situation. Mary decided that when she had finished her sentence she would never allow another human being to abuse her again.

While she was in prison, Mary made the acquaintance of a volunteer from a church in Brooklyn who came every week to visit the prisoners. She took the time to listen to Mary's story, and Mary began to feel close to her. She encouraged Mary to write, and when Mary was released from prison she helped her find transitional housing. Mary had abandoned the church many years before, but she decided she wanted to try her volunteer's church. It was a progressive church, "with every kind of person—black and white together." Mary described her earlier experience: "Every time I went to church I saw all these people gettin' up and gettin' the Holy Spirit." Mary got out of her chair and waved her arms in the air to show me how they moved. "Where was He? Where was He? Try as I might, I couldn't find the Holy Spirit, so I gave up. I'm tryin' to find Him now."

I asked Mary how she got through what she has had to endure in her life. She quoted something her mother often told her: "If you can't make it with, make it do without." Mary said she didn't know if her mother invented that phrase, but it has been her motto all her life. "Oh, and dancing" Mary flashed me a big grin and shimmied her shoulders. "People tell me I should have been a dance teacher."

Mary only came for a few sessions, because her health began to fail. At the end of our last session, she said: "I wish I had met you a long time ago." I thanked her and felt tears well up in my eyes. I knew at that moment that I had connected on an indescribable level with another human being— someone I would likely never have met had I not chosen to do this work.

CULTURAL IMPLICATIONS

A structuralist understanding of the self locates its basic elements, such as personality traits and unconscious drives, within the individual,[17] whereas narrative therapy (NT), a poststructuralist approach, sees the self as shaped by social forces. Derald Sue and David Sue point out that when a sense of self is shaped by forces such as racism and sexism (I would add age-ism), an important focus of multicultural NT is to help clients "resist the internalization of negative cultural messages."[18] Janet E. Helms includes

Caucasian clients whose identities are influenced by the experience of power and privilege.[19] When cultural imbalances are present in the therapeutic relationship, Walter and Fox refer to the therapist as an "outsider witness" (see chapter 4, for a discussion of the role of "outsider witness"). Pamela Semmler and Carmen Williams write that NT allows us to help clients reauthor problem stories and create new stories based on strength and resilience. Multicultural awareness is crucial to this process.[20]

Every narrative, whether clinical case or oral history, contains an element of the counterfactual question: "What if it hadn't happened this way?" This dichotomy often moves us to pay more attention to the negative—what Ann Weick et al. call the "problem-deficit orientation" in social work.[21] Narrative intersubjectivity allows us to assist clients in the creation of strengths-based narratives, as we model for our clients new ways to share in the cocreation of stories and authenticity in avenues of communication.

GROUP THERAPY

Intersubjectivity takes on a new dimension in group therapy. Jose M. M. Rodriguez, citing Colwyn Trevarthen, talks about primary and secondary intersubjectivity, as a means of explaining the need for human interaction in groups.[22] Primary intersubjectivity is the interaction of a baby and its mother or caregiver; secondary intersubjectivity originates in the theory that the brain is a social organism[23] and that the group process becomes a laboratory for improving communication. The group process is one of cocreation on a larger scale, and it allows for the complex integration of multiple and diverse narratives in what Rodriguez refers to as "self-restoration." He explains: "This approach requires that the therapist(s) and group members take into account their own script beliefs, their mutual counter transferences, and the way they activate the transference of others. An intersubjective approach also requires the willingness of the therapist(s) and group members to be open and to resonate with the experiences of their group co-members."[24]

Telling stories in group therapy is a challenge. At times, a group member may need to have the floor for a longer period, and the other group members may listen with empathy. But at other times, one participant may be overly inclusive in recounting a narrative, leaving the others bored or irritated. The group leader has many tasks, including time management, helping the group members with emotion regulation, and inspiring mutual caring. Which task should become a priority, what values should be nurtured or contained, and at what point should the facilitator intervene?

I love running groups, perhaps because of the rich interweaving of narratives. At times, I feel as though I am riding a bucking bronco, and at other times, I can sit back and observe as the group is almost running itself. The essential element of the group process is the complex cocreation of the narrative. As group members share their experiences, each individual will react differently to both the content and the delivery of the narrative and may feel empathic, or indifferent, or rejecting, or allied. Others may be uncomfortable speaking up or may shut down and be unable to listen. My role as the facilitator is to create a safe space for each individual and to help the group members find a common thread among often diverse narratives. At times, I will interject something of my own narrative, often to model vulnerability, and hopefully inspire clients who feel stuck. I may model a new kind of narrative, or I may even add humor to bring the group back together when they are lost in their narratives. The intersubjectivity takes place not only between the group leader and the clients but also, and more importantly, among the group members. Ultimately, the group creates a collective narrative.

INTERSUBJECTIVITY

Drawing on examples from my own group practice, I describe two instances in which group members, using intersubjectivity, helped other group members who were "stuck" in negative narratives, free themselves from these damaging, self-critical stories.

ELLEN'S STORY   *Ellen, an eighty-three-year-old soft-spoken widowed woman, was suffering from depression. She rarely spoke in the group unless I called on her during a round-robin discussion. On one such occasion, she told the group she felt as though she didn't belong there, and in fact, felt as though she didn't belong anywhere. The group came together to support her and invited her to share her feelings about not belonging. Ellen began to weep as she spoke, and the woman sitting next to her gently touched her to comfort her; others offered a tissue to dry her tears. No one tried to "fix" it for Ellen, but their body language and encouraging words were enough to help her feel supported.*

This was a "sacred moment," as the group conveyed, without saying so in words, that Ellen very much belonged to the group. Natterson describes these moments as "intersubjective transactions" and posits that they are crucial turning points in the treatment.[25] At the next group session, Ellen participated spontaneously in the conversation and has been more forthcoming about sharing her narrative.

LUCY'S STORY *Lucy, also a widowed woman, was an active participant in the group process. She was a good listener and had no difficulty jumping in to help others feel better about themselves, but she had a low opinion of herself. One would not have guessed this, looking at her physical presentation, as she was always stylishly dressed in a somewhat conservative manner, and appeared to others to be self-confident. One of the areas in which she had a particularly poor image of herself was in her body. She had not put on a bathing suit in years, despite repeated invitations of friends who had vacation homes at the beach. After receiving yet another invitation, Lucy decided to process this with the group. They all reinforced her attractiveness and encouraged her not to let her negative feelings about herself get in the way of her enjoyment. When she accepted her friend's invitation for a weekend at the beach, Lucy returned to the group and announced that she had worn a bathing suit and that what permitted her to do so was that she "heard" the voices of the other group members supporting her all the way.*

The dynamics of self-disclosure in a group setting are different than in individual therapy. The therapist is disclosing to a wider audience and cannot always judge which members of the group will identify positively with the therapist's story. I may share fewer details of my narrative in a group setting, in party because I am careful not to take up too much time when a number of people need to speak. I have also found, however, that I can sometimes open doors for discussion by sharing anecdotes from my life. The response has almost always been positive, and clients have told me they feel it makes me more "human."

The theme of loss is an undercurrent in the stories of many of our older clients. Nancy Kropf and Cindy Tandy speak of loss and grief "robbing" older people of the meaning of earlier narratives in their lives and, sometimes, of their sense of self.[26] By helping older adults integrate positive earlier narratives into their lives at present, and reshape negative narratives into stories of strength, we help them "make meaning" of the continuum of life. Our generosity in sharing our own stories is one way to contribute to this process. As the poet Audrey Lorde (1998) wrote, in a letter to her therapist: "Some part of my journey is yours too."

My social work students always want to know how to "do" this—that is, how to help another, albeit older, person as a professional. I tell them their ears are their most valuable tools. Deep listening, bearing witness, reflecting, and cocreating positive narratives are gifts for older people in our modern society in which ageist stereotypes abound. Being fully present is the heart of narrative intersubjectivity. In the words of Wendy Lustbader: "What if we realized that relationships are the core of care for frail persons? . . . Doing so would tell us what kind of life to lead. Once we begin living in terms of the question, 'Who would take care of me if I got sick?' the whole of life transforms. The question mandates a shift in the order of things, making a life rich with generosity and kindness more desirable than any other kind of fortune."[27]

NOTES

1. Cassandra L, Bransford, "Reconciling Paternalism and Empowerment in Clinical Practice: An Intersubjective Perspective," *Social Work*, 36, no. 1 (2011): 33–41, https://doi.org/10.1093/sw/56.1.33.1

2. Bransford, "Reconciling Paternalism and Empowerment in Clinical Practice."

3. Cathy Siebold, "What Do Patients Want? Personal Disclosure and the Intersubjective Perspective," *Clinical Social Work Journal*, 39 (2011): 151–60, https://doi.org/10.1007/s10615-011-0338-1.

4. Sigmund Freud, "Analysis Terminable and Interminable," *International Journal of Psycho-Analysis* 18 (1937): 373–405.

5. Alberto Stefana, *History of Countertransference: From Freud to the British Object Relations School* (London: Routledge, 2017).

6. Idell Natterson, "Turning Points and Intersubjectivity," *Clinical Social Work Journal* 21, no. 1 (1993): 45–56, https://doi.org/10.1007/BF00754911.

7. Del Lowenthal, "Countertransference, Phenomenology and Research: Was Freud Right?" *European Journal of Psychotherapy and Counselling* 20, no. 4 (2018): 365–72, https://doi.org/10.1080/13642537.2018.1534676.

8. Christin J. Fort, "Intersectionality, Intersubjectivity and Integration: A Two Person Therapy," *Journal of Psychology and Theology* 46, no. 2 (2018): 116–21, https://doi.org/10.1177/009164711876..7987.

9. Micheal L. Miller, "Dynamic Systems and the Therapeutic Action of the Analyst: II. Clinical Application and Illustrations," *Psychoanalytic Psychology* 21, no.1 (2004): 54–69, https://doi.org/10.1037/0736-9735.21.1.54.

10. Jean Baker Miller, Judith Jordan, Irene P. Stiver, Maureen Walker, Janet L. Surrey, and Natalie S. Eldridge, "Therapists' Authenticity," *Work in Progress* 82, (Wellesley MA: Wellesley Centers for Women, Wellesley College, 1999), 3.

11. Penny Summerfield, *Reconstructing Women's Lives: Discourse and Subjectivity in Oral Histories of the Second World War* (Manchester: Manchester University Press, 1998).
12. Glen O. Gabbard, Judith S. Beck, and Jeremy Holmes, *Oxford Textbook of Psychotherapy* (New York: Oxford University Press, 2005).
13. Maureen Walker and Wendy Rosen, *How Connections Heal: Stories from Relational Cultural Therapy* (New York: Guilford, 2004).
14. Siebold, "What Do Patients Want?"
15. Kenneth I. Pargament et al., "Sacred Moments in Psychotherapy from the Perspective of Mental Health Providers and Clients: Prevalence, Predictors, and Consequences," *Spirituality in Clinical Practice* 1, no. 4 (2014): 248–62, https://doi.org/10.1037/scp0000043.
16. Bransford, "Reconciling Paternalism and Empowerment in Clinical Practice."
17. Sarah Walther and Hugh Fox, "Narrative Therapy and Outsider Witness Practice: Teachers as a Community of Acknowledgement," *Educational and Child Psychology* 29, no. 2 (2012): 8–17.
18. Derald W. Sue and David Sue, *Counseling the Culturally Different: Theory and Practice*, 2nd ed. (Washington, DC: Wiley, 1990).
19. Janet E. Helms, *Black and White Racial Identity: Theory, Research, and Practice* (Westport, CT: Greenwood, 1990).
20. Pamela L. Semmler and Carmen B. Williams, "Narrative Therapy: A Storied Context for Multicultural Counseling," *Journal of Multicultural Counseling and Development* 28, no 1 (2000): 51–62, https://doi.org/10.1002/j.2161-1912.2000.tb00227.x.
21. Ann Weick et al., "A Strengths Perspective for Social Work Practice," *Social Work* 34, no. 4 (1989): 350–54, https://www.jstor.org/stable/23715838.
22. Jose M. M. Rodriguez, "Intersubjective Aspects of Relational Group Process," *International Journal of Integrative Psychotherapy* 8 (2018): 26–39.
23. Natterson, "Turning Points and Intersubjectivity."
24. Rodriguez, "Intersubjective Aspects of Relational Group Process."
25. Natterson, "Turning Points and Intersubjectivity."
26. Nancy P. Kropf and Cindy Tandy, "Narrative Therapy with Older Adults: The Use of a Meaning-Making Approach," *Clinical Gerontologist* 18, no. 4 (1998): 3–16, http://dx.doi.org/10.1300/J018v18n04_02.
27. Wendy Lustbader, "Thoughts on the Meaning of Frailty," *Generations* 23, no. 4 (1999–2000): 21–24, https://www.jstor.org/stable/44877540.

7

INTERWEAVING PATHS

Exploring Convergences and Divergences Between Psychotherapy and Oral History

> *Stories can cry out: these things happen; I embody what happened.*
> —ARTHUR W. FRANK, "JUST LISTENING: NARRATIVE AND DEEP ILLNESS"

CONVERGENCES

I chose to work in both clinical gerontology and oral history because I have always loved listening to stories. Over the course of my career as both clinician and oral historian, I have heard hundreds of life stories. These stories have sometimes been stories of suffering and despair, and sometimes stories of joy and happiness, but always stories of survival and resilience. In my work, I have experienced, time and again, the therapeutic value of life review for older adults.

When I was a graduate student in social work, I did my first-year internship in a nursing home. My primary therapeutic role was to listen. From time to time, I was afraid to look through this "window" that opened onto my own aging. One day, a patient said to me: "You can't possibly understand what I am going through. You are young and I am old." To which I replied: "Just stay right where you are and I'll catch up someday!" That was more than a quarter of a century ago, and I'm well on the way.

Aging is a "problem" that most of us will come to know, but aging does not belong only to the old; it is a phenomenon that begins at birth. When we are young, we can distance ourselves emotionally and physically from the aging process. We may even think of aging as a communicable disease. The last of Erikson's Eight Stages of Psychosocial Development is *Integrity vs. Despair*.[1] In this era of scientific research on aging, we often neglect the personal perspective. Narrative provides us a lens through which to understand the subjective experience of aging. Only an individual can truly answer the question: "What makes a life worth living?" The psychologist Arthur Frank has noted that we prefer "hero" and "restitution" stories, in which an individual emerges from a difficult situation stronger in character. But we have difficulty listening to the chaos story, and the narratives of aging may often appear to be chaos stories. We favor the story with a happy ending, but the only ending of old age is death. In the words of François Mauriac: "Old age is marvelous . . . too bad it has to end so badly!"

We age biographically as much as biologically. Gerontologist Polard compared the physical decline of older people as a kind of homelessness: "the body is no longer a comfortable domicile."[2] De Hennezel described old age as a "No Exit."[3] Consider also the saying that "ageism is the new racism." The idea that aging has its own developmental tasks may seem counterintuitive; however, we must consider aging in the context of the life course and consider each individual's life story within the framework of his or her culture.

Human beings, by nature, are storytellers and listeners. Narrative is a fundamental aspect of our lives. The critic Barbara Hardy wrote: "For we dream in narrative, daydream in narrative, remember, anticipate, hope, despair, believe, doubt, plan, revise, criticize, construct, gossip, learn, hate, and love by narrative. In order to really live, we make up stories about ourselves and others, about the personal as well as the social past and future."[4]

Each time someone tells a story it's a different story, because it is told at a different time. Lorraine Hedtke speaks of "the origami of remembering," a process in which memories continue to fold themselves into different shapes.[5] Temporality is a fundamental aspect of narration, and we understand the meaning of time through stories. Jan Baars makes the case that narratives are crucial to the interrelation of lived experience, past, present, and future.[6] He argues that although the study of chronometric time appears to discard traditional narratives, "narratives tend to creep in and remain hidden behind chronometric exactness." How does this differ in the context of psychotherapy and of oral history? In therapy, the narrative is shared in fragments, and it is the role of the therapist to help the client construct a coherent narrative over time. In the oral history interview, it is the interviewee who brings together the narrative fragments and shares them with the interviewer, sometimes within a single session.

Human beings are always creating and being created. The most important narratives for the individual include note only the stories that are told about that individual but also the stories they tell about themselves. In narrative linkage, the narrator assembles spheres of meaning in the context of lived experiences. The meaning emanates from this linkage; from time to time, however, one steps outside one's story to edit it. We come to realize that "the story of my life" can be rewritten many times. This capacity gives us a certain measure of authority over who we are. One is no longer the patient X in this or that room, but rather, an individual. Bruner Jerome wrote, "No story, no life."[7]

When I was very young, long before the age of computers, I had an educational toy that consisted of a piece of cardboard with two electrodes and a red light on the top. A simple circuit board was attached to the back. A list of states was printed on the left side of the toy, and a list of capitals was printed, in random order, on the right. A small metal hole appeared next to each word. The idea was to put one electrode into the hole next to a state, and the other into the hole next to the correct capital. If you succeeded, the red light was illuminated and you earned a point. I had not thought about that toy until many years later, when I first entered the field of social work as a student. There were certain phrases I heard over and over again in my clinical practice classes: "That must have been very hard for you," or "It must have taken a lot of courage to overcome that." These phrases were used to illustrate the strengths-based practice principle: "Start where the client is." Each time I used one of these with my clients, I got a positive response. It was like plugging the electrode into the right hole and watching that red light go on. Clients felt understood. Only once did this backfire. This client, a retired social worker, snapped back at me: "Don't give me that social worker talk!"

For many years, I have worked as a psychiatric social worker in a mental health clinic for older adults, and for a decade, I have taught and supervised graduate students in social work. I tell my students that I chose the field of aging because I have always loved listening to stories. Much of my work as a clinician involves listening to life stories. In 2008, when Columbia University inaugurated the first Oral History Master of Arts program in the United States, I knew it would afford me the opportunity to pursue my passion for life story at the level of academic research.

DIVERGENCES

Although much evidence-based literature has been published on the therapeutic value of life review for older adults, listening as a therapist is not the same as listening as an interviewer. Therapy is a dialogue involving a vast array of interventions, such as reframing and interpretation. The therapist may reflect on body language that suggests emotional content. When Mrs. W, a woman in her eighties who has had a life full of tragedy, tells me with a big smile on her face that her husband abused her, I can ask her what is behind the mask. When Mr. G clenches his fists while talking about how his father constantly criticized him, I can help him get in touch with his anger. As an oral historian, I might ask for clarification; however, it would not be to probe the deeper psychological underpinnings of the narrative, but rather to better understand the historical and sociopolitical context from which their narrative emerges.

INTENT

In her comparison of oral history and psychotherapy, Wendy Rickard addresses the question of "what vital areas of emotional vulnerability the method of pursuing knowledge through oral history can obscure, leave uncontained, or, at worst, damaged."[8] Raphael Samuel, an oral historian, talks about the "secret, unofficial ambition" of oral history, which is to "break down the divisions between history and anthropology, and psycho-analysis . . . between past and present, between outward history and inner thought."[9] At the same time, Salvador Minuchin wrote about "the oral history of family therapy."[10] In discussing his views on the significance of personal and family history in psychotherapy, Minuchin makes a case for the social construction of history that could easily have been articulated by an oral historian: "History, or 'the past,' is by definition a construction. There are the facts, which are more or less objective; but their grouping, the way they are highlighted, and the shadows that are left are the product of the historian's present position. The mores of his time, the ideologies fashionable at the moment, and current constraints all contribute to the 'proper' interpretation of recorded events—'proper' meaning, in this context, 'correct at this historical juncture.'"

When I first conducted oral history interviews, I struggled with their difference from clinical interviews. Although I never presumed them to be clinical work, I wondered about "plugging in" some of the framing comments so basic to psychotherapy. I wondered if it would be presumptive to help an interviewee feel understood by saying: "That must have been very hard for you." Perhaps not, but, unlike that of the clinician, the role of oral historian is not to help the interviewee interpret and process the narrative, but rather to let the person's story stand as one's legacy.

Drawing on three case examples, in this chapter, I illustrate how these two disciplines, in both their methodology and their outcomes, may diverge and converge. In the first case of Mme. D, oral history developed adjunctively to my work as a therapist. In the second and third examples, my experience and prior role as a therapist with these people influenced the way in which I conducted their oral histories.

MME. D   The first time I met Mme. D, a retired teacher in her eighties, was in her apartment in Paris. She had given me permission to interview her, although she found it difficult at first to understand why anyone would be interested in her story. Mme. D had had some experience as a radio journalist and was worried that I would ask her a series of questions she would be unable to answer. I tried to put her at ease by explaining the difference between a journalistic interview and an oral history, and when she began to tell her story, her anxiety subsided. The first interview was somewhat formal. Mme. D told her story in a factual, chronological manner, in the context of her career and the historical times in which she lived.

Mme. D had grown up near the German border, and the specter of World War I colored her childhood. Despite her father's humble origins, he had become a much-decorated soldier, and his war stories had a profound impact on the family. It was not until the second interview that Mme. D mentioned her mother's sudden descent into a deep depression when Mme. D was only ten years old, from which her mother would never recover. This depression would mark Mme. D for life. Mme. D spoke with deep sadness, but said that she does not cry easily about emotional issues. Toward the end of the second interview she said: "If I knock into something, I cry; I call for my mother; but if I face an ordeal I become hardened, completely hardened." At this point, I reflected to Mme. D that she must have learned at an early age to protect herself. I had begun to slip into the language of therapy. As an oral historian, it was not my place to reflect on the etiology of Mme. D's difficulty. Fortunately, her response to my statement was positive, yet shortly thereafter, she decided it was time to end the interview. I sensed that what she had told me about her mother was acutely painful, and she did not want to go on. Nevertheless, a strong bond had begun to develop between us, and when it was time for me to leave, she embraced me warmly, saying that the experience of telling her story was therapeutic.

The third interview had a different tenor than the others, and Mme. D seemed eager to continue telling her story. She had invited me to have lunch with her before the interview, and the conversation during lunch was a prelude to what she would talk about in the interview. She spoke of her lifelong struggle with feelings of personal inadequacy (she felt competent in her work life), and her years of psychoanalysis. When it came time to begin the interview, Mme. D referred to the recorder, with humor and affection, as "the instrument of torture." I decided to begin the interview by asking her about her experience with psychoanalysis. She spoke openly and in depth about her experiences, and in the middle of the interview, she said she would like to tell me something about her mother that she had not shared in the previous interview. In the second interview, she had told me that her mother had become depressed almost overnight when Mme. D was ten years old; this time, however, she said her mother had been depressed from the time Mme. D was born and was unable to nurture her as she had nurtured her older siblings. She talked in detail about her mother's situation. Her mother had been publicly disgraced when the family applied to an exclusive boarding school for Mme. D's older sister, who was denied admission to the school because of her mother's "transgressions" with men before she was married. In fact, the school, which catered to the upper classes, used this as a pretext in which to exclude this family of humble origins.

Mme. D asked me if I thought she was betraying her mother by revealing this secret. The family had kept quiet all these years, closing in on itself for protection. At that moment, I felt I was being called on to be a therapist and found myself taking the strengths-based approach of a therapist to alleviate Mme. D's self-doubt.[11] I told her that rather than characterizing it as a betrayal, I felt she was giving voice to something important that her mother had never been able to say. Mme. D said that, in reality, she felt a sense of liberation in talking about her mother's experience, yet wondered about the possibility of betrayal.

This interchange illustrates the therapeutic power of narrative, yet, at the same time, the interview was not meant to be a therapy session. As the interview progressed, there were several moments in which I had to consciously direct the course of the interview to prevent it from veering off in the direction of therapy. The more Mme. D began to find her voice, the more she looked to me to help her sort out this painful material, and the harder I had to work to be the oral historian and not the therapist.

Intersubjectivity is at the core of both the oral history interview and the psychotherapeutic relationship (see chapter 6). Oral history and psychotherapy share this core organization. So then, how do the oral historians know when they are slipping into therapy? By the same token, how do clinicians recognize when a client's construction of a narrative may be an objective factual diversion from therapeutic dialogue? The ever-present challenge of this intersubjectivity shapes the outcome in both disciplines.

MARION'S STORY: LIKE A SERIES OF PHOTOGRAPHS   I had been seeing Marion for individual therapy for about a year, when the subject of her writing her life story came up. I don't remember who brought it up first, but I recall that it emerged seamlessly from the conversation we were having. Marion, a widow in her seventies, had been seeing another therapist for many years, but felt the treatment had come to a standstill. Marion wanted a different approach. She was depressed and felt she lacked a sense of purpose. Previously the head of a highly successful international business, Marion's business folded five years earlier, because she could no longer compete with the flood of goods manufactured in China. The business had originally belonged to her father, and after his death at a relatively young age, Marion assumed the leadership and built it into a multimillion-dollar venture. By the time she came to see me, most of the money was gone. But the real pain of Marion's life happened long before the collapse of her business.

We talked on and off for a year about how Marion could begin to write. She wanted to write, but felt blocked, and said she wouldn't know how or where to begin. I finally suggested helping her record her story, and she said she would very much like to try this. Once again, I was both stepping outside, and expanding, the boundaries of my clinical work, but I felt confident that Marion and I would be able to navigate this. I had heard bits and pieces of her story in her sessions, but this was the first time she told it to me as a linear narrative. With the recorder on the table between us, the dynamic changed, and we were engaging in oral history. Yet, because we are also connected by a therapeutic alliance, we had the opportunity to process this experience afterward, which rarely happens following an oral history interview. I will discuss the essence of that conversation, but to help the reader have a deeper understanding of this experience, I will first share some of Marion's story.

Marion, seventy-three-years old, was born in Egypt, the only child of an Italian Jewish father and an Egyptian Jewish mother. Her father owned a textile factory, and in 1956, when Nasser abolished many civil liberties and expelled many Jews and foreign nationals, his business was seized, and the family was forced to leave the country.[12] *Marion, who was seven years old at the time, remembers men with machine guns who came to the door of their home and "escorted" the family to the airport. They were allowed one small suitcase each, and the rest of their property was to be "donated" to the Egyptian government. Marion clutched her favorite doll, one that had been a gift to her from a family friend in Switzerland. When they got to the airport the officials told her they would have to cut the doll open to see if there was contraband inside. Her mother told her to abandon the doll, rather than see it eviscerated. Marion still remembers the feeling of having abandoned her doll.*

The family emigrated to France, and then to South America, where Marion's uncle lived. Her uncle was able to help her father start up a textile business, and he became successful. Unfortunately, he died young, and Marion, who was sent to boarding school in Switzerland, and then to England to study at Oxford, came home to take over the business. She had a flair for design, discovered she was a good businesswoman, and eventually built the business into a very successful international enterprise. However, when Chinese manufacturing began to take over, the business went under, and Marion was not able to salvage it.

Aside from the facts of Marion's story, her emotional life was always complicated. Her mother was a difficult woman, very beautiful and flirtatious, but prone to frequent rages. As Marion's father was often absent because of his work, she took her anger out on Marion. With hindsight, Marion is able to understand her mother's unhappiness, but as a child, she felt there must be something she was doing wrong, to provoke such anger. She tried to be "good," and always think of attending to the needs of others, before attending to her own. Marion married a man much older than she, who was a Holocaust survivor. He, too, was prone to angry outbursts, but Marion loved him deeply and stayed with him. Her greatest regret is that she terminated her pregnancy, because her husband, who had two children from a previous marriage, did not want more children. To this day, Marion feels an emptiness because she did not have a child of her own.

Marion's husband died several years ago after a long illness. She has been trying to put her life back together, but the pandemic has complicated this process. Although she has close friends, her friendships are often fraught, as was her home life, and she sometimes feels upset and disappointed if friends do not understand what she is going through. Therapy has been helpful, and Marion joined one of my Zoom women's groups. Recording her narrative had an interesting effect on her feelings about her story.

When Marion and I discussed the experience of recording her story, she had an interesting response, a different kind of response than I have had from most of the people I have interviewed, whether as a narrative therapist or as an oral historian. Marion said she felt distant from her story, as though someone else were telling it. Throughout the recording, she felt as though she were looking at her life as a series of photographs. Because of my dual role, I was able to utilize this information in our therapy sessions, to gain a deeper understanding of Marion's reactions to the traumatic events of her life, and to help her connect to her own narrative.

BILL'S STORY: A LEG UP   These oral history interviews are not at all the same as our clinical work together, but instead they complement it, as the stories shared within the walls of a treatment room now breathe in a larger arena. Whether stories of suffering or joy, in an oral history interview with a client, I am witness to the linkage of narrative fragments, told to me over the course of many fifty-minute therapy sessions, into the flow of a life story. One such recent experience is the story of Bill, a man who had no legs. I would like to add a comment on the importance of humor, as a form of narrative resilience. Bill used humor, both in his therapy sessions and in an oral history interview, not as a diversion but as a vehicle for narrative engagement. His humor not only helped him cope with his disability but also served to put the listener at ease. It was a measure of Bill's generous spirit.

I first met Bill, now in his early seventies, when I substituted briefly for a colleague who was on sick leave. She was running a group for older men and women who were suffering from depression. Bill was in the group, and I was struck by his honest, and often humorous way of speaking. He asked me if I would take him on for individual therapy, and we formed a strong therapeutic alliance. As I listened to his stories, and how he reveled in talking about his long career as a costume person in the theater, the more I thought about doing an oral history interview. I had a strong feeling it would bring him great joy, and enrich our therapeutic work together. I was an interviewer for an ongoing oral history project about older people in the arts, with a focus on those who came to New York from elsewhere. Bill met the criteria and was very enthusiastic about being interviewed.[13] Here is Bill's story:

Bill was born in a small town in Maryland. He developed an interest in the theater when he was in high school, he but never imagined he would one day be the supervising costume director for a number of major Broadway shows. After high school, he decided to move to New York. He knew if he stayed in the small town where he grew up, he would end up in a "dead-end" office job, and "be bored out of my mind." But the other reasons he shared are that he identifies as a gay man, and felt he would feel more comfortable in a cosmopolitan city, and he wanted to try his hand at becoming a performer. He studied dance and acting, but soon realized he did not have what it takes to be a performer on Broadway, so he went into backstage work. He had learned to sew from his mother, and his talent as a costume designer was soon recognized. Bill went on to have a long, fulfilling career in costumes. He traveled the world, and got to know many of the greats in the theater. But Bill had diabetes, and he did not take care of his health.

A number of years ago, Bill had to have one leg, and then the other, amputated. Although he struggled with depression over these losses, his indomitable spirit won out, and Bill learned to walk with prostheses, using only a cane. He went back to work. He likes to tell the story of a colleague who couldn't reach something one day, on a high shelf in the costume department. She asked if anyone could give her a leg up. Bill, rising to the challenge, removed one of his prostheses and handed it to her. He truly gave her a "leg up."

OTHER PROFESSIONAL VOICES ON CONVERGENCE AND DIVERGENCE

For decades, historians ignored the rich findings that psychology can bring to historical research and, within the field of history, oral history was regarded as a lesser, unreliable, source of information. A few historians argued for incorporating a psychological lens in historical research, but it was not until the mid-1980s that several noted historians began to look at how psychology and oral history could deepen our understanding of history. Among the first to publish on this subject was Charles Morrissey who wrote the following:

> Oral history can fill gaps in archival collections and resolve ambiguities which would frustrate historians who lacked living witnesses to query. It can often provide explanations about human motivations (the persistent question "Why?" is the most important one an oral historian can ask), and it can recapture the emotional tenor which enveloped issues in the past. Additionally, it can serve in lieu of archival sources when knowledge is sought about undocumented aspects of the past (intense personal relationships, for example), and about people ignored to date by record-keeping and record-retention practices (women, racial and ethnic minorities). It can create documentation about people who don't leave records (children, illiterate adults) behind them.[14]

Valerie Yow, in her comprehensive comparison of oral history and psychotherapy, makes the point that oral historians and clinicians rely on the same tools—body language, facial expressions, and gestures—but the primary avenue of communication in both disciplines is the spoken word.[15] Both oral historians and clinicians learn to listen carefully to detect the feelings underlying the words, to understand hidden meanings, and to be alert to what is left out of a narrative. This requires not only careful, attentive listening, but also self-reflection on the part of the interviewer or clinician. Therapists are trained to be attuned to their own reactions to clients' narratives, whether we call it countertransference or intersubjectivity, and through the influence of psychology, oral historians are now paying more attention to this process in their work. Looking at the ways in which differences between the interviewer and interviewee—differences such as race, gender, age, socioeconomic background, and culture—may affect the interview has been a foundation of psychotherapy for some time and is becoming more prevalent in oral history. I have written about the richness of my experiences as an "insider/outsider" while working on an oral history project I conducted at a senior center in East Harlem, where all of the participants were Latino, and I am not.[16]

Donald Spence also reminds us of another common challenge—that is, rather than appearing tongue-tied or incoherent, narrators "may be lulled by the demand to be verbal in place of being accurate."[17] How does this reflect the accuracy of memories? Alessandro Portelli, asked: "Should we believe oral sources?"[18] He answered that the importance of oral testimony may not lie in its accuracy and adherence to fact, but in its departure from it, "as imagination, symbolism, and desire emerge."

Portelli's work, among others, has liberated historians from a "just the facts" approach. This is what historian Susan Matt calls history from the "inside out."[19] I have found, however, that whether we use the discipline of listening to narrative as an oral historian or as a psychotherapist coming alongside the aging process, the words of Carol Staudacher express the significance of what we strive for when listening to the stories of others: "Each time I tell my story, I remove one small bit of hurt from inside me. I ease my wound."[20]

NOTES

1. Erik H. Erikson, *Identity and the Life Cycle* (New York: Norton, 1980).
2. José Polard, "Home: écouter un sujet âgé dans son environnemen" (lecture at the Fourth Conference on Aging, *La cause des aînés: Pour vivre autrement . . . et mieux*, Paris, June 12, 2010).

3. Marie De Hennezel, "La vulnérabilité dans l'accompagnement de fin de vie" (lecture at the Fourth Conference on Aging, *La cause des aînés: Pour vivre autrement . . . et mieux*, Paris, June 13, 2010).
4. Barbara Hardy, "Narrative as a Primary Act of Mind," in *The Cool Web: The Patterns of Children's Reading*, ed. Margaret Meek, Aiden Warlow, and Griselda Barton (London: Bodley Head, 1977), 13.
5. Lorraine Hedtke, "The Origami of Remembering," *International Journal of Narrative Therapy and Community Work* 2003, no. 4 (2003): 58–63, https://search.informit.org/doi/abs/10.3316/INFORMIT.661383982613964.
6. Jan Baars, "Critical Turns of Aging, Narrative, and Time," *International Journal of Ageing and Later Life* 7, no. 2 (2012): 143–65, https://doi.org/10.3384/ijal.1652-8670.1272a7.
7. Jerome Bruner, "Narratives of Aging," *Journal of Aging Studies* 13, no. 1 (1999): 7–9.
8. Wendy Rickard, "Oral History—'More Dangerous Than Therapy'? Interviewees' Reflections on Recording Traumatic or Taboo Issues," *Oral History* 26, no. 2 (1998).
9. Raphael Samuel, "Myth and History: A First Reading," *Oral History* 16, no. 1 (1988).
10. Salvador Minuchin, "My Many Voices," in *The Evolution of Psychotherapy*, ed. Jeffery K Zeig (New York: Routledge, 1987).
11. In a strengths-based approach to therapy, the therapist builds on client's past successes to help the client address challenges in the present.
12. Valerie Yow, "What Can Oral Historians Learn from Psychotherapists?," *Oral History* 46, no. 1 (2018): 33–41, https://www.jstor.org/stable/44993454.
13. Lauren Taylor, "Resilience: Elder in East Harlem," in *Say It Forward: A Guide to Social Justice Storytelling*, ed. Cliff Mayotte and Claire Kiefer (Chicago: Haymarket, 2019).
14. Charles T. Morrissey, "Public Historians and Oral History: Problems of Concept and Methodology," *Public Historian* 2, no. 2 (1980): 22–29.
15. Yow, "What Can Oral Historians Learn from Psychotherapists?"
16. Taylor, "Resilience: Elder in East Harlem."
17. Donald P. Spence, *Narrative Truth and Historical Truth: Meaning and Interpretation in Psychoanalysis* (New York: Norton, 1982), 182.
18. Alessandro Portelli, "What Makes Oral History Different?," in *The Death of Luigi Trastulli and Other Stories: Form and Meaning in Oral History* (Albany: State University of New York Press, 1991), 42–54.
19. Susan J. Matt, "Current Emotion Research in History: or, Doing History from the Inside Out," *Emotion Review* 3, no. 1 (2011): 117–24, https://doi.org/10.1177/1754073910384416.
20. Carol Staudacher, *A Time to Grieve: Meditations for Healing After the Death of a Loved One* (London: Souvenir, 1995), 61.

8

RECOGNIZING RESILIENCE

Compassionate Listening to Trauma Narratives

> *Chaos stories can be heard most clearly in the response they elicit in listeners: when the listener feels sucked into a whirlpool and only wants to get away from the story, then a chaos story is being told.*
>
> —ARTHUR W. FRANK, "JUST LISTENING: NARRATIVE AND DEEP ILLNESS"

BACKGROUND ON PTSD

Ellie picked up a kitchen knife. She would either kill him or kill herself. She had come home from school and Mom and Dad were not home yet. Ellie knew that he, the uncle who lived upstairs, would soon come for her. She braced herself, and put down the knife. He did the same thing to her older sister, but her sister wouldn't talk about it. They never told their parents, because they loved their aunt, the wife of their abuser, and they knew their parents would ask the couple to leave the home they shared. Ellie was sixteen when she picked up that knife. The abuse had been going on for over a year, and would continue until she left home a year later. She is now in her eighties. Like many survivors of childhood sexual abuse, Ellie hid a part of herself, not only from others, but also from her own consciousness, and turned to alcohol to numb the pain.

The now familiar term, posttraumatic stress disorder (PTSD), was first recognized as an official diagnosis in 1980, when it was added to the third edition of the *Diagnostic and Statistical Manual*, the DSM. But its recorded history long predates inclusion in the DSM. Likely a fundamental aspect of the human psychological experience, the earliest documented case of

PTSD was documented by Herodotus in 440 BC.[1] Until relatively recently, PTSD was thought to be primarily a disorder brought on by war trauma, commonly referred to as "shell shock" or "soldier's heart." Today, the diagnostic criteria have been expanded to include specific symptoms in an individual who has experienced any type of major traumatic event. We must take care, however, not to assume that a diagnosis of PTSD represents a client's personal narrative. As Judith Johnson reminds us: "At times of severe personal crisis, a person's problems often become the focus. Individuals can be reduced to diagnoses, taking away their sense of agency. Stripped of the acknowledgement of their unique skills and knowledge their stories and identities become thin and problem-riddled."[2]

In his seminal article, "Just Listening: Narrative and Deep Illness," Arthur Frank speaks of stories as "relationships to be entered," rather than material to be analyzed.[3] He describes three kinds of narratives, and puts each in a cultural context. The "restitution story" is the culturally preferred narrative of illness and suffering in North America. It tells of a suffering individual's being restored to health through treatment. These stories lack, however, the subjective experience of the client; instead, the clinicians are the "experts" of the stories, and their subjectivities determine the outcome. When restitution is not possible, the narrator may turn to the "quest story," in which the sufferer tries to learn something from the suffering and that suffering takes on new meaning. We can tolerate that kind of narrative, but the one most feared in our society is the "chaos story," as it theoretically cannot be told. As soon as the chaos story becomes a narrative, it is no longer a story of total chaos. Frank sees each of these stories as pathways of entry into the therapeutic relationship.

The trauma narrative is most often a chaos story—that is, fragmented and unsequenced. Diane Benjamin and Lori Zook-Stanley posit that seeking help is a "last-resort act of desperation," which can make the client more vulnerable to shame and put the client in a one-down position. Cultural context often supports this notion. The authors ask us to regard the act of seeking help as an "intentional and generous invitation" and to explore how hearing this invitation might shape our responses as clinicians. They point out that "people all over the world are responding to trauma in skillful and knowing ways," and that we can invite these diverse responses into the treatment room, thereby "dissolving the isolating and individualizing effects of trauma."[4]

In this chapter, I examine the salient characteristics of narrative therapy (NT) within a range of diverse experiences of trauma. Using older adults' narratives, I explore the following elements: (1) refraining from exploration to avoid "flooding," (2) dissociation, (3) recognizing inner strength,

(4) vicarious traumatization, (5) caring and connection, and (6) coconstructing and presence.

REFRAINING

THE GUN *I was eight or nine years old. I don't remember how Jane happened to come over for a playdate. I didn't particularly like her. I had never asked her over before. I had never been to her house to play. Maybe our mothers had arranged it.*

There she was. And bored. There wasn't anything she wanted to play with. So we walked around the house.

In my parents' bedroom, there was a small table next to the bed. On the table was a small lamp, an alarm clock and a small gun. All of a sudden, Jane whirled around and was facing me, pointing the gun at my middle.

"Stick 'em up."

Everything froze. The room froze. I froze. I knew I was going to die. I don't remember feeling frightened. I just remember feeling frozen, immobile, impotent. Even Jane froze. She was waiting for my response. She had found something she wanted to play and I was supposed to play it with her.

It was one of those experiences when time stopped and just hung there. Time, also, was frozen.

Then, I could hear my voice, calm and measured. "That is a real gun."

Very slowly, as if she too was frozen in time, Jane walked back to the bedside table and replaced the gun.

I don't know what happened next. Maybe I remember sitting in a corner of the sofa in the living room. Jane sat at the other end. She had kicked her shoes off and they lay in the middle of the rug. She was bored. Maybe this is what happened next. Or maybe it's the storyteller in me that is saying this . . . Or maybe it's my storyteller again, trying to make the story come out alright.

When coconstructing narratives, one of the challenges faced by the therapist is to refrain from going too quickly in exploring issues that might retraumatize the client. The narrator of this story would go on to experience other serious traumas. It is imperative that we allow clients to go at their own pace. In midlife, this client went back to school to become a social worker, which she describes as having liberated her from the yoke of her trauma. She chose to work with the mentally homeless, and she listened to their stories. Now, at eighty-eight, she volunteers in a community program, helping young children whose fathers are in prison. She is passionate about listening to what the children say and finding ways to help them express themselves and develop a stronger sense of self. She knows what it is like to be an unheard child. Jane's mother, always critical and blaming, never validated Jane's distress.

DISSOCIATION

The Long Road to Recovery
Placeholders for my identity:
What I have been, what I can be, what I hope to be.

—ALMA, CLIENT

In her seminal work, *Trauma and Recovery*, Judith Herman describes the shame and isolation of the trauma survivor.[5] Such was the case of Alma, whose history of childhood molestation and abuse, led her to desperate attempts to protect herself in adulthood. The protective fortress she built around herself, both physically and emotionally, kept her imprisoned for many years. Although she had a successful career earlier in her adulthood, she had to stop working when her anxiety began interfering with her functioning. She became a hoarder, and cut herself off from many social connections. When she first came to see me, she was isolated, and mired in the chaos of her living environment. Her apartment was in need of repairs, but Alma was afraid to let anyone in. Over the years, she has worked hard and consistently in therapy to move beyond her fears, and she is truly on the road of recovery. One of the most powerful interventions in her healing journey has been her writing, which she has generously shared with me and has given me permission to include her own writing in the narrative.

ALMA'S STORY

Alma, a seventy-six-year-old African-American woman, was an only child, raised by her mother and stepfather. Alma never knew her biological father. Her stepfather was a harsh man, and every day, when Alma came home from school, he made her clean the house. After she was done, he would run his finger over the furniture and complain that she had not done a good job. His punishment was to take her to a hallway, an impersonal space in the apartment, and molest her. And then he paid her.

Alma was a diligent student. She attended college, and then earned advanced degrees. She landed a job working as a producer of television news and had several romantic involvements. But all the while, she felt like an outsider, looking in at her own life. Alma describes it this way: "There's also an element of dissociation. I don't really know how to be in the process. There's a level of disassociation when I don't want to do something. My body just shuts down. I have built up all these systems in my head to deal with it."

Dissociation is one of the hallmarks of PTSD, but Alma is learning to use mindfulness to recognize it. In her own words: "The work I'm doing, it's a new way of thinking about my place in the world. I've got to make sense of it. I'm trying to stay in the moment. How do I want to be living now? What can I do about it?"

Alma's living space, and what it represents, has been one focus of our treatment. I asked her to tell me the story of her clutter. She replied: "That's a good one. There's a timeline to it, and how it developed. I need to pay attention to that as I write the story." Alma has developed insight into the expression of despair that her clutter story is telling her: "I was made to clean the house every day after school. I had no choice. I had to do it. Here I don't have to do it, but there are outside forces, pushing me to do it like the landlord. Water was pouring down on me, and I knew the ceiling was collapsing. But no one would listen. I can never be whole to really deal with this as I am always involved in my survival. Putting that aside, when all the clutter is gone, I have to face the underlying problems. The way I'm living now is that I'm blocking my own choices, and I want to stop doing that. That's the work I'm doing, and it's good to recognize that."

How does recovery happen? What is our role in this process, and what role does narrative play? What we have learned about trauma is that it disconnects and disempowers the survivor.[6] Consequently, the role of the therapist must be to help the survivor create new and trusting connections. Herman feels strongly that recovery cannot take place in isolation and that medical treatment models fail to address this fundamental necessity. As Herman has written: "Repeatedly in the testimony of survivors there comes a moment when a sense of connection is restored by another person's unaffected display of generosity. Something in herself that the victim believes to be irretrievably destroyed—faith, decency, courage—is reawakened by an example of common altruism. Mirrored in the actions of others, the survivor recognizes and reclaims a lost part of herself. At that moment, the survivor begins to rejoin the human commonality."[7]

At times, we may feel burdened as the sole person in a client's life who can provide this validation and connection. But as we and our clients work together to create new narratives of safety and possibility, greater networks of trust and connection can grow. Johnson alerts us to the missing pieces of a story, which she calls "gateways" to deeper, hidden stories.[8] These missing pieces often contain the keys to an individual's "hopes and dreams, their visions for the future, and what they value and treasure in life." This concept brings us back to Michael White's thesis about the pain resulting from trauma as a testimony to what was lost.[9] But we must tread lightly when eliciting hidden stories, as they can also unlock a Pandora's box.

RECOGNITION

ACQUIRING A TOOL BOX Everlee picked up the phone and called 911. Her life had become unbearable, and she decided to end it. Multiple traumas throughout her life had created a domino effect, one after another. White states that many trauma survivors have "lost touch with a sense of personhood."[10] This sense of personhood is intrinsic to being human, but trauma can diminish it to such an extent that life seems meaningless. As she would later recognize, taking an overdose of medication was a cry for help; had she really wanted to die, she would not have called for an ambulance. Somewhere inside her there was a ray of hope. Everlee's road to recovery was long and arduous, but she stayed the course, and I stayed it with her, helping her coconstruct and reconnect with her strengths through individual NT.

EVERLEE'S STORY Everlee's creativity as an artist, musician, and writer, as well as her faith, have helped her heal. Here she tells the story of her recovery.

I'll start with when I first took myself, after twenty years of depression, to get tested for Prozac. At the time I worked in an office but felt quite unable to comingle with others around me. I was very imprisoned within myself. I also would become anxious in a crowded train and in a full airplane. I would exit both. Prozac was recovery then. Today there are times I can feel like a new person as I did after taking Prozac daily and life becomes easier. Inevitably that newness wears off and other unknown complications arise, which require tenacity, compassion, and patience to find the solution. My recovery today has become a spiritual program as well as continuing to take my medication, which at one point I thought I didn't need anymore. I tried to kill myself and after being alive I thought I would see a big sign, from God, telling me the answer to my life. It wasn't there, so recovery became as well as returning to medication, accepting being here and accepting change. It means learning how to value my life, not comparing myself with others who I think have success, accepting my talents, and continuing to hone them as well as enlarge them. I also know I have to keep my support connections open, even though that still may be difficult for me. Isolation is different for me now because aging makes it a new ball game. It's a big change. So I have acquired a tool box and I've learned that yesterday's triumphs may not carry over into the next day. I may plummet, which means I have to use my tool box. The solution may be a crayon, a nap, moving my body, saying a prayer, playing or listening to music, writing, calling someone to hear a voice, taking a bath, finding a way to laugh, or practicing gratitude and forgiveness. I'm learning how to add in enjoyment, how to expect the Good, and to love and appreciate other humans, those I don't know as well as others I do know that show how much they care about me.

VICARIOUS TRAUMA

There were times when Everlee was angry at me, and abruptly cut me off, but she learned that I wouldn't abandon her, and she returned to try again. Herman cautions us that as the client becomes engaged in the treatment, the wish to be rescued by the therapist may emerge, but the client is bound to be disappointed.[11] The struggle and rage that ensue may replicate the trauma. We may, in turn, find ourselves feeling angry and frustrated, or anxious and vulnerable. This is vicarious traumatization, which is not the same as countertransference or burnout.[12] Although it is beyond the scope of this chapter to discuss this topic in depth, it is important to recognize that listening to trauma narratives can have a transformative effect on us and on our work. Charles Figley, who has written extensively on compassion fatigue, talks about the dilemma of remaining objective while being compassionate:

> There is a cost to caring for those with chronic illness just as there is a realization that these clients will never fully recover. As psychotherapists, we learn to be on the one hand objective and analytical in our role as helper. We must put our feelings aside and objectively evaluate our clients and administer the best treatments according to best practice guidelines. But on the other hand we cannot avoid our compassion and empathy. They provide the tools required in the art of human service. To see the world as our clients see it enables us to calibrate our services to fit them and to adjust our services to fit how they are responding.[13]

Listening to trauma narratives transforms us. As Karen W. Saakvitne and Laurie A. Pearlman explain, "Trauma work can have serious and lasting effects on workers' sense of safety and well-being."[14] The cumulative effect of listening to clients' experiences of trauma has the potential to make workers feel as though the world is no longer a safe place. Images, retained from clients' narratives, have become part of my emotional fabric—the woman who heard the screams of victims of the Holocaust, the man whose father (a policeman) sodomized him with his nightstick, the woman whose husband held a knife to her throat. In contrast, as Shantih E. Clemans has written, there can be "rich emotional, psychological, and spiritual rewards" for social workers helping trauma survivors. "Having the opportunity to help a client through a traumatic terrifying life event can foster feelings of purpose and personal satisfaction in workers." The following narratives illustrate this possibility in my own work.[15]

CARING AND CONNECTION

Connection strengthens the life in us. Sometimes the life in us is strengthened by discovering that others need us. Other times we are strengthened by discovering beyond a doubt that our love matters to someone more than we realized possible or that someone loves us just as we are.

—RACHEL NAOMI REMEN, *MY GRANDFATHER'S BLESSINGS*

Irene Stiver makes the distinction between "caretaking," which implies a custodial and unequal relationship, and "caring," which is an investment in the feelings of another, "with no implication of status of equality."[16] Stiver goes on to say that in traditional models of therapy, and even with the modern advances in treatment, caretaking is considered to be more acceptable for a therapist, than caring "too much." Stiver makes it clear that she is not advocating emotional involvement with a client to gratify the therapist's needs, but rather, "caring about." Caring is fundamental to the treatment of trauma, but it requires that we stay the course, even in the face of a client's difficulty accepting our caring. Benjamin and Zook-Stanley address this in their article on working with trauma survivors: "Sometimes kindness can burn and hurt. If one is left in the freezing cold for a period of time, it can be excruciatingly painful and burning to help the body and limbs come back to warmth and circulation."[17]

Perhaps the most critical element of caring in narrative work with trauma survivors is to bear witness, to remain present with clients, as parts of themselves previously frozen, or hidden, are awakened, and to remind them that any emotional pain they may be experiencing has deep meaning and purpose for their healing. At first, clients may be uncomfortable with a new and different perspective, as change may evoke anxiety in and of itself.

The web of our life is of a mingled yarn, good and ill together: our virtues would be proud, if our faults whipped them not; and our crimes would despair, if they were not cherished by our virtues.

—WILLIAM SHAKESPEARE, *ALL'S WELL THAT ENDS WELL*

Shakespeare's words express magnificently the basic tenets, and the challenges, of NT for the treatment of trauma. White, considered the founder of NT, posited that the ongoing pain resulting from trauma is a "testimony to the significance of what it was that the person held precious that was violated through the experience of trauma." He goes on to say: "The steps that people take in the midst of trauma, and in its aftermath, that are invariably disqualified or diminished, are founded on knowledge of life and on practices of living that have been developed in the history of the person's life, in the history of their relationships with others. In our work it is possible to create a context whereby these steps, and the practices and knowledges which they represent, can become known and richly acknowledged."[18]

COCONSTRUCTION AND PRESENCE

The story that follows is a narrative of the strength found from both loss and resilience. It is a coconstruction, and it represents an invitation by the client to allow me to accompany her on her journey to recovery. The road is not an easy one, and the journey is sometimes delayed, but we have made a commitment to travel together, wherever it may take us.

OUR LOVE IS HERE TO STAY The following story grew out of a therapeutic dialogue, and this is the sequel to a story I wrote several years ago. Joe was a client and Phyllis was his wife. Joe and I had worked together in treatment to coconstruct a narrative about his journey from deep depression to emotional health. I wrote of his remarkable recovery in my chapter "Sharing a Narrative Meal."[19] I have also had the honor of working with Phyllis, his widow.

Since Joe's death, Phyllis has been on her own journey to recovery. There are still days when she is blanketed in grief, but she is also discovering untapped creative elements of her being. Her drive to reinvent herself is one of the foci of our sessions, and she is determined to live her life to the fullest. Phyllis described this time as a "new chapter" in her life.

The advent of the coronavirus limited what she could do in person, but she mastered Zoom and opened herself to new learning, including taking an online writing class. Her writing sparked in me the idea of a shared written narrative, linking with the narrative work of her deceased husband. In the age of COVID, this sharing is fostering a deep therapeutic connection. It is also a legacy for Joe, her late husband.

I was finishing dinner late one evening when I received a call from Phyllis. Her husband, Joe, had been my long-time client, and I had worked briefly with Phyllis as well. It was not unusual for Phyllis to call and cancel appointments for him, especially when he was recovering from a seizure, but the tone of her voice told me something dire had happened, Joe was dead. He died of a massive heart attack on the way to sing at an open mic. Singing was what had helped him recover from a suicidal depression, and music had given new meaning and purpose to his life.

Phyllis and Joe's interracial marriage was an act of courage at that time in the history of our country. Joe's best friend cautioned him against marrying a black woman, and Phyllis's family was concerned about their daughter marrying into a white world. But their love was stronger than caution, and they went ahead with the marriage. Not too long afterward, their daughter was born. The marriage was rocky, and at one point they separated, but they came back together and remained together until Joe's death.

Phyllis and Joe met in an acting class. Joe grew up in a mining town, but when the coal industry tanked, the family moved and eked out a living on a peach farm. Poverty had been part of his narrative for most of his life, and he carried a bitterness with him that ultimately led to thoughts of suicide. He had come to New York hoping to find success on the stage, but his epilepsy got in the way, and he was forced to take a series of dead-end "day jobs" to help support the family. He began to feel that death was the only way out. His wife and daughter insisted he get help.

It was his love of singing that ultimately helped Joe recover from depression. Through music, and with the support of his family, he found new meaning in his life. *Our love is here to stay* became their theme song. Joe created more than one autobiographical show, where he told his story in song, and he was working on a new idea when he died. He was going to call the new show *Yesterday and Tomorrow*. Even though for Joe there was no tomorrow, the grief of losing Joe has opened up new tomorrows for Phyllis.

Phyllis wrote the following piece about how she met Joe. In it, she shares a memory she holds dear. This is an example of White's belief that we can help clients heal from trauma by helping them give voice to that which they value.[20]

1961 NEW YORK   *I was working at a nine-to-five job—as we in the theater would say—a between job until I could get another acting job. This lasted for over a year as I remember.*

At this time I was living in Westchester with my parents and making that commute to midtown every day. Arising at some ungodly hour in the morning, I didn't mind waking up early, and catching a train at a certain time every day in order to hopefully be on time for work. Oft times not, because of the train schedule or the weather, not. The week usually passed uneventfully or so I thought.

It was just monotonous, but at least I had a job.

Finally, the week ended and it was TGIF or Thank God It's Friday. Time to go to the favorite watering hole or bar and unwind and see and hear what the latest news was in the theater world.

This particular watering hole we called "The Theater Bar," located at the time on 45th Street between Broadway and Eighth Avenue. It was a place that all, and I do mean all, of the struggling actors I knew would come and hang out to get the tips on auditions, who was working or not, who had landed and agent and better than that, had actually signed a contract to be represented by said agent. This, of course, is what we all wanted to have happen to each of us.

It was an exciting time for me because I was around my peers, we were all going through much of the same experience. The support and encouragement were always to be found among this group of friends and I truly mean that.

We were all in the early stages of development in this business and so in turn we were all there to nurture each other to keep going 'cause we were sure one day we were going to succeed.

During this time, there was a guy I was dating of whom I was very fond of. We would meet there on a regular basis discussing how our auditions had gone or not. Both of us working at nine-to-five jobs for the time being until that big break which we knew was inevitable.

I can remember the smells and the food of our watering hole. I especially loved the liver and onions with mashed potatoes and string beans. Which was fairly cheap for the owners knew that on the whole we were just trying to make ends meet and here was a place we could come to and not spend beyond

what we could afford at this time. They were pretty understanding, I must say.
I know that is why we all kept coming back.

It was a very special time and a special place in my lifetime. To be always
etched in my memory.

By the way, that guy that I was dating, we got married.

Much of our work with trauma survivors involves bearing witness to suffering. We need to be present, but not allow ourselves to be engulfed by the client's trauma narrative. This is a delicate balance, and the work of helping people heal from trauma can be painstakingly slow. Early in my career, I did not understand that encouraging a client to tell a trauma story all at once could lead to flooding and cause the work to shut down. This happened with a new client who had survived the horrors of a war, and after telling me the terrifying details of her survival, got up and abruptly left the session. She never came back.

The healing narrative is, by nature, a narrative of connection. Jean B. Miller speaks of the trauma survivor's "condemned isolation" and asks us to consider what will lead to a growthful connection, and what interferes with it. She underscores that it is only through deepening connection that our clients can heal, but she cautions us that many of the forces that interfere with connection reflect patterns of culture: "Culture has everything to do with psychological growth and development. . . . A culture that does not provide a growth-fostering impetus for everyone sets in motion forces that can end in psychological problems — and the therapeutic relationship, itself, reflects the surrounding culture in both obvious and subtle ways."[21]

Beyond listening, we provide this healing connection in many ways, which we will explore in the next chapter. I conclude by sharing one such way, poetry, written by a trauma survivor, who now is connected and able to feel joy in being alive.

VERY READY

There is always a road
of chords that stretch and bend
leading to an array of sunflowers and poppies
that pulsate
their bold hues of light
And love

Above the road
Clouds of truth, goodness
and beauty gather
around in celebration of
Your life
Your august life with its own language
silly sometimes
pellucid at others

Today, feel the hours falling
into place
happily whispering and
spinning
Your name

—AZURE (AUGUST 2022)

NOTES

1. Marc-Antoine Crocq and Louis Crocq, "From Shell Shock and War Neurosis to Posttraumatic Stress Disorder: A History of Psychotraumatology," *Dialogues in Clinical Neuroscience* 2, no. 1 (2000): 47–55, https://doi.org/10.31887/DCNS.2000.2.1/macrocq.

2. Judith Johnson, "Awakening to Hope Through Narrative Practices," *International Journal of Narrative Therapy and Community Work* 1 (2018): 49–56, https://search.informit.org/doi/abs/10.3316/informit.477108620072932.

3. Arthur W. Frank, "Just Listening: Narrative and Deep Illness," *Family Systems and Health* 16, no. 3 (1998): 197–212, https://doi.org/10.1037/h0089849.

4. Diane Benjamin and Lori Zook-Stanley, "An Invitation to People Struggling with Trauma and to the Practitioners Working with Them," *International Journal of Narrative Therapy and Community Work* 3 (2012): 62–68.

5. Judith L. Herman, *Trauma and Recovery: The Aftermath of Violence—From Domestic Abuse to Political Terror* (New York: Basic, 1992).

6. Michael White, "Working with People Who Are Suffering the Consequences of Multiple Trauma: A Narrative Perspective," *International Journal of Narrative Therapy and Community Work* 1 (2004): 44–75.

7. Herman, *Trauma and Recovery*, 214.

8. Johnson, "Awakening to Hope Through Narrative Practices."

9. White, "Working with People Who Are Suffering."

10. White, "Working with People Who Are Suffering."

11. Herman, *Trauma and Recovery*.

12. Richard E. Adams, Joseph A. Boscarino, and Charles R. Figley, "Compassion
Fatigue and Psychological Distress Among Social Workers: A Validation
Study," *American Journal of Orthopsychiatry* 76, no. 1 (2006): 103–8, https://
doi.org/10.1037/0002-9432.76.1.103.
13. Charles R. Figley, "Compassion Fatigue: Psychotherapists' Chronic Lack of
Self Care," *Journal of Clinical Psychology* 58, no. 11 (2002): 1433–41, https://
doi.org/10.1002/jclp.10090.
14. Karen W. Saakvitne and Laurie A. Pearlman, *Transforming the Pain: A Workbook on Vicarious Traumatization* (London: Norton, 1996).
15. Shantih E. Clemans, "Understanding Vicarious Traumatization: Strategies for
Social Workers," *Social Work Today* 4, no. 2 (2004): 13.
16. Irene P. Stiver, "The Meaning of Care: Reframing Treatment Models," 1985,
http://www.wcwonline.org/pdf/previews/preview_20sc.pdf.
17. Benjamin and Zook-Stanley, "An Invitation to People Struggling with Trauma."
18. White, "Working with People Who Are Suffering."
19. Lauren Taylor, "Sharing a Narrative Meal: The Therapeutic Use of Narrative with Older Adults," in *Narrative in Social Work Practice: The Power and
Possibility of Story*, ed. Ann Burack-Weiss, Lynn S. Lawrence, and Lynne B.
Mijangos (New York: Columbia University Press, 2017).
20. White, "Working with People Who Are Suffering."
21. Jean B. Miller, introduction to *How Connections Heal: Stories from
Relational-Cultural Therapy*, ed. Maureen Walker and Wendy B. Rosen
(New York: Guildford, 2004).

9

DISCOVERING NARRATIVES BEYOND WORDS

Exploring Diverse Modalities for Deeper Connections

> *Storytelling reveals meaning without committing the error of defining it.*
>
> —HANNAH ARENDT, *MEN IN DARK TIMES*

The stories of my clients are preserved in memory, in progress notes, and in always confidence. When I choose to reiterate them, names and details have been withheld or modified so that the people are unrecognizable.

This chapter is a compilation of vignettes using different modalities from my clinical work in the field. I have chosen to present cases from my work in older adults' homes, as this aspect of my work has enabled a degree of creativity with narrative therapy (NT) that is not possible within the confines of a clinic treatment room. The stories in this chapter reflect a range of narrative modalities: (1) with words and imagery, (2) without words, illustrating the power of presence, (3) through writing, (4) with art, (5) with meaningful artifacts, and (6) through motion. In this chapter, I also highlight deepening the therapeutic rapport, using presence, self-disclosure, and shared connections, within these different narrative modalities.

WORDS AND IMAGERY

HOME WORK: BEING PRESENT WITHIN THE OLDER ADULT'S ABODE   Even before the pandemic, a frequent part of my work was bringing therapy to older adult clients in their homes. Seeing the surroundings in which an older adult lives brings a different perspective to the work and to the narrative. Sometimes I was astonished by the beauty of an adult's home, but more often I was struck by the years of accumulated belongings, sometimes a much-loved source of comfort, and sometimes creating an almost impenetrable barrier between the clients and their emotional and physical freedom. Although outside the official realm of my clinical work, going into older adults' homes has required me to figuratively stretch the walls of the treatment room, drawing on collaborative creativity and on my humanity.

At times, in a client's home, I have been called on to help with concrete tasks that may be outside the realm of my official title of "psychiatric social worker." I have helped a client pin up a dress, brought a client a newspaper, and mailed a letter. These are choices I have made, and it required a clear sense of my own boundaries and comfort level. In some cases, there were touching moments that would not have been possible in a treatment room. A client who was nearly blind offered to make me a cup of tea on a cold day. I gladly accepted, and watched as the client poured half a cup of sugar into a mug, and then filled it with only a few drops of water, as she could not see what she was doing. She stirred the mixture lovingly, and handed me the mug. I sipped it slowly as we talked, knowing that to leave it would have been an affront to the client.

There are difficult moments as well. One such occasion, at the end of my work day, as the client and I stood up to part, she sank slowly to the floor. She was not injured but could not get up on her own. I tried to help her, but she was too heavy. I called downstairs to her doorman, but he said he was not able to leave his post. The client had a life alert button, which she pressed. As she had no family or close friends, the system alerted the police. As the minutes passed, and the sun began to set, I decided I would sit on the floor with the client, so that she did not feel alone. Although I missed an appointment of my own, I knew this was more important.

PONCHOS FOR THE AFTERLIFE   I can't really remember the first time I met Sam, which is unusual for me. I have a reputation at the agency for being able to recall, in great detail, everything about my clients. Sam's wife Martha had been in the hospital, and the nurse who tended to her when she came home thought Sam was depressed. I like working with couples and, although Sam was the client, I knew there would be marital issues leading to the wife's involvement as well. The location was convenient—only a few blocks from the agency. The building was a middle-income high rise, with long halls, shiny green and black tiled linoleum floors, and cinderblock walls.

I rang the bell and was greeted at the door by Sam, a short, stout man, with a shock of white hair and a thick white mustache. "Come in, come in," he said, graciously. The apartment was tidy, with teak Danish modern furniture upholstered in burnt orange and ochre. Sam directed me to the dining table, set in an alcove. One of the walls of the alcove was painted burnt orange to match the furnishings. Two large Japanese prints of cranes adorned the wall at the back. The other wall was mostly windows, with a door leading to a bare concrete terrace. There were a few plants on a shelf under the window and several stacks of books. A woman in a white uniform sat in a chair by a door leading to the terrace. The door was ajar, letting in a warm breeze. Sam introduced me to her. She was the home health aide, and her name was Elizabeth.

Sam's wife Martha was in her wheelchair at the side of the table by the windows. Now sixty-eight years old, in her thirties she had been in a car accident that had left her disabled. Large glasses slid partway down her nose. Her fingers were gnarled. Sam introduced her to me and she greeted me in a gravelly voice, with reserved suspicion. Sam sat down at one end of the table, and I sat down across from him. "What can I do for you?" he asked. Before I could answer, Martha started to shout at me: "No one can do a damn thing for *me*, and don't think that just because you're a social worker you can! I know—I was a social worker too, and I retired because I *wanted* to—not because I *had* to. How do you think I feel, trapped in this body?" It would be a long struggle before Martha accepted me into her home without hostility, but eventually she began to rely on me for help.

For a long time before this, I really struggled to know why Sam had been referred to me, and what help I could give. The visiting nurse thought he was depressed, but he didn't think so and neither did I. He was very philosophical about everything—until his circulatory system began to betray him. Sam was growing weaker and had developed renal insufficiency—eventually he would need dialysis. I began to see how profound the emotional toll on the couple was. Martha was labile and would scream at Sam, or cry uncontrollably, with no perceivable provocation. Sam, stoic on the outside, was now growing more depressed. What troubled him the most, he said, was the loss of Martha's keen intellect. Whereas he had been her caretaker for so many years, she had been his intellectual muse. Sam spoke admiringly, and nostalgically, of Martha's former brilliance. She could no longer keep up with him. Yet, despite their despair, the bond between them was still vibrant. This couple had survived unthinkable travails together. How would they survive now? And, how could I help them face the inevitable?

When Sam first began dialysis, he was able to obtain an electric scooter to make his trip to and from the dialysis center more manageable. Until Sam began to fail, he was proud of his red scooter. Once he was caught in a downpour, and he thought it would be a good idea to have a poncho. I saw Sam and Martha the next day, and the following dialogue ensued. It is a narrative of despair, loss, and love.

SAM *Do you have any idea where I could get a poncho? If I had a poncho, I wouldn't get wet when I go to dialysis on my scooter in the rain. The other night I got soaked, and boy was that unpleasant!*
MARTHA *Sam doesn't want just any old poncho.*
SAM *I'd like the kind I had in the war.*
THERAPIST *Perhaps you could try an Army-Navy store.*
SAM *That's a good idea, but where do I find one?*
THERAPIST *Maybe you can order one by phone.*

Martha's bony, crippled hand inched along the table toward the telephone. She made growling noises. She pounced on the phone and wrestled it to her chest. Her determination to fight for her life was evident in this gesture.

Sam waited on the other side of the table for the inevitable eruption. Martha screwed up her face and clenched her teeth. Out came a stream of invectives, directed mostly at Sam.

MARTHA *I can't take it anymore. Do you know what it's like to be trapped in this body? I'm ruining your life. I know you hate me!*
SAM *(rolling his eyes)*
I'm facing my death, Martha.
MARTHA *I know Sam. You look like hell!*

Sam looked away, and then shot a glance at me, as if to say: "You see what I'm living with?"

Martha began to cry.

SAM *Look, Martha, I've decided to make the best of what little time I have left to live. I'm trying to make it bearable for the two of us. Okay?*
MARTHA *I'm too old and too tired for this.*
SAM *Old and tired, yes, but not too old or too tired. Now Martha, just stop it!*
MARTHA *(still sniffling)*
I guess I'm just the apotheosis of kvetch [embodiment of complaining].
She turns to the therapist.
How many of your elderly clients have used that phrase before?

SAM *Martha is very good at putting words together. She used to write wonderful poetry.*

MARTHA *I can't write anything anymore.*

Martha turned to the therapist.

MARTHA *Who are you here for—Sam or me?*

THERAPIST *On paper, I'm here for Sam; but in reality I'm here for both of you.*

MARTHA *(nodding approvingly)*

Good!

THERAPIST *(To Sam)*

I guess this isn't the first time you've faced death, Sam.

SAM *It wasn't the same then. I was a different person—hell, nineteen years old. What did I know? I lived from one day to the next. My goal was just to survive the next day.*

THERAPIST *Did you think about going home?*

SAM *(shaking his head)*

Nah. I didn't want to go home. My mother was an awful woman. When I finally did get home, I changed into civilian clothes and gave her the lace handkerchiefs I'd brought her from Europe. She didn't think they were good enough! After the war I didn't have shell shock—I had home shock.

MARTHA *(looking at Sam with admiration)*

Sam was in continuous combat during the war. He landed at Normandy on D-Day. Because he was so short and he could run so fast they sent him to the front as a scout.

THERAPIST *(to Sam)*

Tell me about the poncho.

SAM *(relaxing his face into a smile)*

It wasn't an ordinary poncho. It closed securely at the neck and you could snap two ponchos together to make a tent. You see, I made a bed of pine branches, wrapped myself in a blanket, covered it with the poncho, and then a layer of snow. The poncho kept the snow from melting on me, and the snow kept me warm. I could hear the shells exploding around me, but I felt secure. I looked up at the stars. It was wonderful.

While Sam is talking Martha's chin drops onto her canary-yellow sweater. She falls asleep.

SAM *(looking at Martha with frustration)*

Martha has the attention span of a two-year-old.

The session was coming to an end, and I had to leave for another appointment.

THERAPIST *(standing up)*
I have to go now. I'll see you next week.
MARTHA *(waking with a start)*
Could you do us a favor? Find Sam a poncho.
THERAPIST *Ponchos for the afterlife?*
Martha and Sam laugh.
MARTHA *That would make a good title for a book.*

PRESENCE

SONG WITHOUT WORDS The day after my mother died, I received a call from a coworker of hers. I had met Mrs. S. numerous times, and when I saw her name on my phone, I answered by saying: "I guess you heard about my mother." She sounded perplexed and said: "I'm looking for a Lauren Taylor. Dr. L. gave me her name." I realized that just a few days earlier I had received a call from Dr. L., a psychiatrist with whom I work, asking me if I would have time to see a new client. The client had been suffering from Parkinson's for years, and his wife had asked Dr. L. if he knew of a therapist who could visit her husband at home to give him extra support. Dr. L. told me they were a lovely couple, but that the husband's illness was putting a strain on the couple's relationship. When I realized why Mrs. S. was calling me, I explained that I was, in fact, the person she was trying to reach, but I was also the daughter of her coworker who had died the day before. Mrs. S. asked me if I thought this connection would pose a problem for me, even though I had never met her husband. I said it would not, and Mrs. S. said that it was fine with her as well, but asked that I not mention my mother who, in fact, had met her husband many times.

Parkinson's affects different people in different ways. Allen had been living with the disease for many years, but had none of the flailing or jerking motions we often associate with Parkinson's. Instead, it had diminished his ability to speak, and he suffered from some cognitive impairment. His wife complained that he had become irritable and uncooperative. When I first began working with Allen he could still say a few words, and occasionally, he would utter a complete sentence. Once when I greeted him and asked how he was feeling, he smiled and said: "Well, I didn't get into any mischief today."

As normal conversation with Allen was not possible, I had to think of creative ways to use narrative in our work together. Allen could not verbally tell me his life story, but I could help him find other modalities to discover new meaning of the life he had lived, and was still living. To that end, I asked Mrs. S. if she had some family photos I could use. For the next few months, I was able to engage Allen by asking about the stories behind the photos. Although Allen could not construct a complete sentence, he was able to relate enough through individual sounds and nods of the head to help me understand the stories behind the pictures. I asked him if he would like me to write down these stories, and he indicated he would. This became an important part of our time together. He relished the process, and especially enjoyed it when I read to him what I had written about his life.

Toward the end of his life, Allen lost all ability to speak. Instead, I talked to him for the hour we spent together each week. He often sat in his wheelchair across from the west-facing windows of his dining room, and I noticed he seemed fascinated by the setting of the sun, and by the reflection in the window of the chandelier over the dining room table. In my effort to keep him engaged in the therapy, I began taking pictures of the sky and the reflection as the sun began to set. With each phase of the sunset I showed Allen the picture I had just taken. He was delighted, and indicated as best he could that I should take more pictures.

Although very little conversation transpired in my narrative work with Allen, I felt a deep connection with this client. When he died, I had the feeling that I had helped him reconstruct a meaningful life story, a "song without words."

SHE WAS NOT AT ALL WHAT I HAD EXPECTED   I work with my students to raise their awareness of their biases. That keeps me thinking about my own. Sometimes, for example, a name alone can evoke an image, such as a woman with an Irish-sounding name, who lives on the East Side of New York, is homebound, and has a long history of depression. I imagined a small, frail, white-haired woman. On the phone, her voice was friendly, so I harbored no concern about being greeted with hostility. All I knew about her, besides her name, was that depression had been her constant companion since the death of her parents, who died within three months of one another, when she was only twenty-five. She had tried many treatments to rid herself of this albatross, but none had really touched it. She had become attached to the social worker with whom she had been working for the past six months and was ambivalent about making this change. As she said to me, right after I introduced myself: "I can't believe I have to start all over from the beginning." But at the same time, she expressed gratitude that I had been able to arrange to see her only a week after the other social worker had left. That is the nature of ambivalence.

My first surprise was the building in which she lived. I had pictured a walk-up, or perhaps a small apartment building with the fire-escape in front. As I walked east, about as far as one can go in New York without ending up in the river, I realized that I was in a swank neighborhood and that perhaps I should leave my preconceived notions behind. As I was greeted by the doorman of her luxury building, I knew there was another story than the one I had imagined. I rang the bell.

Margaret looked anything but frail. Her walking was labored, the result of numerous back surgeries, but she had a robust appearance. Her straight hair, medium-brown, was cut even with her chin. As I would write in a psychosocial assessment: "Neatly groomed, dressed in slacks and sweater, client looks younger than stated age." The apartment was well-appointed and stylish. Margaret sat at one end of the couch and motioned for me to sit down at the other end. She quickly realized I had to crane my neck to talk to her, and she asked me if I would prefer a chair. I readily accepted. She sighed and, after having expressed her feelings about starting over, she asked: "Where do I begin?" Before I could answer, she began telling me the story of her life. She seemed to have resigned herself to the idea that her depression was caused by her parents' deaths and that there was no way to change this because death was a hard, cold fact. Margaret had *become* her depression. Despite the rote quality of her narrative, I felt the spark of connection igniting between us—the so-called therapeutic alliance.

Six months earlier, I left the clinic where I had worked for many years, to take a university-based position as project manager of a multi-million-dollar research study on complicated grief in the elderly. I left behind the work I came to realize I love the most—listening to old people tell their stories. Although I decided to leave the project and return to the clinical work I loved, I had learned a lot about complicated grief. Although people suffering from complicated grief appear to be depressed, the syndrome does not respond to treatments for depression. If there is coexisting depression, which is often the case, the depression may disappear, but the complicated grief remains. Complicated grief shares some of the hallmark symptoms of PTSD, and some people suffer from it for decades. This is what moved the director of the study to develop a treatment designed specifically for complicated grief. Her pilot studies on younger people showed the treatment to be very effective. Her new study was designed to test this treatment on older adults. It suddenly dawned on me that Margaret was suffering from complicated grief. I wanted to share this information with her, but I knew I had to go slowly. After all, this was our first time together. Maybe she wouldn't be interested. I casually mentioned that I had worked on this study, and perhaps, down the road, we might look into the possibility that . . . And then, something amazing happened.

Margaret paused her narrative and said: "You know, your name sounds very familiar. When you worked on this study, were you up at the Psychiatric Institute? And did you attend your first staff meeting up there on a Thursday? It must have been in January or February. You told the staff about your clinic, right?" I could feel the crescendo of anticipation inside me that one feels when reading a good mystery story. Where could she have gotten this information? When I said yes, Margaret's demeanor became animated. "Son of a gun!" she said. "I was part of a depression study up there. I worked with Dr. M and Sara. I don't remember her last name. Lovely woman." When I mentioned Sara's last name, Margaret became even more animated and said: "That's right. You know her too? She was very helpful to me. The problem is, my depression didn't get better. So, the day after that meeting you attended, Dr. M referred me to your clinic! And he mentioned that you had told the staff about it. I can't believe it! And now you're here. It feels like this was meant to be!" Margaret thought for a moment and asked: "This complicated grief you mentioned. I'd be interested in finding out more about it." I told her about the director's findings, and it was as though a light went on for her. "I think that's what I have," she said. "How can I learn more about it?" I asked her if she would like to read some articles. She said she would. I promised to bring them the next time.

It was time to go. Margaret walked me to the door, and when I said goodbye, she smiled broadly and said: "I still can't believe it. I think this is going to work out well." I felt as though I had opened a door for her that had been sealed tight for decades. Walking to the bus stop after the session, I was filled with joy. I was happy to be back at the clinic doing the work I love. But as a teacher, I had to ask myself the same question I would ask my students. How would I have opened that door for Margaret without the key I now possessed? At that moment I decided not to analyze it, but rather, to let it be whatever it was. I couldn't help but recall the words of a wise woman who said to me, when I was struggling with my decision to leave the project: "Remember, the Chinese word for *crisis* is *opportunity*."

Self-disclosure has remained a controversial topic in therapy, since the term was coined by the psychologist Sidney Jourard in 1958. Self-disclosure must be used with care and sensitivity. The "golden rule" of self-disclosure is that it must be used in the interest of the client, and not for the benefit of the therapist. Not every therapist feels comfortable with self-disclosure, and not every client wants to hear about the therapist's experiences. Yet, many therapists, myself included, consider self-disclosure a critical element in developing a human connection to strengthen the therapeutic alliance.[1] Cristelle Audet and Robin D. Everall, in their study of self-disclosure, found that early self-disclosure, especially in the first three sessions, contributed to "an atmosphere of comfort and general ease," and "balanced the asymmetry caused by the one-way exchange."[2]

One caveat is that cultural norms may make self-disclosure inadvisable. Bryan Kim et al. sought to determine how therapist self-disclosure would be perceived by Asian-American clients, paired with Caucasian therapists.[3] One hypothesis was that modeling self-disclosure might encourage clients to open up and could diminish the perception of the therapist as an agent of an oppressive system. What he discovered was that, consistent with Asian cultural norms, clients responded more positively to disclosure about problem-solving strategies, than about the therapist's emotional experiences. If used with care, however, self-disclosure is a valuable tool in fostering a therapeutic connection. NT places a high value on therapist transparency.

WRITING

THE GIRL FROM BROOKLYN   Sometimes when I came to visit, Jane called to me from the other end of the apartment, letting me know that the door was open and I should let myself in. At other times she came to the door, dragging her bum leg as she walked. Jane has multiple sclerosis. She has good days and bad days. One couldn't help but notice her shiny red electric scooter parked near the entryway. Once she sat down you would never have known she has a disability. When Jane told a story, her speech was punctuated with the words: "I don't know what to tell you," and "I don't know what to say." She didn't mean it literally; it was just part of the rhythm of her narrative.

I was always struck by her beauty—the kind of beauty that must have turned a lot of heads when she was younger—perfect features, thick raven hair, peaches-and-cream skin. It was hard to believe she was well over seventy. Although she grew up poor, her husband made a fortune, and she got used to living in luxury. She had money worries later, but you could tell she still felt at home in a mink coat. What stood out the most, however, was her warm and welcoming demeanor. I was her therapist, but she called me "Sweetie," which felt completely natural coming from her.

Jane was born in Brooklyn, the younger daughter of Russian-Jewish immigrants. Her father had trouble holding a job, but there was always food on the table, and Jane's mother held the family together. Jane met her future husband in high school, when she was only fifteen. They were inseparable, although Jane said he was more like a brother than a boyfriend, and she got married at nineteen to get out of the house. It was difficult at first, because they lived with his mother, who was not well. When her mother-in-law died, they got their own place and started a family. Jane's husband went into business and Jane worked alongside him. The business flourished, and the couple bought a magnificent home in a wealthy suburb, although Brooklyn was always close to Jane's heart. Jane was a gregarious person, and they soon had a circle of couples with whom they socialized regularly. Like many of their friends, when the children were grown, Jane and her husband sold their house in the suburbs and moved back to the city. A group of the wives—Jane among them—eventually divorced or widowed but remained close friends.

When Jane was in her early fifties, she discovered that her husband was "running around" with other women. Jane got fed up and asked him to leave, and although they lived separately for a couple of years, he always returned home for holidays, remaining devoted to his daughters. It was during this separation that she fell in love with Frank, even though after a couple of years, she asked her husband to come back. She felt it would be better for the girls to have their father at home, especially as her younger daughter was a difficult child, and Jane was having a hard time taking care of her alone. Jane put her foot down about her husband's running around, and he agreed to stop. She, however, continued to see Frank, until she developed multiple sclerosis.

You know my friend Ethel—the one who has Parkinson's—she introduced us. I guess he just came along at the right time. Sixteen years we were together. I'm glad I listened to my friend Judy, the older woman I told you about. She was very wise. When my husband and I got back together, she told me not to let Frank go." I asked Jane if the affair helped her stay in her marriage. She said: *"You bet! You think I could have survived without sex for sixteen years?*

Seven years before he died, Jane's husband, Alan, was diagnosed with cancer. At first, he responded well to the treatments, but eventually the cancer metastasized, and, despite her own disability, Jane became a full-time caretaker. Several times, when Jane was home taking care of him, the phone rang but there was no response at the other end of the line. Jane is almost certain it was Frank. On occasion, she has thought of calling him, but she doesn't even know if he is still alive. "Besides, if he is still alive, he would be an old man by now."

When I began working with Jane, she was still deep in grief. Although her husband was not an easy man to live with, Jane missed him, and she missed having someone to lean on. We talked about what might help her in her distress. Jane said she had always wanted to write. She loved to tell stories of the neighborhood in Brooklyn where she grew up and found she loved to write about it. Each week Jane read me her latest creation, which she embellished with a spoken narrative. As our work progressed, Jane became more and more engrossed in her writing, and it sustained her. She decided her goal was to publish her stories and, after many months of trying to find a publisher, she called me excitedly to tell me the book was coming out in print. She handed me a copy with an inscription, in which she thanked me for believing in her. I cherish it to this day.

ART

RUTH'S QUILT

Life is less a quest than a quilt. We find meaning, love, and prosperity through the process of stitching together our bold attempts to help others find their own way in their lives. The relationships we weave become an exquisite and endless pattern.

—KEITH FERRAZZI, *NEVER EAT ALONE*

When I rang the bell I could hear the clip-clop of a walker, as Ruth struggled to get to the door. After she greeted me, I waited patiently while she arranged herself in a large, overstuffed chair in her living room. She groaned as she moved, obviously in pain. When she was seated, Ruth positioned a tray table, covered with her latest quilting project, over her lap. I remained standing until she was seated, in case she needed my assistance. I sat down opposite her in a wooden rocking chair fitted with flowered, chintz cushions. Her old, black rotary phone, her tissues, her pencils, and her books, were piled within arm's reach on an old, dark wooden side table. Although the apartment was sunny and tidy, it showed signs of wear. There were spindly plants by the windows, which looked out on a small concrete terrace. The terrace was devoid of any furnishings, except a white molded plastic chair.

Ruth was not a conventionally attractive woman; her body became misshapen as a result of a childhood spinal injury. Her face was what one might call homely. Perhaps she had compensated for her appearance by developing a bitingly sarcastic wit. I suspect that Ruth had offended more than one person in her life, but as I learned through her narrative, she was very loyal to her friends.

She was born in Czechoslovakia, and her mother had died in childbirth. Ruth's father was in the army, and could not care for his infant daughter, so he gave her to her mother's sister to raise. Ruth's aunt already had a child—a daughter who was fourteen years older than Ruth, but her husband had died, and the aunt decided to move with the children to America. She arrived in the United States with little, and set up shop as a dressmaker in a small apartment in the Bronx.

When Ruth was three years old, she fell down the steps as she followed her aunt downstairs to the laundry room. Ruth was unable to walk properly after the accident. Her aunt, who was a resourceful woman, heard that a famous orthopedist was coming to New York from Europe. She wrote to him, and he agreed to examine Ruth. He diagnosed Ruth with a fractured spine, and put her in a body cast. For the next four years Ruth remained imprisoned in plaster. Because her aunt had to go to work every day, Ruth's cousin stayed home and took care of her. It was from this cousin that Ruth learned to read, to do needlework, and to sew. Ruth developed a passion for travel books, and she vowed that someday she would be free as a bird and would explore the world.

When Ruth was seven, the cast was removed. The doctor pronounced her cured, but she had to learn how to walk again. Her aunt sent her to a farm outside the city, thinking the fresh air would be good for her. By the end of the summer, Ruth could climb a tree and ride a horse. In September, she returned home and attended the local public elementary school, feeling a whole new world of learning had opened up to her.

One of the great regrets of many older adults with whom I have worked is that they did not have the opportunity to go to college. This was certainly true of Ruth, as she was expected to work as soon as she graduated from high school. She got a job as a secretary and continued throughout her life to work at jobs that did not utilize her vast intellect. Her goal was to save enough money to travel.

Eventually Ruth was able to realize her dream. She developed an interest in bird-watching, and her interest led to involvement in a variety of bird-watching organizations and extensive travels to far-away and often exotic places. Although she had little success with men at home, partly as a result of her self-consciousness about her appearance, she was able to free herself of self-doubt when she traveled. She told me of several love affairs, including a passionate romance with a man who worked on a river boat she took through the Amazon.

As Ruth grew older, her childhood back injury reappeared in the form of chronic pain. By the time I first met her, she was unable to walk without a walker. By the end of her life, she was not just homebound, but her world revolved around the immediate vicinity of her seating arrangements. She began to despair, and depression became her constant companion. Thankfully, however, her childhood years of occupying herself with needlework expanded her involvement in the world and became her salvation. Ruth began to make quilts, and she made some of these quilts for children who had been less fortunate than she.

When Ruth learned that was celebrating its twenty-first anniversary, and that there would be a party with door prizes, she set about making two large quilts to donate to the cause. Each week when I arrived at her apartment, she showed me what she had accomplished, and quilted as we spoke. The first quilt was a magnificent work, in the traditional style of early American quilts, with intricate circles of patchwork in shades of peach, rose, blue, and green on a cream-colored background. I could picture it gracing the walls of a large, elegant loft. The second quilt was very different, created from our interactions.

During out interactions over the years, Ruth learned some things about me too. She knew I had children, and she often asked after them. She had volunteered at the local library, and had accumulated a collection of books the library had discarded. Ruth seemed particularly interested in hearing about my daughter's passion for reading. She would occasionally pass along a book she had read that she thought my daughter might like. I accepted these small gifts as a way to esteem Ruth's kindness and support her generative desire to create a legacy for her passion of reading.

Ruth showed me the pattern she had chosen for the second quilt. It was a rectangular design with a narrow patchwork border and an appliqué in the center of a young girl walking in the rain, holding an umbrella and reading a book. The girl appeared completely absorbed in her book, as she splashed a puddle with her red rain boots. This could have been my daughter. Ruth worked on this quilt for many weeks, finishing it just in time to donate it for a raffle for the anniversary gala. I yearned to choose the winning number for this wonderful work of art, but I didn't win.

One day when I came to Ruth's door she did not answer. I called the friend she had listed as an emergency contact and learned that she had been taken to the hospital during the night, delirious from a high fever. There was an infection in her spine, and she would not be back home for two weeks. I spoke to her in the hospital, and she said she did not want any visitors but promised to call when she came home. The next time I went to see her, I knew this might be our last time together.

When I came to see Ruth, I was happy to see that she seemed a little better. I felt optimistic, but this was the optimism of false hope. When it was time for me to go, she took a shopping bag from next to her chair and pressed it into my hand. It was stuffed with tissue paper so I could not see what it contained. I asked her if I should open it then, but she said I should wait until I got home. I followed her instructions, and when I unwrapped the paper, I discovered a repetitive scaled-down replica of the second quilt, with every detail of the original, only in miniature. The next day Ruth's friend called to tell me that Ruth was in the hospital and that she had asked me to come and see her. When I entered her hospital room, she reached out and took my hand, too weak to speak. She died later that night.

MEANINGFUL ARTIFACTS

A SHARED CONNECTION: BOX OF MEMORIES

Our lives are ceaselessly intertwined with narrative, with the stories we tell and hear told, those we dream or imagine or would like to tell, all of which are reworked in the story of our own lives that we narrate to ourselves.

—MICHAEL WHITE AND DAVID EPSTON,

NARRATIVE MEANS TO THERAPEUTIC ENDS

She was a tiny woman, four-foot ten at most. I had been working with her for a couple of years, making weekly visits to her well-appointed apartment; it was impeccable, with paintings and sculptures from her many travels with her late husband artfully displayed. Our clinic psychiatrist, who also visited her from time to time, once remarked that it made him think of someone waiting to die. He was right. She had already made one suicide attempt in recent history, and it would not be her last. Ever since the death of her husband, some eight years prior, depression had become her constant companion. She once said to me:

> *Being depressed is like wanting to get away from this world; wanting to lose oneself in sleep; waiting for the end of the day when you know you are going to sleep and don't have to think about it anymore; missing the things that you're used to and not really enjoying whatever is left; just pushing through.*

Anna was born in Ukraine, the youngest of four daughters of middle-class Jewish parents. Religious and political persecution forced her family to flee, first to Romania and then to the United States. Unlike her older sisters, who maintained their European customs until they died, Anna quickly assimilated into American culture in the Bronx. By the age of eleven, under the tutelage of one of her aunts, she had become involved in leftist politics. At fourteen, she left school and went to live in a mining town in Pennsylvania to help organize a union. Although she became deathly ill because of the harsh living conditions, she threw herself into the politics of the Left, and at age seventeen was sent to Russia to work for the Communist Party. There she fell in love with a Russian soldier, but when the Party got wind of this forbidden romance, she was forced to leave Russia and go to California. Although she never got over him, Anna came back to New York to help a friend start a leftist publishing house where she met her future husband, who shared her political views and had gone to Spain with the Lincoln Brigade. They married and had two daughters. Anna's husband became a successful accountant, which eventually enabled the couple to purchase a large apartment, build a vacation home, and travel extensively. Their older daughter, who never married, became a lawyer; their younger daughter became a teacher, married, and had two children. Anna and her husband were very close to their grandchildren. After the first suicide attempt, Anna promised her grandchildren that she would not try again. Several years later she broke her promise.

During one of my visits, Anna asked me to help her pull down a box from the top shelf of the closet in her bedroom. It was an old hat box, made of round cardboard and covered with paper decorated in cabbage roses. It reminded me of the hat boxes on the shelf in my grandmother's bedroom. Only my grandmother's hat boxes were filled with hats, in shades of blue and aquamarine (my grandmother's favorite colors) which she wore stuck through with a hatpin. When Anna opened the box there was no hat under the wads of newspaper she removed. Instead, there was another box, a small square box that, long ago, must have contained a piece of jewelry. She carefully removed it and motioned to me to follow her back into the living room. Inside this box was some tissue paper, yellowed by the passage of time, which concealed two small photos. The first was a smiling young man in an army uniform. The second was eighteen-year-old Anna in his arms. As she handed me the photos, she told me that she had never shown them to anyone before. As we shared this most intimate moment, I could feel her yearning, and like the physics of a sympathetic vibration, I could also feel my vibration resonating.

I have always kept a box of memories in my closet. Mine looks like a small valise covered in dark green plaid fabric, with gold-colored clasps and a dark green handle. There is a place to lock it, but I never had the key. It's something women used to use when they traveled, long before the days of miniature plastic bottles, to store their cosmetics and perfumes. I knew it had a specific name, but I couldn't remember it. I called my mother, who was almost ninety at the time, older than Anna. She thought for an instant, and said: "It's called an etui." I don't know where my etui came from. Perhaps it belonged to my grandmother. It was my own box of memories.

MOTION

STORIES OUTSIDE THE BOX: LAUREN'S DANCE

> A narrative is like a room on whose walls a number of false doors have been painted; while within the narrative, we have many apparent choices of exit, but when the author leads us to one particular door, we know it is the right one because it opens.
>
> —JOHN UPDIKE, MORE MATTER

Telling a story is a process of selection, as is writing a narrative. We may decide, according to the circumstances and the audience, what to include and what to leave out. We may choose to omit family secrets, regrets, or painful memories, sometimes to protect the listener, and sometimes to protect ourselves. A narrative is elastic and fluid, and it can be molded and shaped any way we please, but sometimes we become stuck in a story that defines us such that we feel we cannot escape. NT can be the key to opening the door to a new perspective.

I have so many stories that I can't possibly include all of them here. One last one, however, stands out for me as a story "outside the box."

"You're going to work with *her*?" asked a colleague. "I don't envy you!" Jill had the reputation of having alienated anyone who had been put in the unfortunate position of trying to help her. I couldn't wait to meet her—just the kind of challenge I love.

Faded beauty. That's how you might describe her. You could tell that Jill had been a dancer and choreographer. The remnants of this life were still evident in the way she moved her now-misshapen body. Her bleached blond hair was tied back in a low pony-tail, and over her simple black knit dress she wore a calf-length fur coat. She greeted me almost in a whisper, her voice hoarse from cigarettes. Her tongue made little, repetitive movements when she spoke, most likely a touch of tardive dyskinesia[4] from her years on heavy psychotropic medications. Her anxiety level was off the charts, and when she was anxious, she screamed at people who happened to get in her way.

In our first session I said to her: "An image comes to mind when I listen to you speak. I picture you in a cage, desperately beating your fists against the bars trying to get out. Is this how you feel?" She seemed instantly intrigued, as though someone had finally understood her dilemma.

"You were a dancer and choreographer," I continued. "Could you think about choreographing a dance so that you could gracefully exit the cage?"

She looked at me as though something that had long been extinguished illuminated her eyes. "Yes, I like that idea."

Jill's drinking had spiraled out of control after her mastectomy, several years before our first meeting. The last piece she had choreographed for a public performance was for an event marking the anniversary of the September 11 terrorists attacks. She had lost touch with her body and hadn't even realized that her illness had had a profound effect on her body image. She just knew she couldn't get motivated to do anything physical, and she hated the way she looked. It would have been all too easy to fall into the trap of suggesting she try this or that, to get her over the hump of her resistance. I knew that the more I gave her suggestions, the more she would resist: "Why don't you try just doing five minutes a day?" or "Perhaps you could put on some music and see if it inspires you." I knew from past experience that suggestions such as these are doomed to failure.

Often these attempts to help on the part of the therapist create resistance in the client. David Burns suggests a different approach:

Ah, resistance! Haven't we all, at times, blamed our clients for it, suggesting that they secretly don't want to get better and are, in some way, purposely sabotaging us? But what if the problem is really with *us*, that we've become so single-minded in our attempts to be helpful, that we tend to ignore the aspects of our clients' inner ecology triggering the resistance? And what if the negative thinking patterns, feelings, and behaviors that keep them stuck have powerful, unconscious advantages serving vital, even life-preserving purposes? Finally, what if their resistance to change reveals something positive, beautiful, and even healthy about them—something that we've overlooked? If so, we might want to view resistance from a radically different perspective.[5]

I began to feel stuck in my ability to help Jill overcome her inertia, and she felt mired as well. Jill had spent years teaching dance and choreography at a number of prestigious universities. Teaching had been her passion. One day, a light bulb went on in my head to use affirmation of Jill's talents to validate her and support her continuing her narrative: "Jill, I can tell by the way you speak about teaching that you must have been a very good teacher."

"Yes," she replied, "I was good; I was very good."

I continued, using a strengths-based approach to play the role of being helped rather than helper, and said casually: "Perhaps sometime you could show me some of the things you did as a teacher."

She said she would, but time went by and nothing happened.

Nearly six months later, Jill arrived at my office carrying a CD/cassette player. It was the same blue and white model that I had next to my bed. She took a cassette out of her bag, and put it in the machine. "I choreographed a dance for you," she said. "I'm calling it 'Lauren's dance.' But first we're going to do a warm-up, so take your shoes off and let's get down on the floor."

And I did.

Just as I initially felt that I was at an impasse in my work with Jill, she too had felt trapped in a negative narrative, in a symbolic "narrative cage." Instinctively, I knew that the only way to reach her was to find a way to help her out of the cage, which is what I did when we sat down on the floor for the warm-up. Now she had agency, as she led me through the movements leading up to the dance. In his richly detailed article about dance movement therapy and narrative, Christian Kronsted writes about "enactivism," a theory of embodied cognition, which posits that cognition arises through a dynamic interaction between an organism and its environment, by the active exercise of that organism's sensory motor processes.[6]

Had I been unwilling, or unable, to get down on the floor with Jill, I would have had to find another way to help her out of the "cage." There are times when thinking outside the box in designing creative interventions, allows us to reach certain clients who might otherwise be deemed "resistant." In the case of Jill, my intervention gave her an opening to share her considerable expertise with me and to shine once again as a teacher. In Jill's case, we were each, in that moment, both student and teacher, sharing a connection through movement that enabled Jill to step out of her cage with grace. There is a saying, attributed to Buddha Siddhartha: "When the student is ready, the teacher will appear."

NOTES

1. Jeffrey E. Barnett, "Psychotherapist Self-Disclosure: Ethical and Clinical Considerations," *Psychotherapy* 48, no. 4 (2011): 315–21, https://psycnet.apa.org /doi/10.1037/a0026056.
2. Cristelle. T. Audet and Robin D. Everall, "Therapist Self-Disclosure and the Therapeutic Relationship: A Phenomenological Study from the Client Perspective," *British Journal of Guidance and Counselling* 38, no. 3 (2010): 327–42, https://doi.org/10.1080/03069885.2010.482450.
3. Bryan S. K. Kim et al., "Counselor Self-Disclosure, East Asian Client Adherence to Asian Cultural Values, and Counseling Process," *Journal of Counseling Psychology* 50, no. 3 (2003): 324–32, https://psycnet.apa.org /doi/10.1037/0022-0167.50.3.324.
4. Tardive dyskinesia is an uncommon side effect of certain medicines, especially antipsychotic medications to treat mental illness. People who develop this drug-induced movement disorder cannot control their facial movements and may develop facial tics like lip-smacking, tongue thrusting, and rapid blinking.
5. David Burns, "When Helping Doesn't Help: Why Some Clients May Not Want to Change," Psychotherapy Networker, March/April 1, 2017, https:// www.psychotherapynetworker.org/article/when-helping-doesnt-help.
6. Christian Kronsted, "The Self and Dance Movement Therapy: A Narrative Approach," *Phenomenology and the Cognitive Sciences* 19, no. 1 (2020): 47–58.

10

CHARTING UNEXPLORED ROUTES

Narrative Road Maps to Rediscover Our Beginnings

THIS BOOK IS ABOUT the therapeutic value of narrative for older adults in two very different parts of the world. My contributions are based on my long career as a psychiatric social worker in an outpatient geriatric mental health clinic in New York City. My training has been rooted in Western psychological thinking, focusing on the needs of the individual, before the needs of the community. Fortunately, the field is evolving, and more attention is being paid to the importance of community, and to the cultural norms that affect the individual in the context of community. Narrative therapy is a powerful tool that allows us to connect with others, across cultural divides.

EAST AND WEST

In the 2019 film *The Farewell*, a Chinese-born, American-raised, young woman, goes to China because her grandmother is dying. While she is there, she discovers many differences between her cultural lens and the lens of her relatives who have stayed in China. Her uncle sums it up, when he says to her: "There are things you must understand. You guys moved to the West a long time ago. You think one's life belongs to oneself. But that's the difference between the East and the West. In the East a person's life is part of a whole—family, society."

As a therapist, one cannot possibly have lived all the experiences of one's clients. Clients will sometimes ask the intake department in the clinic to match them with a therapist who shares an aspect of their identity of experience, be it racial, religious, or gender. This is not always possible, and the therapist must be prepared to bring this into the open and to find common ground through which to form a therapeutic alliance. Assael Romanelli, a narrative therapist, writes: "As a listener there is a high probability you won't share the same reality as the speaker. You might not own the same objects, live in the same area, or know the characters in the teller's story."[1] But he goes on to make a distinction between "hearing" and "listening," positing that deep listening can help us connect with clients whose experiences are often quite different from our own. Regardless of differences and similarities, telehealth has affected the way in which we hear and listen. This will be addressed in chapter 16.

A narrative approach can open the door to treatment for individuals whose cultural norms may not be consistent with models of Western psychotherapy. Narrative therapy is client-centered and nonjudgmental, and it involves active listening in which the client is the "expert." When using a narrative approach, I listen intently for four significant elements in a client's story: regrets, re-membering, restoring, and turning points. I will touch on each of these elements briefly, and my work with the clients discussed in the following chapters incorporates these four elements. This aspect of cross-cultural narrative work has a positive impact on the therapeutic alliance and on treatment outcomes. Nevertheless, the work is not always easy. One of my colleagues, Nelson Ho, who identifies as Asian-American, generously contributed his thoughts about the challenges of working with a population that has traditionally been mistrustful of outside help:

> As a bilingual clinician, working in two senior centers in Manhattan's Chinatown, some of my clients are naturalized citizens who speak Cantonese. I am a first-generation Asian American male in my mid-thirties. These intersecting identities have an impact on my awareness, and I am beginning to recognize the stigma involved in even broaching the mental health topic, especially in the geriatric immigrant population. I strongly feel that a factor that comes into play is how families in China have traditionally dealt with mental health issues. According to Dr. Fong on Psychologytoday.com "hospital-based service model and institutionalization and psychiatric and pharmacological treatment were mainly provided" in China for those with mental health issues. I think part of the stigma comes from not wanting to be called "crazy" as mental health connotes something that needs fixing via receiving treatment in a hospital. Or not wanting to seem "weak," or even perhaps in some Chinese cultures, poor mental health means "spirit possession." Another factor is how assimilated the person and his/her family is to the American culture. If good mental health/wellbeing is seen as an

important value for the family culture, then anyone in such a family suffering from depression, anxiety, or another serious mental health issue, would be more likely to seek help. My entryway into talking about mental health with my Cantonese-speaking clients is focusing on physical health, medical concerns and linking their current physical health to their mood, thoughts and feelings. In Eastern philosophy or spiritual practices such as Taoism, Hinduism, Buddhism, the mind, body, and spirit connection has always been an important discussion and links well into a person's lifestyle. I usually try to find out more about my client's family.

Nelson's difficulty treating Chinese mental health, even as a professional with some understanding from inside the community he serves, highlights the potential challenges for those of us who are not members of a particular cultural group. Yet, as we will see as this book unfolds, creating a safe space for people to tell their stories, and truly listening to what they have to say, are invaluable gifts in every culture that we can offer to help people heal.

REGRETS AND RE-MEMBERING

"Getting old is a fulltime job," said my client Mike, with a chuckle, "I'm just busy staying alive." Although he was able to say this with humor during a recent session, there was a time when Mike had been so filled with regret about his perceived mistakes of the past that he was unable to see beyond his disappointment. Providing him with the opportunity to share his story with me enabled him to acknowledge that his life had been more than just a series of mistakes. It also enabled me to help him recognize the resilience he had demonstrated in overcoming numerous challenges, including losing his parents at a young age, which had left him emotionally adrift to make his way in the world with little guidance.

For the majority of my career, I have worked in an outpatient not-for-profit mental health clinic for older adults. As a distinct organization in the community, one of its missions is to support older people who wish to age in place. This program allows them to continue receiving quality mental health services, even if they are homebound. Many of our clients suffer from depression and anxiety, but I have often thought that if we hung a banner over the front door of the clinic to express their emotional plight, it would read: "REGRET." Narrative therapy can help clients recognize that the paths not taken are a part of their life stories and that the road maps they used in the past may, in fact, have gotten them where they needed to go at a time when they were unsure or unsafe. These road maps may no longer serve them in the present, but they constitute the guideposts of a life narrative.

Re-membering is a term coined by Barbara Myerhoff.[2] It was first introduced by Michael White in the context of narrative therapy, which enable him to see beyond the regret and appreciate the life he had lived.[3] Re-membering encompasses multiple layers of storytelling and is different from simply remembering. For Myerhoff, re-membering is the active unification of figures from one's life, rather than passive reminiscence. It can link an individual to a larger world, in terms of shared experiences, in what White refers to as the "club of life." Shona Russell and Maggie Carey highlight the importance of the hyphen in re-membering, "as it draws our attention to the notion of membership rather than to a simple recalling of history." Re-membering offers the possibility of reorganizing the membership of the "club of life," through therapeutic conversations, and gives more importance to the members of the club who have been the most significant in providing support. Russell and Carey, quoting Jill Freedman, write: "Holding particular people in one's heart and mind as a personal team, and owning their experiences of oneself, allows people to know themselves in a community of choice, rather than one of chance. This can make all the difference."[4] As White has written:

> Re-membering conversations are shaped by the conception that identity is founded upon an "association of life" rather than on a core self. This association of life has a membership composed of the significant figures and identities of a person's past, present, and projected future. Re-membering conversations provide an opportunity for people to revise the memberships of their association of life: to upgrade some memberships and downgrade others; to honor some memberships and to revoke others; to grant authority to some voices in regard to matters of one's personal identity, and to disqualify other voices with regard to this.[5]

One of the narrative exercises I share with clients is to ask them to look at their hands, and tell me the story of what comes to mind. Often this leads to a rich narrative, and connection to past and future generations. "My hands remind me of my grandmother's hands." "My hands held my children, and now their children." Sometimes the narrative evokes work and creativity, sharing and caring, or historical events in an individual's life. "My hands helped till the soil on the farm." "My hands played the piano." "My hands helped a wounded soldier." When I do this exercise with a group, I write down each phrase as it is spoken, and then read this collection of phrases back to the group as a poem. People are amazed and thrilled that this is what they have unwittingly created. Here is a poem written by one of my groups.[6]

MY HANDS

My hands are my identity
They have personality
and scars
Hands in general, but mine in particular, remind me of my mother, a caregiver
Of being present
My hands remind me of my impulsivity
Of connection
My hands are tired
I see lines
Hard-working hands
Friends tell me my hands are beautiful
I cherish my hands
I used them to save my friend's life
When my marriage fell apart, I took off my wedding ring
and bought one of my own
My hands are connected to my culture
They represent the immigrants
My hands have helped me get where I am today
I see journeys
I have been through a lot
When I look at my hands, I see gifts of feeling and creativity
When I look at my hands I see strength, power, and beauty
I see love
My hands are
Soft
Strong
Large
Small
My hands are my destiny
My hands are part of me
They're mine!

This poem evokes so many rich themes: identity, caring, connection, motherhood, marriage, culture, creativity, work, and strength. The beauty of this exercise is that with each group of participants, the narrative will be different. This exercise can be done with an individual as well as with a group. Hands evoke many elements of re-membering, and this exercise helps those people whose hands can no longer function as they used to appreciate the history they are holding. One of my clients referred to her hands as "a reference library."

RE-STORYING

One of the principal goals of narrative therapy is to assist our clients in developing a sense of agency, helping them revise unhealthy or unproductive narratives, and guiding them in transforming themselves from victims to agents of change. The following examples illustrate some of the ways in which I have used a narrative approach in that process.

IRIS'S STORY

When Iris told me she was a "bad kid," made to sit almost daily in the corner in the classroom with a dunce cap on her head, I was able to help her understand that her "bad" behavior was her way of expressing what she dared not express at home, and that the humiliation she suffered only reinforced her "bad" behavior. Once she understood this, she was able to have compassion for the child inside her who had been made to suffer and to symbolically remove that dunce cap, re-storying herself as a normal and intelligent child who needed to be shown love, offered a supportive environment, and helped to find constructive ways to express her anger.

ERMA'S STORY

Erma was stuck in a narrative of compulsive behavior. She had been sexually abused as a child and had not known a healthy loving relationships as an adult, although one union had produced a son she adored. By the time I met her, she was obese, in constant pain from spinal stenosis, and socially isolated. Erma was trapped in the story she told herself, in which she was "addicted" to the shopping channel on television and could not control her behavior. Every day she would order things, and the postman, whom she had gotten to know, would bring the packages right to her door. She felt excited by

the new things she received, but once she opened the packages, she realized
she did not need them. She would carefully wrap them up, with the intention
of sending them back. Too ashamed of her behavior to take them to the post
office all at once, she would only put two at a time in the basket of her walker,
and save the others for another day.

Instead of trying to change Erma's behavior, I helped her look at what positive elements it was bringing her. She had grown up poor, so receiving these
"gifts" every day was uplifting. She was socially isolated, so the daily visit
from the postman gave her some social interaction, as did waiting on line at
the post office. Rewrapping the packages involved manual dexterity, a kind
of creativity, and going to the post office got her out of her apartment every
day. Erma was intrigued by this approach to her story, and focusing on the
benefits of her behavior motivated her to change it herself. Her compulsive
shopping naturally decreased, and she began to make collages, instead of
rewrapping packages, as a way to express herself creatively.

MILLIE'S STORY

Creativity is a powerful tool in the process of re-storying. When Millie was
young, she had been a backup singer for a celebrity singer. While on tour, he
seduced her and promised her the moon. But the affair ended badly for Millie;
when the tour was over, he dropped her like a hot potato and went back to
his wife. Millie was devastated and grieved for many years over the loss of this
relationship. Her grief, compounded by unresolved feelings about her alco-
holic father, led her to a suicide attempt, which was a cry for help. She took
a bottle of pills, but then called someone to take her to the hospital. After her
hospitalization, Millie began writing in a journal about her experiences. One
day, she brought me the journal, and asked me to throw it away. She said it
was too painful for her to keep. I suggested instead that I keep it in my desk,
as some day she might be ready to look at it again. Years passed, and Millie
worked hard in therapy on healing. One day, she asked for the journal, saying
she felt ready to look at it again. She thanked me for holding it for her and
read a page aloud in her session. The following week she returned to tell me
she, herself, had decided to throw it away. She was no longer grieving and felt
that part of her life was now in the past. Millie had her memories, but she no
longer needed the journal as a constant reminder of her pain. She literally
threw away the narrative that had bound her in misery for so many years. In
doing so, she felt liberated.

TURNING POINTS

Obstacles do not block the path. They are the path.

—ZEN PROVERB

Changing one's narrative is not an easy process, as we are often ambivalent about letting go of our current narratives—the stories we tell about ourselves, and the stories others tell about us. Yet ambivalence means there is discontent, which can create an opportunity for movement, making change possible. Aptly written by my client, Phyllis:

> *It would be so easy perhaps to remain in this place of darkness rather than light but as of now, I am going forward. I have begun to ask for and get the help I need and will continue to need, in the coming months and possibly years. If that is what it is going to take to help me find my way in this new chapter in my life. It is exactly what I am going to do.*

Helping someone rewrite a life narrative can be exhilarating. One of my clients likened it to baking bread:

> *You know how you make bread? You knead it and then cover it and set it aside to proof. Well, I feel like I'm proofing.*

Another compared it to giving birth:

> *It feels like labor pains; as though I'm about to give birth to something important.*

Whatever the metaphor, narrative therapy can help clients find alternatives to stories that have kept them from recognizing their strengths, give value to stories that were not previously heard or acknowledged, and allow us to honor the experiences of those who endeavor to share their stories with us.

In the next section, we will recognize the power of stories for groups and communities in an Asian context, focusing on the use of metaphor as more than a literary device—as a tool to give us the buffer of externalizing while deepening meaning in our lives.

NOTES

1. Assael Romanelli, "Deep Listening to the Heart of the Story," *Psychology Today*, September 3, 2021, https://www.psychologytoday.com/us/blog/the-other-side-relationships/202109/deep-listening-the-heart-the-story.
2. Barbara Myerhoff, "Life History Among the Elderly: Performance, Visibility, and Re-Membering," in *Remembered Lives: The Work of Ritual, Storytelling, and Growing Older*, ed. Barbara G. Myerhoff, Deena Metzger, Jay Ruby, and Virginia Tufte (Ann Arbor: University of Michigan Press, 1992), 231–49.
3. Michael White, *Maps of Narrative Practice* (New York: Norton, 2007).
4. Shona Russell and Maggie Carey, "Re-Membering: Responding to Commonly Asked Questions," *International Journal of Narrative Therapy and Community Work* 3 (2002): 23–31.
5. White, *Maps of Narrative Practice*.
6. My thanks to Susan Perlstein, founder of Elders Share the Arts, for introducing me to the concept of a hands poem.

NARRATIVE PRACTICE WITH OLDER ADULTS IN EASTERN CULTURES

11

EMBRACING LIFE'S SEASONS

Rediscovering Wisdom Through the Tree-of-Life Metaphor

IN THE NEXT FOUR CHAPTERS, we will explore the application of group and community narrative therapy (NT), and its potential for enhancing self-worth and quality of life for older adults living with chronic illnesses in the Eastern society of Hong Kong. Chapters 11 to 13 introduce metaphorical frameworks used in our group practice, including the Tree-of-Life, the Recipe-of-Life, and the Train-of-Life metaphors. Chapter 14 discusses the potential of community NT practice through "narra-drama," which is a novel approach to facilitate narrative justice and advocacy. Chapter 15 summarizes the power of unleashing corporate narratives in group and community practice.

MS. YE'S STORY *Ms. Ye, a loving, sixty-nine-year-old grandma of four grandchildren, was a spirited and strong-willed volunteer of a district elderly community center. She grew up in a low-socioeconomic family with five siblings. They lived in poverty, and she eked out a living by working for her father as well as collecting and reselling recycled materials with her siblings. She married in her early twenties. Life became harder still after marriage, as she had to carry her child with her to work. Her husband was unemployed because of health concerns, making her the primary breadwinner. Yet, when sharing her life experiences about how she got through her earlier difficult times, Ms. Ye immediately said, "Your aspiration should stay strong despite [the fact] that you are broken, and stand with a firm and straight backbone." She has learned and attested to this belief after facing various life challenges. This has become her life tenet, which has upheld her through difficult times. While narrating the hardships of her past, she wept and apologized, explaining, "Looking back, there were no more painful tears, the hard days were over; these tears are full of happiness, and gratitude."*

In reflection, Ms. Ye retold the Life Wisdom group that this belief indeed stemmed from the teachings of her father: "Recalling that my father was very strict and our five brothers and sisters all followed his philosophies, we grew up as good citizens. . . .We were grateful that our mother took care of the family well. . . . Although our family was poor, we survived the difficult times because we went through them together."

Ms. Ye gradually became a person with independence and strong willpower. She has lived her life with "no regrets."

As a child, Ms. Ye worked for her father, pouring coal and collecting the kitchen waste for a jumble sale, earning money to help her family, and living a hard life. Thinking retrospectively, her belief in "standing firm in poverty" began to take shape during her earlier years. "Back then, we tried our very best to keep the trolley from sliding down the hilly slope. We tried different ways, using wooden sticks to fasten the wheels, and slowly pushing the trolley full of kitchen waste down the slope step by step. Our brothers and sisters worked together to complete each job assigned to them, and this fostered a rich sense of brotherhood, in understanding and supporting each other through difficult times."

"Standing firm on my feet" was a powerful belief, especially when her husband was seriously ill. "At that time, my husband was ill and could not work. The children were still young, my eldest daughter was only two, and the son was only one year old." Ms. Ye shouldered the financial pressures all on her own. She took her two young children with her on cleaning jobs and did not borrow money from relatives and friends during those tough days. She sold her dowry, some golden jewelry, in exchange for money to support her family.

"I learned that we have to overcome the challenges by ourselves. Moreover, borrowing money always has to be returned to others. If it is returned to relatives and friends bit by bit, the money they get back is not easy to use, and it is hard on the relatives and friends. It is better to sell my dowry. I knew that it was the only way that I would have peace of mind and not owe anyone any favors. Taking life one step at a time, I developed my attitude of "adapting to the environment and looking for changes."

Ms. Ye said, "I am a competent wife and mother. My three children have grown up, and they have all started their own families. I have another wish, which is 'world peace': an era without war, and everyone can live in peace." She hoped to transfer her core beliefs of "Relying on yourself" to everyone, and "Standing firm during difficult times" to her children. Her three children all had the demeanor of Ms. Ye, and they were also practical people who followed the rules, often thought of others, and did volunteer work.

Ms. Ye was able to reconnect with and coauthor her positive beliefs by participating in the Tree-of-Life narrative group to rediscover her wisdom in life: "Standing firm in difficult times" included the belief of "helping others whenever you are able to, having willpower, hard-work, and owing no one any favors (relying on oneself)." Ms. Ye celebrated her life with a smile. She has planted her own "Thanksgiving Tree" with her "hardness and endurance." Being a Buddhist, she described herself as an "ordinary person with a satisfying life," with one dream remaining: "I also look forward to world peace, where all people can live in peace and have happy families."

Older adults generally accumulate valuable wisdom throughout their lives, but neither they, nor others, may recognize the value of this wisdom. This may constrain problem-solving, self-esteem, and relationships with others. In 2016 to 2017, we developed a new group practice using strength- and meaning-based NT called "Rediscovering wisdom in older adulthood: a randomized waitlist control trial of a specific narrative therapy in group practice" for older Chinese living in Hong Kong to help them rediscover their life wisdom. In this study, we recruited a total of 157 older adults who were fifty-five-years-old and older from different regions of Hong Kong. Among the participants, seventy-five of them were randomly assigned to the intervention group and eighty-two participants were assigned to the waitlist control group.[1] In four biweekly sessions, older Chinese adults participated in collaborative narrative conversations in a group of six members, using the Tree of Life (ToL) metaphor, with a narrative practitioner, to reexamine their life experiences and recognize their accumulated life wisdom.

We measured the effectiveness of our program using both qualitative and quantitative approaches. We conducted semistructured interviews with the participants to explore the insight they gained from the program. We used the Brief Self-Assessed Wisdom Scale (BSWS) to measure the perceived wisdom among the participants before and after the program.[2] This scale includes nine items that cover five aspects of the original forty-item Self-Assessed Wisdom Scale (SAWS),[3] including critical life experiences, reminiscence/reflectiveness, openness to experience, emotional regulation, and humor. We collected data according to the following schedule: (1) T0: the baseline level; (2) T1: at the end of the program; (3) T2: four months after the baseline time point; and (4) T3: eight months after the baseline time point. In this chapter, I report the ToL practice protocol as well as its short- and long-term effectiveness.

INTRODUCTION TO THE TREE-OF-LIFE METAPHOR

The ToL metaphor was first founded and used by Ncazelo Ncube in working with vulnerable children living with HIV/AIDS,[4] children who experienced the loss of their parents in war or genocides, and children who encountered other life traumas, such as abandonment in Southern Africa. The ToL metaphor has been widely used clinically, initially with children, and subsequently was extended to young and older adults.[5] The use of the ToL metaphor prevents retraumatizing the participants and helps them reconnect with their abilities, values, and family support, which may help them go through difficult times. Previous studies have been conducted using the ToL metaphor among refugee youth,[6] as well as parents of children with chronic physical health conditions.[7] These studies have worked to help people reauthor their life stories and construct preferred identities. This study demonstrates the first attempt to use the ToL metaphor as a method to illuminate, rediscover, and recollect life wisdom among older adults living in Hong Kong.

The use of ToL is a good fit with the narrative approach to understanding wisdom accumulation over one's lifespan. By examining one's past and present, the many aspects of one's life and self-identity are symbolized, reflected, and embedded in the different parts of the tree. This metaphor can also be used to rediscover and incorporate other elements in the person's life experiences, hardships, and history. It can also be extended from the social support in the clinical setting to a daily life setting. Traditional therapeutic processes often fail to facilitate social connections and interpersonal support that may benefit people outside of a clinical setting. The ToL metaphor allows participants to connect with their origins; reconnect with their personal resources; and rediscover their rooted values, beliefs, and life wisdom that have helped them endure through hardships to validate their self-worth and affirm meaning in life.

As introduced in chapter 1, Hong Kong older adults may have experienced previous traumas, including war and poverty, at an early age. As these adults have grown older, they also may have experienced more common traumas of family life, including marital strife, abuse, divorce, the sickness of the partner, the burden of raising children alone, and blended families. The wisdom accumulated throughout life is often a valuable resource that can help people carry forward when they face difficulties. A recent study found that wisdom can predict greater subjective well-being, autonomy, meaning in life, and physical health.[8] The life wisdom of older adults, once rediscovered, can be beneficial to their daily life adjustment and can be transferred to other people for their betterment as well.

IMPLEMENTING THE METAPHOR IN GROUP-BASED NT

The implementation of the ToL metaphor generally occurs over four two-hour sessions: (1) describe different parts of the tree; (2) create a forest of life; (3) weather the storms of life; and (4) witness a celebration of life.[9]

SESSION 1: DESCRIBE DIFFERENT PARTS OF THE TREE

The aim of the first session is to allow each older adult to establish "a second story" about his or her life. During the process, the practitioner first invites the participants to draw their own tree, which incorporates eight different parts of the tree, including the (1) roots, (2) the ground, (3) the trunk, (4) the branches, (5) the leaves, (6) the flowers, (7) the fruits, and (8) the seeds. Each part of the tree symbolizes different aspects of the person's life (see table 11.1A) and also includes related questions inviting the person to identify different parts of the trees. The therapist/practitioner helps the person reflect on the impacts and importance of different parts of the ToL

SESSION 2: CREATE A FOREST OF LIFE

The aim of the second session is for participants to create a visual "forest of life," share their different stories through the tree metaphor, and identify the contextual factors of the forest in the group. The practitioners first may ask questions associated with the contextual factors, which may affect the forest. The therapist can invite the group members to share details about the trees they draw. Through this process of "telling and retelling," the group members are able to appreciate and reflect on each other's life stories. Table 11.2 lists related questions that invite the participants to disclose details about the forest of life.

SESSION 3: WEATHER THE STORMS OF LIFE

The aim of the third session is to create space for participants to speak about some of the difficulties or hardships that they have experienced as

TABLE 11.1 A. Tree-of-Life metaphoric framework

Session 1: Describe different parts of the tree	
1. Roots	Where the person is from.
	– What is their country of origin or place of birth?
	– What is their family history?
	– What they did/do for a living (i.e., their careers)?
2. Ground	Where the people currently live and their activities of regular daily life.
	– Why do you do activities every day?
	– What has sustained you to do this consistently?
3. Trunk	The strengths, skills, talents, personality characteristics, and problem-solving mechanisms of the people.
	– How did you develop these strengths, skills, and talents?
	– How important are these strengths, skills, and talents in your life?
4. Branches	Hopes, dreams, and wishes that the people have for the direction of their lives.
	– Why are these hopes, dreams, and wishes important to you?
	– What has sustained your hopes, dreams, and wishes?
	– Is there a history behind these hopes, dreams, and wishes?
5. Leaves	People who are or were important in their lives.
	– Why is or was this person important to you?
	– What was special about this person to you?
6. Flowers	Cherished memories of beauty, love, connection, and fulfillment of the people.
	– Why are these cherished memories to you?
	– What is special about these memories to you?
7. Fruits	Gifts that the people have been given. These may be material gifts or acts of love and caring from others.
	– Why do you think the person gave you this?
	– What did they appreciate about you that would have led them to do this?
	– What do you think you might have contributed to their lives?
8. Winged seeds	Legacies of the people.
	– Why do you think these legacies are important?
	– What care and support do you think you need to ensure that these legacies are carried forth?

well as how they made it through the storm. After discussing how people weather the storms that inevitably come, the session ends by inviting the group members to imagine a time when their trees encountered storms and other challenges. As discussed in chapter 4 on working with groups, mutual aid is necessary for this metaphor narrative group to work well. By the third session, if enough mutual aid has not cultivated, group participants will have difficulty sharing deeper thoughts and feelings with each other. To

TABLE 11.2 Forest of life

Session 2: Create a forest of life

1. Invite the people to stick their trees to one of the walls, creating a beautiful forest.

2. Invite a few people to share the stories of their trees in front of the group.

3. Ask volunteers to come up to the front of the room. Demonstrate that like their trees, they can also stand tall with a sense of pride.

4. Invite three or four people to share with the group their hopes and dreams:

   a. Telling questions:

   - What is the history of the hopes and dreams that have been expressed?
   - How did you manage to hold onto these hopes and dreams, to keep them alive?
   - Who else in the family or in your life knows about these hopes and dreams?
   - What does it mean to the person to be talking about her/his hopes and dreams in these ways?

   b. Retelling prompts:

   - Draw attention to the dreams and hopes that they have for their lives.
   - Acknowledge their connections to those who have taught them a lot of things in their lives, and continue to care and support them in different ways.
   - Acknowledge that some of these precious people have died, but they still hold them in loving memory for the many wonderful things that they did.
   - Speak of how the relationships that they shared with them still support them in many ways as they continue to live their lives.

5. Discuss and reflect on the following:

   - What do these trees have in common?
   - What are the differences?
   - How can they support each other as trees belonging in the same forest?

continue to foster this type of mutual aid, the therapist may ask emotionally "safer," fact-based questions, and some examples are included in table 11.3. Along with these safer questions, table 11.3 also provides examples that require more vulnerability if the group is ready to go deeper. The purpose of all of these questions is to let the participants know that life challenges are inevitable, that no one should be blamed for the challenges they face, and that they do not have to face these challenges alone. If enough mutual aid has been cultivated, the group may then discuss the ways that the trees can protect themselves when the storms come. Throughout this process, the therapist may encourage the group members to reconnect with their personal resources, such as their rooted values, strengths, and friends that may support them through the difficulties.

In sharing the storms of life, participants can freely identify an earlier hardship that they have overcome and share coping strengths and beliefs that have been unearthed in the process. These are unique outcomes of

TABLE 11.3 Storms of life

Session 3: Weather the storms of life

1. Create space for the people to speak about some of the difficulties they may be experiencing in their lives (but in ways that would not be retraumatizing).

   a. Find ways that they can collectively speak about some of the shared experiences.

   b. Acknowledge the effects of harm on their lives (never to blame the people for this harm).

   c. Unearth and acknowledge some of the skills and knowledge that the people demonstrate in trying to respond to the hazards in their lives.

   d. Help the people to grow *mutual aid* in their interactions, so that their own skills and knowledge can be more visible to oneself and the group.

2. Assemble the people to resume the conversations about trees and forests:

   a. Acknowledge that we have lovely trees that have strong roots and beautiful leaves and fruits.

   b. As beautiful as our trees and forest are, can we say that they are free from danger?

   c. Invite the group to mention some of the potential dangers that may threaten these beautiful trees.

   d. List the potential hazards (e.g., burning of trees, cutting trees down, kicking trees, too much rain, lightning, aging).

   e. Name these problems and challenges, and discuss the effects of such hazards on their own lives: feelings and thoughts collectively (naming without shame or creating any sense of being defined by others).

   f. Discuss ways that they may respond, using examples, such as how animals respond to storms when they are in a forest (tap into their knowledge).

   g. Discuss ways that they can protect themselves and respond to the storms of life.

3. Divide the people into groups of five to spend time reflecting on the following questions:

   a. When do storms feel like they are never ending?

   b. When do our lives feel like they are free of storms and that calm is restored?

   c. What do we do when the storms have passed?

reauthoring conversations. When the participants documented these strengths in their ToL drawings, they named these strengths, just like the aerial roots stemming from the branches of older trees, like the Banyan tree.[10] As the aerial roots grow older and become stronger, they develop into prop roots that mature into thick, woody trunks, which, with age, can become indistinguishable from the primary trunk. This professionally facilitated NT group, like a cultivated forest, provides emotional safety and support for the participants to positively improve their perceived wisdom, which like the prop roots, will uphold them and become beneficial to their general physical and mental health, as well as validate their life wisdom.[11] As a result, we added one more component to the ToL metaphor (i.e., aerial/prop roots), which furthers the rediscovery of their life wisdom through this NT group practice (see table 11.4).

TABLE 11.4 B. Additional parts of the tree

Aerial/Prop Roots	Discuss the strengths that the participants have identified and lived through as a result of earlier life challenges. These may include values, beliefs, and commitments in life that they have recognized or acknowledged and testified.
	- What upholds you during these trying times?
	- When did you first realize these strengths? Can you tell us a related story?
	- How have they supported you subsequently?

SESSION 4: WITNESS A CELEBRATION OF LIFE

The fourth session features a certificate-giving ceremony and the last step of the therapeutic process: "certificate and songs." This is the opportunity for group members to review each other's knowledge, strengths, skills, talents, hopes, and dreams unearthed in this process. Family members and friends are invited as the audience and witnesses and are given the opportunity to listen, acknowledge, and receive this "life wisdom" as it has manifested through outsider witness practice (as discussed in chapter 4). The audience members will listen to participants' conversations about their life narratives and collectively witness and document their strengths. In this way, the valuable relearning of their life wisdom is also transferred to each participant's family and friends, as well as to other participants' family and friends. The audience members are invited to retell what they have heard to participants and to acknowledge the usefulness of their responses to hardships they may face in their life. Through this process of "tellings, and retellings," it is expected that both the participants and audience and witnesses will reconnect more deeply with the "wisdom" they have learned from the past and to celebrate with the participants as they acknowledge the benefit of this wisdom. The therapist/practitioner may also invite the audience members to write a letter to their family to extend support to them. This process is described in table 11.5, which includes questions for this celebration of life.

Throughout this program, the older adults gave their trees different names, such as the Gratitude Tree, Happiness Tree, Responsibility Tree, and A Powerful

TABLE 11.5 Celebration of life

Session 4: Witness a celebration of life
1. Record their hopes, their dreams, and their skills.
2. Invite a range of outsiders to witness the certificate-giving ceremony.
3. Write a letter to the person's family to extend support to them.

Tree of Life. Their tree names allowed for a rich recollection of the thoughts, feelings, and experiences of the transformative NT group process. When facing past, present, or future difficulties, older adults can use this group to reconnect with their life wisdom: to hold on to what they have learned from their tough lives and to cope with the difficulties and traumas.

STUDY RESULTS OF TREE OF LIFE

Based on the quantitative results of this study,[12] we observed that the older adults in the NT groups showed significant improvement in the various outcome measures, including a sense of mastery ($F = 3.54$, $p < 0.03$), self-esteem ($F = 2.70$, $p < 0.49$), hope ($F = 3.15$, $p < 0.03$), meaning in life ($F = 3.28$, $p < 0.02$), wisdom ($F = 7.21$, $p < 0.001$), and well-being ($F = 6.67$, $p < 0.001$) compared with the control group, which indicated that the group NT using the ToL metaphor strengthened the older adults' connections with their critical life events, and helped them appreciate their effort in making important decisions in their lives.

Based on the qualitative interview responses of the participants,[13] we identified a total of six themes, including the following: (1) insight into their abilities, intentions, and problem-solving capabilities; (2) a sense of purpose and commitment to preferred identities; (3) realization of personal values and beliefs; (4) increasing a sense of agency and level of acceptance; (5) maintaining hope in times of challenges; and (6) cherishing life as a journey to consolidate their wealth of wisdom for the common good. The following is the narrative of Mr. Cheung's life story after rediscovering his wisdom during the ToL program.

MR. CHEUNG'S STORY

REDISCOVERY OF HIS LIFE WISDOM *Mr. Cheung, a sixty-eight-year-old widower, is retired and lives alone. Mr. Cheung has refreshed his memory of his parents' teaching, and their love that continued to support his personal growth throughout his life. His parents had high moral standards for him and his siblings, and educated them to be honest, conscientious, hardworking, and down-to-earth and to support each other. He felt that it was difficult to repay the kindness of his parents. His father was engaged in trade in Hong Kong, and when he (father) was stagnant in his business in his old hometown, he was criticized as being a capitalist. After the liberation and liquidation, his father accepted the reality that he was sent to the countryside to do farming work. Mr. Cheung also remembered that his father cared about them. In the summer, the brothers and sisters gathered around the table to do their homework, and his father fanned them one by one. The mother had a compassionate heart and cared for the family. When the mother saw that children were in need, she always helped them.*

EXTERNALIZING PERSONAL TRAITS   *Mr. Cheung knows that his belief in life comes from his family's education. As a man, he knew he must develop a man's spirit, including being strong, accepting reality, relying on oneself, not sighing, not complaining when wronged, and not being afraid of hardships. After returning to Hong Kong from mainland China, life was difficult. In order to survive, Mr. Cheung worked two jobs and never complained. He endured hardship, fought hard, and seldom shed tears. He feels that he endured every hardship and that only cried when his parents and his wife passed away, because he loved his parents and his wife dearly. When his wife passed away, his eldest child was only twelve years old, and all three boys burst into tears. Mr. Cheung passed on the spirit of manhood and his attitude toward life to his sons. He is not afraid of hardships, working diligently to adjust to reality and has placed high demands on himself. He tries his best to do the best, reflecting on himself for improvement, and having a clear conscience.*

REAUTHORING HIS LIFE EXPERIENCE   *Mr. Cheung recalled his wife's advice before her death: "Tell him to quit smoking, and ask him to start and establish a new family." He did follow all of his wife's wishes, except for remarrying. Mr. Cheung chose not to marry again, for the sake of his family and for his son. Following the teachings of his parents, he has developed the characteristics of conscience, responsibility, love, and gratitude. Mr. Cheung gets along with his son like a friend, with a strong, persistent, and realistic attitude to overcome different difficulties.*

He said that if his dad knew that he had inherited his virtues, he would say, "You deserve it; you are a good boy."

Mr. Cheung would answer his father, saying, "That's how I should behave."

Mr. Cheung also said with great emotion: "The poor's children will mature earlier than the children of their same age group."

In the eyes of the team members, Mr. Cheung is "a good father, a good husband, and a filial son." Mr. Cheung said both he and his sons are ordinary people, who have grown through hardships to become mature "successful people."

REDISCOVERING HIS LIFE WISDOM *Mr. Cheung misses his wife and believes that he is fortunate to have had a lovely and wise wife, three sons who behave well, and a happy family, which he nurtured together with his wife. When narrating his life experiences, Mr. Cheung affirmed that from his father, himself, and his sons, all three generations have lived through life challenges to become tough and resilient. His father's teaching, carefully backed him up like his golf caddie, giving advice and providing moral support to him. In drawing and consolidating his "Gratitude Tree," Mr. Cheung celebrated his "Tree of Life," which has grown wide and deep over the years through the aerial and prop roots, which are labeled "positive attitude," "giving your best," and "growing from errors." He realizes and recollects this life wisdom, and finds comfort. Now his three sons are academically successful, with university and master's degrees, and they have all married. Looking back on his life, Mr. Cheung said, "I've lived life to its fullest, and it's very comforting to witness that my sons have become good citizens to the society."*

Mr. Cheung concludes that he has fulfilled his wife's advice, because he is a "person who faces reality" and has planted a "strong tree." Mr. Cheung also added a note next to the Tree of Life: "This tree is an organic jujube tree in the Northeast, and you can safely pick and eat it." It can be seen that Mr. Cheung is a caring person who cares about the needs of others.

PASSING DOWN HIS WISDOM OF LIFE *Mr. Cheung passed on his "down-to-earth, hard-working spirit" and his ability to "grow from errors" to the new generation of young people, saying that success requires hard work.*

CONCLUSION

From these quantitative results, we can observe that the older adults' perceived wisdom had increased after the program. Moreover, the results of the interview also revealed improvement in self-agency and self-perceived competencies. We verified that the group narrative practice using the ToL metaphor allowed the older adults' life wisdom to be recorded, which preserved their dignity as they aged. This process resonated with the active aging concept (chapter 1) by enhancing older adults' mental health and quality of life. This intervention significantly improved self-perceptions of wisdom compared with baseline and with the control group, and demonstrated positive effects in the short and longer term. NT should be employed to help older adults recognize the value of their wisdom, enhance their self-worth, and increase participation in family and community activities.

In this chapter, I focused on the use of the ToL metaphor framework in serving older adults living in Hong Kong in narrative group practice. This metaphoric framework uniquely related to the individual within their support systems and provided opportunities for these individuals to share their trauma without retraumatizing them. In next chapter, I provide guidance in the use of the "Recipe of Life" metaphor, which I have adapted and tailored to accommodate the local Hong Kong culture.

NOTES

1. Esther Oi-Wah Chow and Sai-Fu Fung, "Narrative Group Intervention to Rediscover Life Wisdom Among Hong Kong Chinese Older Adults: A Single-Blind Randomized Waitlist-Controlled Trial," *Innovation in Aging* 5, no. 3 (2021): igab027, https://doi.org/10.1093/geroni/igab027.
2. Sai-fu Fung, Esther Oi-Wah Chow, and Chau-Kiu Cheung, "Development and Validation of a Brief Self-Assessed Wisdom Scale," *BMC Geriatrics* 20, no. 1 (2020): 1–8.
3. Jeffrey Dean Webster, "An Exploratory Analysis of a Self-Assessed Wisdom Scale," *Journal of Adult Development* 10, no. 1 (2003): 13–22, https://doi.org /10.1023/A:1020782619051; and Jeffrey Dean Webster, "Measuring the Character Strength of Wisdom," *International Journal of Aging and Human Development* 65, no. 2 (2007): 163–83, https://doi.org/10.2190/AG.65.2.d.
4. Ncazelo Ncube, "The Tree of Life Project: Using Narrative Ideas in Work with Vulnerable Children in Southern Africa," *International Journal of Narrative Therapy and Community Work* 1 (2006): 3–16, https://doi.org/https://search .informit.org/doi/10.3316/informit.197106237773394.
5. David Denborough, "Stories from Robben Island: A Report from a Journey of Healing," *International Journal of Narrative Therapy and Community Work* 2 (2004): 1–10; David Denborough, *Collective Narrative Practice: Responding to Individuals, Groups, and Communities Who Have Experienced Trauma* (Adelaide SA: Dulwich Centre, 2008); and Janelle Dickson, "The 'Mighty Oak': Using the 'Tree of Life' Methodology as a Gateway to the Other Maps of Narrative Practice," *International Journal of Narrative Therapy and Community Work* 4 (2009): 9–23.
6. Deborah A Stiles et al., "Researching the Effectiveness of Tree of Life: An Imbeleko Approach to Counseling Refugee Youth," *Journal of Child and Adolescent Trauma* 14, no. 1 (2021): 123–39.

7. Jessica Haselhurst et al., "A Narrative-Informed Evaluation of Tree of Life for Parents of Children with Physical Health Conditions," *Clinical Child Psychology and Psychiatry* 26, no. 1 (2021): 51–63.

8. Monika Ardelt, "Disentangling the Relations Between Wisdom and Different Types of Well-being in Old Age: Findings from a Short-Term Longitudinal Study," *Journal of Happiness Studies* 17, no. 5 (2016) : 1963–84.

9. Denborough, *Collective Narrative Practice*.

10. Chow and Fung, "Narrative Group Intervention to Rediscover Life Wisdom."

11. Andrew W. Bailey and Keith C Russell, "Volunteer Tourism: Powerful Programs or Predisposed Participants?," *Journal of Hospitality and Tourism Management* 19, no. 1 (2012): 123–32; Rachel V. Costa and Kenneth I. Pakenham, "Associations Between Benefit Finding and Adjustment Outcomes in Thyroid Cancer," *Psycho-Oncology* 21, no. 7 (2012): 737–44; Webster, "Measuring the Character Strength of Wisdom"; Chow and Fung, "Narrative Group Intervention to Rediscover Life Wisdom."

12. Esther Oi-Wah Chow and Chau-Kiu Cheung, "Contribution of Wisdom to Chinese Elders' Well-Being," *Innovation in Aging* 1, Suppl. 1 (June 30, 2017): 605, https://doi.org/10.1093/geroni/igx004.2117.

13. Esther Oi-Wah Chow, "Rediscovery of Older Adults' Life Wisdom: Application of Narrative Therapy Using a Tree-of-Life Metaphor," *Innovation in Aging* 4, no. Suppl. 1 (December 1, 2020): 835–835, https://doi.org/10.1093/geroni/igaa057.3059.

12

HEALING JOURNEYS

The Recipe-of-Life Metaphor for Chronic Pain Recovery

MS. CHAN'S STORY   *Ms. Chan, seventy-eight years old, has been bothered by chronic pain in her right arm for more than eight years. In recent years, her pain has worsened. She is often woken up by her pain during the night and cannot sleep well. She described the "taste" of her pain as spicy and bitter, that there were many chili peppers sticking to her arms. Sometimes the pain was so extreme that she would lose her appetite.*

Although the pain has bothered Ms. Chan, she was still actively facing her life. When the pain visited her, she would use Chinese medicine, painkillers, pain relief patches, and ice patches to soothe her pain. She also has tried to distract herself from the pain by engaging in some daily life activities, such as cooking. Ms. Chan has used her experiences in living with pain to compose her "life recipe". The ingredients in her recipe include "optimism, persistence, patience, responsibility, never give up, and positivity." She has named her recipe "tips for taking responsibility in living with the pain".

Ms. Chan told us that she was a nurse before she moved to Hong Kong to take care of her mother who had a stroke. She brought her daughter with her, moving into her brother's home. She took care of her mother and her family with all her heart. To save money to further support her family, she only ate the cold and leftover food, and she took extra side jobs, like making plastic flowers and watchbands. She was once also a part-time nurse, and she sent the money she earned to her husband to support his needs in mainland China.

From Ms. Chan's narrative, the group members witnessed that she was a person with "consideration, filial piety, love, and strength." From her warmth in retelling her story, it was evident that she was a person full of affection. Ms. Chan said that she learned to be considerate to others from her mother, and she believed that her mother would be glad to see that she has inherited this quality from her and become someone who loves and cares for others.

Older people in Hong Kong most commonly experience chronic musculo-skeletal pain in the joints.[1] In general, people age sixty and over tend to be more susceptible to chronic pain, which may seem an inevitable part of the normal aging process.[2] Joints, knee, back, shoulder, and muscle pain are the most common types of chronic pain reported.[3] Continuous pain restricts a person's mobility and negatively influences their mental health and social functions, with significant physical, psychological, and social impairments. For instance, chronic pain was found to be associated with an enhanced risk of depression,[4] increased recent suicide attempts, increased use of tobacco, and painkillers misuse.[5] The prevalence of depression among people living with chronic pain in Hong Kong was found to be 5.6 times higher than among their pain-free counterparts, and 71 percent of those living with chronic pain in Hong Kong experience anxiety or depression, or both conditions. A local survey reported that 38.3 percent of respondents experienced negative effects on their work, and more than 70 percent felt that pain interfered with their daily life.[6] Moreover, people in chronic pain are more likely to feel a sense of isolation that may further intensify their negative emotions.[7] Often a domino effect continues with isolation further negatively influencing the person's social interactions, which then continues a vicious trajectory that negatively affects a person's mental health and social adjustment.[8] In general, the effects on daily life are felt on an individual's mood, mobility, and work performance.

Chronic pain not only affects physical functions but also has an influence on the mental health and social adjustment of the person experiencing pain. Thus, it is important not to focus merely on the physical pain symptom reduction but also to assist the person's psychological and social adjustment to chronic pain.[9] Previous research using group and community narrative therapy (NT) has suggested that this type of therapy is helpful in assisting the participants to develop personal strategies in coping with the pain, investigating cures and relief for their pain, and negotiating their interpersonal relationships after they encounter the pain.[10] The existing medical care system in Hong Kong mainly focuses on treating a person's physical symptoms but not their psychological and social adjustment.[11] We conducted a group narrative practice using the Recipe-of-Life metaphor to build a mental and social support system for older adults with chronic pain and for their caregivers.

METAPHORIC FRAMEWORK: RECIPE OF LIFE

From Ms. Chan's story, we can observe that her values and beliefs in "being considerate to others" and "being responsible for her family" were unearthed during the group therapeutic process.[12] In this group narrative practice, we used the Recipe-of-Life metaphor as a medium to help the group members unfold their stories of living with pain. The Recipe-of-Life metaphor was first introduced by Natale Rudland Wood as a response to children and young people who experience homelessness in shelters in Australia.[13] Inspired by her own interest in cooking, Wood found that foods not only link with personal memories but are also associated with a person's tradition, history, and culture. Therefore, making use of a recipe metaphor in a counseling setting may be a powerful medium to link a person with his or her experiences, personal strengths, and social support system. In addition to applying the Recipe-of-Life metaphor to work with vulnerable children, this metaphor has also been applied to work with adult women who have encountered gender violence in their families,[14] and older adults living with chronic pain in Hong Kong.[15] In this chapter, we introduce how to implement this metaphoric framework in NT and present qualitative evidence on the effects of this metaphoric framework when working with older adults living with chronic pain in Hong Kong.

RECIPE OF LIFE: NARRATIVE METAPHOR GROUP FOR OLDER ADULTS COPING WITH CHRONIC PAIN IN HONG KONG

PARTICIPANTS

We recruited thirty participants from two not-for-profit organizations that serve older adults in Hong Kong. The participants were recruited based on the following inclusion criteria: (1) have been diagnosed with at least one type of chronic pain for more than three months; (2) are at least sixty years old; (3) do not have active psychotic symptoms; and, (4) are willing to commit to actively share their experiences in the NT group.[16]

OUR STUDY DESIGN

As suggested by David Denborough, it is important that the selected metaphor fit the local cultures.[17] In Hong Kong, it is easy for people to find foods from both the Eastern and Western cultures, and it is also common for people to share foods.[18] Therefore, the use of the Recipe-of-Life metaphor can easily connect the participants with their day-to-day experiences. In our project, we invited the participants to name their "pain" with different flavors and link it with related foods. The program duration was two hours each week for six weeks.

IMPLEMENTING THE RECIPE-OF-LIFE METAPHORIC FRAMEWORK

The practice of this metaphoric framework often starts from the discussion of favorite food and important memories brought by the foods. The practitioners may also bring some food samples to help the participants to recall the memories of food through aroma and tastes. This can be especially helpful when working with people who have memory problems, such as Alzheimer's disease.[19] The practitioners may help people think of the recipe for their own lives, which may include the recipe for happiness, recipe for life challenges, and the like. This process often includes the inquiry about the following: (1) ingredients; (2) source of the ingredients; (3) method; (4) techniques and tips; and (5) ritual.[20]

INGREDIENTS   The ingredients for life recipes include personal qualities, abilities, resources, and social support that help people endure hardship. For example, ingredients may include confidence, humor, acceptance, or family support, to name just a few.

UNINVITED INGREDIENTS: THE THREATS AND CHALLENGES IN LIFE   In situations in which participants face a specific threat or life challenge, the practitioner may introduce "uninvited ingredients" to represent the unwelcome elements in a person's life. For example, in Meizi Tan's experiences working with women who experience domestic violence in Singapore, she made use of "bacteria" to symbolize the social discourses that have caused the women's self-doubt and reduced their confidence after they experienced domestic violence.[21] These uninvited ingredients can be used to externalize the problem and enable people to freely discuss the effects of the problems on their lives.[22] The practitioner and the participants may work collaboratively to figure out ways that the ingredients in their life recipe may help them deal with the uninvited ingredients.

SOURCE OF THE INGREDIENTS   The practitioner then traces back to the origins of these life recipe ingredients with the participants. The practitioner may ask questions like: "Where are the ingredients from?" "What's your earliest memory about the ingredients?" "What do you think is the reason that other people have given you this ingredient?" and "Do you share these ingredients with others?" The inquiry of the origin of the ingredients helps participants connect with the important people in their lives, their family and cultural histories, and their personal beliefs.[23]

METHOD   Next, the practitioner and the participants explore the methods of using the ingredients. Several questions that may facilitate this process include "When do you use these ingredients?" "How do you use them?" "What happens after you use the ingredients?" and "Would you change the combinations and sequence in using the ingredients?" The purpose of these questions is to discuss how the ingredients (resources in life) can be put into practice to benefit the persons' lives.

TECHNIQUES AND TIPS   In the next session, the practitioner helps the participants consider the techniques they discover when making the recipes as well as the tips they would share with people who want to use their recipes. This is a process of "enabling contribution,"[24] in which the participants are able to share their life wisdom with others. Enabling contribution helps participants strengthen their preferred identity.

RITUAL   Finally, the practitioner and the participants discuss who they would like to invite to their meals as well as whether they follow any special rituals when enjoying the meal. This is a process of re-membering conversations in which the participants select and connect with the people they would like to share their life recipes with and may seek support from.[25]

Similarly, this Recipe-of-Life practice follows the strategic procedures included in NT (see chapter 3), which are as follows: (1) externalizing conversation (deconstruct), (2) reauthoring (coconstruct), and (3) re-membering conversation and outsider witness practice (thickening and reconstruction). This Recipe-of-Life metaphor can be applied to the NT session plan for "Life as a Tasty Journey." The examples of the NT questions are presented in tables 12.1 to 12.4.[26]

At the beginning of the first session, the therapist adopted the questions as listed to *externalize* the lived experience and impact of the pain. Because this was the first session, the therapist began to welcome and engage participants collectively, establishing equality between therapist and participants through group sharing of individual disclosures of the experience of living with various types of pain. Individual and group contracts were completed,

TABLE 12.1 Life as a Tasty Journey: Session 1

Session 1: My journey started with heart-warming foods

1. What kinds of taste would you identify to represent pain? (spicy)

2. Which type of ingredient would you choose to represent this taste? (red chili)

3. When did "the chosen ingredient" (red chili) first appear in your life?

4. How did (red chili) affect your daily life?

5. What is living with (red chili) like for you and your family?

6. Did it affect your relationships with others? With whom? In what way?

7. Does the (red chili) come in various sizes? With different degrees of spiciness?

8. How would you name this (red chili) if you have to give it a name?

TABLE 12.2 Life as a Tasty Journey: Sessions 2 and 3

Sessions 2 and 3: Searching for and making a "Spiritual Recipe"

1. When the stroke (use the name given to red chili by each participant; i.e., the pain) appears, what kind of ingredient did you use to relieve the spiciness?

2. What makes you persist in making yourself a favorable dish despite the stroke (use the name given to red chili by each participant)? Please share with us those ingredients (i.e., personal qualities, values, and core beliefs) you have added to reduce the spiciness of the red chili.

3. Please try to list ingredients and give weight to each, like a recipe.

4. Did this special ingredient (i.e., "seasoning") help you? Tell us a story about how this seasoning has made a difference in your life.

5. After telling this story, can you tell us what kind of person you are? What is your preferred identity?

6. Has your feeling toward the (use the name given to red chili by each participant) changed?

7. How will you name the (use the name given to red chili by each participant) now?

TABLE 12.3 Life as a Tasty Journey: Sessions 4 and 5

Sessions 4 and 5: Mixing my "Spiritual Recipe" and collecting more recipes

1. When did you first notice yourself possessing this special ingredient (quality)?

2. Who have you acquired this ingredient (quality) from?

3. Please tell us a story about this ingredient (quality).

4. Did the quality reflect who you were? Name your preferred identity.

5. How would the person who taught you the values respond when she or he knows you have adopted this value?

TABLE 12.4 Life as a Tasty Journey: Session 6

Session 6: Sharing and appreciating a collection of recipes

1. Participants shared their life wisdom about pain relief, which contributed to a group declaration and camaraderie.

2. Participants celebrated their spirit of fighting against the pain, and they hoped these qualities would help others.

with agreement to adopt a collective metaphoric framework in the session (i.e., "life as a taste journey"), experiencing tastes at various stages. Participants were invited to describe and externalize pain by giving their pain a name. Participants were given a set of cards that contained vocabulary words highlighting different types of tastes, such as, sour, sweet, bitter, and spicy. They were asked to identify one taste to represent their experience with pain and to choose a food ingredient to symbolize the pain as an externalization. Some examples of the ingredients used to externalize the pain included spicy (e.g., red chili), sweet (e.g., mandarins), sour (e.g., lemon), and bitter (e.g., bitter melon).

The aim of the next two sessions was to *reauthor conversations*—that is, to thicken a new alternative storyline. Questions were used to identify the sparkling (eureka, or "Aha") moment when participants were empowered and took charge of the problem or challenge. Most participants could name their pain (e.g., chili, the unpleasant food ingredient) in the session and identified the sparkling moment or unique outcome, unearthing their personal qualities and beliefs that had sustained them during previous difficult times (the favorable seasoning that counteracts red chili), which gave rise to the "spiritual seasonings of life." As they developed these spiritual seasonings of life, they named the tastes of the pain and gave tentative names to the seasoning. Successful stories that participants preferred to live in, including their "preferred identity," emerged during these conversations. Participants wrote the story of strengths, added flavor to the chosen food ingredients, made and named their personal seasoning, and listed the ingredients. Eventually, individuals' recipes of life were produced in the session. Meanwhile, an in-group witness practice was also conducted. Other participants were invited to be the witnesses when an individual participant disclosed his or her seasoning formula. By inviting the participants in the process of renaming the red chili, participants came to realize the magnitude of changes as they gained insight from these reauthoring conversations.

The aim of sessions 4 and 5 was to *thicken the identity*. Each participant came with earlier "life associations," telling stories from which he or she acquired their core values, personal qualities, and preferred identity and used these details to fine-tune the sauce of their lives. Through these *re-membering* conversations, they reconnected significant others to their present lives, reconstructed and thickened their identities, and solidified their core values.

The aim of this sixth and final session was to conduct definitional ceremonies and in-group *witness practice*. Participants were invited to present their personal seasonings, drawings, and sealed bottles, which represented

TABLE 12.5 Themes and illustrative cases

Theme 1: Identification of personal qualities and capabilities	Description of Pain and Beliefs	Qualities and Capabilities
Ms. Leung	Treated chronic pain as an **unwelcome "friend"** and managed this "friend" well with her life motto: "taking it easy."	While narrating how she got along with this friend, she obtained the insight that her core belief of **"trying her best"** is very important to her and has supported her in facing life–and-death experiences when she worked as a nurse in her earlier years.
Ms. Wong	Associated the taste of pain as "bitter" and revealed the prominence of her major strength, "staying calm," in supporting her through this bitter journey living with this **"bitter melon"** in reauthoring conversations.	Her self-narrative was full of **"tranquility,"** and this personal quality developed when she was very young and remained in force after she underwent both her own and her husband's stroke rehabilitation.
Ms. Shek	Externalized pain using **"green chili"** to describe the discomfort in her left shoulder and her weak legs, which often restricted her daily functioning. Green chili has given her a difficult life for the past five years and made her feel miserable at times.	She has tried to take good care of herself, supported by her belief that "persistence is essential for life management." She followed her doctor's instructions. In reauthoring conversations, this belief fused with her belief that "life is a series of exercises" that helped her in most of her painful experiences. Hence, she named her 'spiritual seasoning of life' **"bravery,"** which included "physical exercises, positivity, tolerance, persistence, belief and slowing down."

Theme 2: Validation of preferred identity	Core Beliefs and Character	Preferred Identity
Ms. Cheung	Was upheld by her core belief of **"trying her best"** and **"taking it easy"** during difficulties, and this was witnessed by group members. She was happy to apply these beliefs again to her current life situation.	Through revisiting various critical instances, she now sees herself more as a **"challenger,"** and her relationship with pain as a lifelong friend, growing together as companions. She developed self-acceptance, and as a result her self-relationship and relationship with chronic pain were altered and enriched.
Ms. Ma	Recalled her characteristic of being calm in re-membering conversations. She was encouraged when the group members were impressed by her **"calm"** quality and her preferred identities as a **good daughter** to her mother, a **good wife** to her husband, and a **responsible person** to herself.	She was happy to bring this quality with her all the time. Her self-relationship and chronic pain relationship were strengthened. She sees her self as a caring wife to her husband and someone who enjoys peace of mind.

Theme 3: Fusion of spiritual seasoning of life	Seasoning	Results
Ms. Lee	Stated that the seasoning was enriched with **"1 tablespoon of calmness," "1 cup of gratitude,"** and **"2 teaspoons of optimism."** These ingredients were recollected through dialectical conversations among group members.	She could handle the green chili and became less fearful of it by mixing **"1 more cup of bravery"** and **"1.5 more cups of tolerance".** Ms. Lee proposed to combine all these ingredients into a small bottle, and keep it in the refrigerator, which is good for a lifetime. The findings suggest that her self-relationship, chronic-pain-relationship, peer relationships, and social relationships had been reconnected when their preferred identities were restored.
Ms. Lim	Experienced pain relief at the final session during the definitional ceremony. Her perspective has been expanded after recollecting her values/beliefs with group members.	On top of **"1 tablespoon of persistence, 1.5 tablespoons of tolerance, 1 cup of activeness, 1.5 cups of responsibility,"** more ingredients were added into the **"spiritual seasoning of best and ease."** They are **"1 tablespoon of openness,"** and **"1.5 tablespoons of friendliness,"** which helped her become happier and more pleasant. Each of these ingredients helped her to accept pain as a lifelong friend, and surprisingly her self-reported degree of pain had decreased substantially. She even suggested "living with pain" as the name of the group. She was then living with happiness, not with pain as she had done prior to participating in the group.
Ms. Kwong	Named her spiritual seasoning of life **"serenity,"** which contained **"2 teaspoons of independence, 1 tablespoon of persistence, 1.5 tablespoons of confidence, 1 cup of healthy habits, knowledge, and good memory."**	She observed that the Serenity Seasoning had made the bitter gourd less sour than it was when she joined the group. She took additional seasoning ingredients from other group members, felt better, and felt full of ideas for preparing a bitter gourd dish in the future.

a symbolic collection of life experiences and emotional ingredients, such as calmness, gratitude, and bravery, that they had shared and developed through group discussions. Definitional ceremonies were conducted using photo records, in-group witness practice, and a collective declaration to document their individual spiritual seasoning of life. The group renamed their experience of "living with pain" as "living with pain happily." Participants were invited to display their special pass; read a farewell letter, the group declaration, and the final spiritual seasoning of life; and evaluate the group's goals.

When applying this metaphoric framework, after the recipe is done, the practitioner may invite the important people that have been identified by the participants to conduct an *outsider witness* process,[27] which Wood has called "the presenting and re-presenting of the recipe."[28] Through the telling and retelling process (present and re-presenting), personal strengths and preferred identity can be strengthened. We conclude with the lived experiences by applying this Recipe-of-Life metaphor in work with older adults who have chronic pain and their caregivers in Hong Kong.

OUR PROJECT OUTCOMES

During this program, participants used different foods to represent their pain. For instance, some said that their pain was sour as lemon, kiwi, and orange; some said that their pain was spicy as chili pepper or bitter as the bitter gourd. From the interview results of the participants, we observed the following positive effects of the program: (1) rediscovery of personal competence; (2) validation of preferred identity; and (3) fusion of spiritual seasoning of life. Each theme with case examples are given in table 12.5.[29]

The participants reported that the program enabled them to realize that despite facing challenges, they still had strengths. They found that after rediscovering their personal qualities and competencies, their personal power became stronger while the power of the pain grew weaker. In spite of the initial problem-saturated life stories, these participants were able to reconstruct a strengths-based identity after completing the program. In addition, the participants were also inspired by other group members' life recipe ingredients and wanted to add those ingredients to their own recipes. Some participants reported that the program enabled them to "live with happiness rather than pain" as they perceived themselves more capable of enduring their pain.

The following is another case illustration of this process and the effects of group NT using the Recipe-of-Life metaphoric framework. Ms. Zeng's story and the group members' responses to her story demonstrate how this therapy incorporates NT strategies (externalizing, reauthoring, and re-membering conversations and outsider witness practice).[30]

MS. ZENG'S STORY   *Ms. Zeng has lived with chronic pain for six months. The pain in her left body was caused by strokes and it restricted her mobility, especially in her left arm. She described her pain as spicy, like a small chili pepper. She recalled that she learned the symptoms of strokes from her experiences in taking care of her husband and other family members. When she first noticed her stroke symptoms, the first thing she did was to prepare food for her husband so that he could be fed while she was treated in the hospital. She calmly revealed the news of her stroke diagnosis to her youngest daughter and consoled her not to be afraid. Even in her toughest time, she still cared for her family and remained calm and strong.*

Ms. Zeng said that her characteristic of "staying calm" originated from her father's teaching, further influenced by her mother. Her father was a calm person, while her mother was submissive and expressed few personal opinions. Being the eldest daughter in her family, Ms. Zeng believes that she had to be like her father, and she calmly has taken on responsibilities when facing different life situations. During the program, she made up her own recipe for life named "staying calm." The ingredients included self-help, persistence, getting rest, knowledge, and good memory.

From her story, the group members found that Ms. Zeng was very responsible in her social roles, including being a good wife and a good mother, and that she reacted calmly in challenging situations. "Staying calm" and "don't worry" were her father, Mr. Zeng's mottoes, which she used to tackle several difficulties in her life with a positive attitude. After hearing her story, the group members refined her "recipe of life" to include components, such as "strong, brave, happy life, believe in herself, try her best to overcome challenges." Ms. Zeng also accepted the group members' suggestions and included these new ingredients in her recipe. With the support of her life beliefs and the encouragement of the group members, she has found her pain to be more tolerable.[31]

Moreover, Ms. Zeng's life recipe included "confidence, open-mindedness, endurance, strength, acceptance, and being positive" to support herself during the challenging time. Just like Ms. Zeng, other participants in the program also developed their own recipes of lives, recording the values that helped them endure hardships. For example, Mr. Yip's recipe for his chronic pain included "courage to try, persistence, perseverance, being positive, never give up, and distract himself from the pain," which helped him endure the difficult times in his life.

As the program came to an end, each of the participant's recipes was made into a Celebration of Life certificate, which was a reminder of their abilities in overcoming hardship.[32]

CONCLUSION

Chronic musculoskeletal pain is prevalent among older adults, especially in Hong Kong, causing physical, psychological, and social impairments. Not bounded by cultures and age, we recognized that food and cooking would be a good starting point as externalization in therapy. Therefore, by adapting a cooking-related children therapy first applied in Australia, the Hong Kong version of the Recipe-of-Life metaphor was tailor-made to target older adults with chronic pain.

This metaphoric framework helped the participants distance themselves from their chronic pain and reauthor their strengths-based identity in an interesting way. Through this program, the participants increased their self-control and power over their chronic pain. Despite their initial problem-saturated life story, they were able to rediscover the values and social supports that helped them endure tough times, and they learned that they could apply these supports in the future. The group setting also provided mutual social and mental support for participants to form a social cure community.

This Recipe-of-Life metaphor can be applied to using diverse metaphors with people and groups of different needs and backgrounds as a way to acknowledge problems while also helping participants reauthor narratives using a strengths-based approach.

NOTES

1. Regina W. S. Sit et al., "Management of Chronic Musculoskeletal Pain in Hong Kong," *Hong Kong Medical Journal* (*Xianggang yi xue za zhi*) 28, no. 3 (2022): 201–3.

2. M. Stompór et al., "Prevalence of Chronic Pain, Particularly with Neuropathic Component, and Its Effect on Overall Functioning of Elderly Patients," *Medical Science Monitor* 25 (2019): 2695–701, https://doi.org/10.12659/msm .911260.

3. Chi Cheung et al., "Changes in Prevalence, Outcomes, and Help-Seeking Behavior of Chronic Pain in an Aging Population Over the Last Decade," *Pain Practice* 17, no. 5 (2016): 643–54, https://doi.org/10.1111/papr.12496.

4. Ho-Jin Lee et al., "Prevalence of Unrecognized Depression in Patients with Chronic Pain Without a History of Psychiatric Diseases," *Korean Journal of Pain* 31, no. 2 (2018): 116–24; and William H. Roughan et al., "Comorbid Chronic Pain and Depression: Shared Risk Factors and Differential Antidepressant Effectiveness," *Frontiers in Psychiatry* 12 (2021): 643609.

5. Roughan et al., "Comorbid Chronic Pain and Depression."

6. Chi Wai Cheung et al., "Changes in Prevalence, Outcomes, and Help-Seeking Behavior."

7. Sarah Bannon et al., "The Role of Social Isolation in Physical and Emotional Outcomes Among Patients with Chronic Pain," *General Hospital Psychiatry* 69 (2021): 50–54.

8. Esther Oi Wah Chow, *Narrating Faith. Love. Hope: A Practical Manual on Narrative Therapy* (敍出信。愛。望: 敍事治療實務手冊), 2nd ed. (Hong Kong: City University of Hong Kong, 2016).

9. Brandon A. Kohrt, James L. Griffith, and Vikram Patel, "Chronic Pain and Mental Health: Integrated Solutions for Global Problems," *Pain* 159, no. Suppl. 1 (2018): S85; Eloise C. J. Carr, Graham McCaffrey, and Mia Maris Ortiz, "The Suffering of Chronic Pain Patients on a Wait List: Are They Amenable to Narrative Therapy?," *Canadian Journal of Pain* 1, no. 1 (2017): 14–21.

10. Laurel Phillips, "A Narrative Therapy Approach to Dealing with Chronic Pain," *International Journal of Narrative Therapy and Community Work* 1 (2017): 21–30, https://doi.org/10.3316/informit.768720305988235.

11. Chow, *Narrating Faith. Love. Hope.*

12. Chow, *Narrating Faith. Love. Hope.*

13. Natale Rudland Wood, "Recipes for Life," *International Journal of Narrative Therapy and Community Work* 2 (2012): 34–43.

14. Meizi Tan, "Recipes for Life: A Collective Narrative Methodology for Responding to Gender Violence," *International Journal of Narrative Therapy and Community Work* 2 (2017): 1–12.

15. Esther Oi Wah Chow and Doris Yuen Hung Fok, "Recipe of Life: A Relational Narrative Approach in Therapy with Persons Living with Chronic Pain," *Research on Social Work Practice* 30, no. 3 (2020): 320–29, https://doi.org/10.1177/1049731519870867.

16. Chow and Fok, "Recipe of Life: A Relational Narrative Approach."

17. David Denborough, *Collective Narrative Practice: Responding to Individuals, Groups, and Communities Who Have Experienced Trauma* (Adelaide, SA: Dulwich Center, 2008).

18. Chow and Fok, "Recipe of Life: A Relational Narrative Approach."

19. Wood, "Recipes for Life."

20. Wood, "Recipes for Life."

21. Tan, "Recipes for Life: A Collective Narrative Methodology."

22. Tan, "Recipes for Life: A Collective Narrative Methodology."

23. Wood, "Recipes for Life."; and Tan, "Recipes for Life: A Collective Narrative Methodology."

24. Denborough, *Collective Narrative Practice.*

25. Denborough, *Collective Narrative Practice.*

26. Chow and Fok, "Recipe of Life: A Relational Narrative Approach."

27. Chow, *Narrating Faith. Love. Hope*; and Denborough, *Collective Narrative Practice*.
28. Wood, "Recipes for Life."
29. Chow and Fok, "Recipe of Life: A Relational Narrative Approach."
30. Chow, *Narrating Faith. Love. Hope*.
31. Chow, *Narrating Faith. Love. Hope*.
32. Chow, *Narrating Faith. Love. Hope*.

13

RIDING THE RAILS OF RECOVERY

The Train-of-Life Metaphor for Stroke Rehabilitation

ALONG WITH THE Tree-of-Life and Recipe-of-Life metaphors, the Train of Life can also help groups and communities externalize their identity apart from diverse life situations. This metaphor can be particularly helpful when a patient is facing a difficult life situation and trying to view life as a trajectory of stations.

MS. YEUNG'S STORY: FROM A HARD LIFE TO "EASY" *Ms. Yeung, an eighty-year-old woman, was single and never married. For many years, she felt that her life script was burdened by setbacks.*

Being an elite gymnast for the China National Team, her childhood was filled with daily practices. In one of her practices at the age of ten, she severely injured her right knee, which threatened to end her career. It was a huge shock for her, but she was determined to pursue gymnastics. Throughout the months of medical treatments, she continued her gymnastics training. During three years of medical treatment and retraining, she never gave up her career despite the severity of the injury.

Looking back, Ms. Yeung was proud of how she handled this life challenge: she never complained about how the pain tortured her, and she continued to have hope in her future even though she had to give up her life's dream of becoming a champion gymnast.

After she completed her high school studies, she found a job as a salesperson for a Chinese machinery company, which required long working hours. She was proud that she continued this type of work despite the sustained physical pain since her childhood injury, as well as other pain and health issues that had developed in later stages of her life, including cervical spondylosis, which was caused by prolonged head-down typing over a thirty-five-year career. As she grew older, she was diagnosed with glaucoma and has had a constant stinging pain in her right eye.

She also has had trouble stretching her back, which she believed to be the consequence of gymnastics training and long hours of work. Her head and neck have suffered from a lack of cervical support. Because the upper part of her body has tilted forward, she has lived with constant pain all over her body.

Ms. Yeung's story reveals her toughness in dealing with the challenges in her life journey. In narrative practice, we can make use of common communication skills to adopt the Life as a Journey: Train-of-Life metaphor to Ms. Yeung's story.

METAPHORIC FRAMEWORK: TRAIN OF LIFE

This chapter introduces the Train-of-Life metaphoric framework for group narrative therapy (NT). We first illustrate the practical applications of the Train-of-Life metaphoric framework by sharing the therapeutic process applied to a group rehabilitation program. These sessions were developed through real-life scenarios for stroke survivors to help them cope with and adjust to their recovery. We used and evaluated this metaphoric framework in fifteen NT groups with 101 stroke survivors. We compared results with fifteen psychoeducation groups (comparison group; n = 92) in a randomized controlled trial.[1] This framework was found to be an effective alternative practice to psychoeducation therapy.[2] It offers a means for participants to deconstruct the impact of their stroke experience, reauthor their lives, and reconstruct their identities with new hopes and dreams.

DEFINITION

The Train-of-Life metaphoric framework was chosen mutually by the therapist and the group participants collaborating on the storyline development. To apply this metaphoric framework, the therapist invited participants to imagine constructing a train journey that consisted of different life stations (i.e., events from the participants' past and present experiences) to eventually reconstruct the life stations they imaged in their future. During these therapeutic conversations, when participants first introduced themselves to the therapist, almost all of them presented their stories according to a problem-saturated perspective. Helping people externalize their chronic illnesses (e.g., chronic pain and stroke) is a process of deconstruction. By visualizing the series of life events as part of a continuing train journey, group members are able to depart from their previous life stations and move toward coconstructing new stations in the future. According to previous research, narrative group practice has been effective in enhancing survivors' illnesses knowledge, mastery, self-esteem, hope, meaning in life, and life satisfaction.[3] In this chapter, we introduce a method to implement the Train-of-Life metaphoric framework and present quantitative evidence of its effects among older adults surviving from stroke in Hong Kong.

STEPS TO INTEGRATE THE TRAIN-OF-LIFE METAPHORIC FRAMEWORK

The following section is organized by stages to deconstruct, reconstruct, and coconstruct the relationships between stroke survivors and their challenging life situations, after reconnecting them with their purpose and meaning of life. In applying therapeutic conversations, primarily using questions, these conversations can be conducted in the six steps shown in table 13.1.

Table 13.2 outlines the session plan for implementing the Train-of-Life metaphor in working with groups and individuals.

STAGE 0. PREGROUP INTERVIEW: PREPARATION BEFORE PRACTICE Building rapport, the relationships and interactions between participants and the therapist play the most important roles at the beginning of group therapy.[4] At this preliminary stage, the pregroup interviews, the goal is to align appropriate expectations between the person and the therapist. Engagement with

TABLE 13.1 Train-of-Life dialogue

SIX STEPS OF TRAIN-OF-LIFE DIALOGUE	NT STRATEGIC STAGES
1. Engage participants to establish a harmonious station (i.e., a here and now life station).	• Current construct (narrative) exploration
2. Unfold the experience with stroke: • Viewed as an externalized entity from a previous life station • Viewed from the perspective of each of the participants	• Deconstruct problem-saturated narratives
3. Speak directly with stroke.	• Reconstruct
4. Coconstruct the train carriage.	• Coconstuct
5. Plan for a future life journey with stroke (i.e., the next life station).	• New construction celebration
6. Celebrate the unlocking of a new journey.	

TABLE 13.2 Session plan for the Train of Life

SESSION	GROUP NAME OR THEME	OBJECTIVES	STEPS
0	Pregroup interview	• Build rapport • Engage individual participants • Get background information • Provide group details to potential participants • Address concerns • Contract with participants individually	
1	When I had my first encounter with stroke	• Get to know each other • Introduce group objectives and contents; establish individual and group expectations • Set group goals and rules together to establish a trusting and supportive group atmosphere • Understand the impact of stroke on the group members	1. Ask participants to provide a self-introduction 2. Warm up 3. Establish group rules 4. Invite group members to share their stories of stroke 5. Write down individual goals of attending the group 6. Give a name to the collective journey with stroke (collective metaphor) 7. Round up
2	When we met with a stroke	• Externalize the problem • Promote mutual understanding and support with the group members	1. Introduce the content of session and read welcome letter 2. Warm up 3. Name the stroke and the life station with it; evaluate the relationship with stroke (externalizing conversations) 4. Invite group members to share and give feedback (outsider witnesses) 5. Round up
3	When we live with stroke	• Externalize the problem • Promote mutual understanding and support among group members, increasing sense of belonging and cohesion	1. Review the content of last session 2. Warm up 3. Name the stroke and the life station with stroke; evaluate the relationship with stroke (externalizing conversations) 4. Invite group members to share and give feedback (outsider witnesses) 5. Round up
4	When we talk to stroke	• Personify the character of stroke by medical professional • Talk with "Stroke" directly by asking structured questions about medical knowledge of stroke • Evaluate the relationship with stroke	1. Review the content of last session 2. Warm up 3. Talk with "Stroke": invite a medical professional to play as a "Ms./Mr. Stroke" and have the group members ask questions freely 4. Round up

SESSION	GROUP NAME OR THEME	OBJECTIVES	STEPS
5	**When I fight against stroke**	• Hold reauthoring conversations: discover unique outcomes and ask landscape-of-action questions and landscape-of-identity questions • Coconstruct the new storyline combating with stroke	1. Review the content of last session 2. Warm up 3. Discover the instances and events that do not fit with the problem-saturated stories with stroke 4. Explore the values, beliefs, and desires behind the unique outcomes 5. Invite group members to share and give feedback (outsider witnesses) 6. Round up
6	**When we fight against stroke**	• Hold reauthoring conversations: ask landscape-of-action questions and landscape-of-identity questions • Coconstruct the new storyline combating with stroke	1. Review the content of last session 2. Warm up 3. Identify valued identity behind behaviors 4. Name the new life station with stroke 5. Name the collective plan for future life journeys with stroke 6. Invite group members to share and give feedback (outsider witnesses) 7. Round up
7	**The stroke is still there, but we are always smiling**	• Thicken the alternative stories: re-membering conversations • Discover the participant's contribution to the figure's life and the implication of this contribution for the figure's identity	1. Review the content of last session 2. Warm up 3. Auction results: review the results they have shared and ask them to bid on things they value, including people, objects, beliefs, expectations, and life goals 4. Invite group members to share and give feedback (outsider witnesses) 5. Round up
8	**Future life with stroke**	• Evaluate the effectiveness of the group • Summarize the positive effect	1. Review the content of last session 2. Warm up 3. Read the group members' thank-you letter and give feedback 4. Consolidate the preferred storyline and identity: invite the group members to share their expectation of their future life 5. Hold definitional ceremonies: celebrate the grand opening of a new journey with stroke 6. Round up

individual participants begins with pregroup interviews, in which the therapist will:

Ask about the individuals' background information,
Brief them on the details and process of the group work,
Address concerns, and
Contract with the participants individually.

Questions that can facilitate this process include the following: "How is your life being affected by stroke, and how would you describe yourself after stroke?" and "If you could make some changes in your life, what would you want to change?" These questions allow the therapist to better understand the situation and each participant's self-concept, and thus they form a therapeutic alliance between the therapist and participant, so that they can develop a therapeutic goal and plan collaboratively.

STAGE 1: DECONSTRUCTING PROBLEM-SATURATED STORIES Many stroke patients blame their perceived internal failings, especially eating habits and lifestyle, as they face their disabilities, biomedical discourse, and social stigma brought on by the stroke.[5] Losing physical function and freedom, along with a slow and sometimes sporadic recovery process, persons often perceive themselves as "useless" and "worthless" and would internalize the belief of being a "burden" to their family and society. This can cause them to "internalize" the problem and see it as a personal failure, which could eventually become their whole identity and their "internal state of self."[6] Narrative therapists seek to help these participants separate their identities from the problem by deconstructing the problem-saturated stories and creating a therapeutic space for them to develop a different life perspective through externalizing conversations.[7]

The stage of deconstruction of problem-saturated stores consists of the first three successive steps of Train-of-Life dialogue:

1. Beginning from a harmonious station
2. Unfolding the experience in meeting with stroke
3. Dialoguing directly with the stroke

At the first step, beginning from a harmonious station, our goal is to set an equal position between the therapist and the participants as they are going to develop the metaphor together. The therapist respects the persons as the "experts" in their own lives and takes on the role of an empathetic listener while listening to their life stories. In this scenario, the Life as a Journey: Train-of-Life metaphor emerges: therapists and the participants would name the place in which they first met the harmonious station. This station acts as concord life station, which is a hub for sharing and linking the life experiences shared by the participants because they are now on a joint train journey to depart from their past lives in hardships.

The therapist may begin by disclosing his or her pathway leading to this harmonious station. Following are some suggestions explaining how the therapist could start the conversation for Step 1, Beginning from a harmonious station:

1. Here is the ABC Center. Let's call it the ABC Station, where we will meet and begin our journey.
2. Let me share the reason why I came to this station. I come from XYZ (a district) and work to understand the effects of stroke on individuals. I call stroke a "trouble" that has imposed many limitations on older adults and their loved ones (and I share my personal experience in caring for a stroke survivor). This trouble has indeed paved my pathway when working with stroke survivors. I would describe my experience with stroke as my service to those who I care about and respect. Therefore, I came from this Service Station.

Step 2, Unfolding the Experience in Meeting with Stroke, and Step 3, Speaking Directly with the Stroke, share the underlying characteristic of externalizing the problem.

During Step 2, participants are asked to describe and reflect on their experience of living with a stroke. They have to define and give a concrete account of the impact of stroke on their life, including how the stroke has affected their way of living or reactions from themselves and their families. This is followed by an evaluation of their relationship with the stroke. People are encouraged to contemplate and report any positive, negative, or mixed influences on their identity. Participants are then invited to give a self-selected name in describing their life-altering station that they have passed through (e.g., past life station), such as "Station of Darkness." Finally, participants link their individual life stations together by sharing mutual experiences and naming this stroke journey as a group (e.g., the Bittersweet Journey). Following is an example of an externalizing conversation from Steps 2 and 3:

THERAPIST: *What is it like for you living with stroke?*

MAY (PARTICIPANT): *It* [the stroke] *has totally changed my life, as I have become physically dependent on my spouse for personal care. I am not able to move around by myself—I have to walk with aids and cannot even go to the toilet by myself on some occasions. My family members worry about me, and [they] don't allow me to go out alone.*

THERAPIST: *How would you describe this stroke?*

MAY: *It's like a "rope"* [naming of the stroke] *that holds me back at home and restricts my life. I have become a prisoner and a useless person* [a person with a problem-saturated identity].

THERAPIST: *If you have to name this specific experience with stroke as one of your life stations, what name would you give to this station?*

MAY: *I would call this life station "Restriction."*

This series of externalizing conversations allows participants to separate problem-saturated events from their identity. In so doing, they can witness and acknowledge the effects of chronic illness on their lives, thereby exploring their knowledge, skills, and ways of responding to chronic illness and its effects.[8]

In addition, by sharing stories in a group with others who have been through similar experiences, participants can further externalize their problem situations. This helps them understand that they are not alone in their struggles, which encourages them to overcome feelings of isolation, develop mutuality, and form social connection.[9]

THERAPIST: *Now we know where we come from. Indeed, as a group, we share a life experience with stroke. If we have to designate this stage of life experience together as one part of our life journey, how would we name it?*

GROUP: *A Bumpy Railway Line . . . Tunnel of Despair . . . Rehabilitation Railway Line.*

To further externalize the experience of stroke from the participants, they were invited to Speak Directly with the Stroke (Step 3), as personified by medical professionals. The conversation progressed from conveying perceived knowledge of stroke to exploring the emotional aspects of the stroke experience. By enhancing their sense of self-agency and repositioning their relationships with stroke, this process empowered participants to draw conclusions and to find closure with the period in which they felt controlled by the stroke.[10] The practice of direct discourse also fostered feelings of gratitude toward their supporters and toward what they still had and cherished. As participants further separated themselves from the problem-saturated stories and identity (i.e., externalizing the problems), they developed insight into the uncontrollable nature of stroke, such as stroke attacks, and the importance of not letting this experience define their identity or self-worth.

STAGE 2: RECONSTRUCTING ALTERNATIVE STORIES   After successfully externalizing the problem, the group engaged in reauthoring conversations to construct alternative storylines.[11] This process involved discovering unique outcomes, the landscape of actions, and the landscape of identity questions, which constituted Step 4, Coconstructing the Train Carriage in the Train-of-Life metaphoric framework.

Each person was invited to share the characteristics of their train carriage, which carried them away from the plight of the life station at which they first experienced the stroke. To identify the carriage characteristics, narrative therapists helped participants explore some of the forgotten but potentially significant life events and distinct beliefs, qualities, abilities, purposes, and commitments that have been deeply rooted in their identity since their earliest memories.[12] In NT, these components are considered "unique outcomes."[13] This step allowed individuals to discover other ways of living, which empowered them to live out their preferred identities and storylines. Following is an example of a therapist uncovering the unique outcomes of a group member:

THERAPIST: *What helps you to pass through the life station where you met stroke? Tell us the characteristics of your carriage that makes you stronger?*
PETER (PARTICIPANT):   *My train carriage is made up of hard work and persistence . . . through observing diet control and doing exercises regularly . . . it carried me away from the Devil Station, where I was stuck with [the] stroke, and where my life was altered. Also, determination is the fuel that has taken me this far . . .*
THERAPIST: *You have mentioned that being hardworking, persistent, and determined is your main source of energy. When did you become determined? Please tell us a story about your "determination."*

To uncover unique outcomes and create an alternative story, therapists ask questions about the "landscape of action" and "landscape of identity."[14]

Landscape-of-action questions involve inquiries into events and actions about what, where, why, when, who, and how participants are coping with their problem.[15] These types of questions help people link these events to an alternative storyline.

Landscape-of-identity' questions elicit information about the commitments, principles, dreams, hopes, values, beliefs, and purposes that inform the actions that the participants have taken.[16] Landscape-of-identity' questions also invite people to reflect on their identities and others, to relate the alternative storyline to the person's understanding of his or her preferred identity.[17]

The following is an example of landscape-of-action and landscape-of-identity questions that emerged in the process of uncovering unique outcomes:

(Continued from previous conversation)

PETER: *Yes! I got to know "determination" when I was ten. I promised my father to take care of my younger brother and sister when he was chronically ill.*

THERAPIST: *What have you done to know "determination" more?*

PETER: *I know if I persevere and work hard, I will reach my goal one day. That was how I worked full-time to help my mother to raise a family of four, and how I completed my high school education on a part-time basis* [landscape of action].

THERAPIST: *You had to take up such a heavy responsibility when you were very young?*

PETER: *Being the oldest son, I just knew that I have to support my mother to raise the family. We had already lost one parent. I knew that if I worked faster and harder, it would make a great difference* [landscape of identity].

THERAPIST: *Being a good son and a caring brother were important to you since the early stage of your life. It seems that "determination" has helped you to achieve these identities and to fulfil these roles.*

The narrative therapist guided the participants to reflect on and discover instances and events that did not align with the person's problem-saturated stories. This process helped the participants to recognize their will and ability to live a meaningful life, and the existence of infinite possibilities beyond their current seemingly problem-saturated stories caused by stroke. By reconnecting with the values, beliefs, and desires behind these unique outcomes, participants regained their sense of personal agency and worthiness, reconstructed preferred identities, and envisioned possible futures.

STAGE 3A: THICKENING THE ALTERNATIVE STORIES Once an alternative story was reconstructed, the final stage was to thicken their story, which constituted Steps 5 and 6 of the Train-of-Life metaphoric framework. By conducting re-membering conversations, inviting an outsider witness group, and performing definitional ceremonies, we worked to plan for and celebrate the participant's new train journey embracing the stroke.[18]

Narrative therapists believe that the sense of self is socially constructed and exists in relationships with others (i.e., an association of life).[19] Thus, re-membering conversations enrich each person's view of their capabilities, connecting them to significant people in their preferred storylines.

These conversations provided an opportunity for individuals to revise their membership in these associations and describe the alternative stories that have been cogenerated within these relationships.[20] For instance, participants identified and mentioned important people from their past and their positive contributions. The therapist facilitated this process by using a series of re-membering questions to prompt individuals to describe what they, in turn, have contributed to the significant figure's life and sense of identity. Re-membering conversations like this created opportunities for individuals to view their lives through the eyes of these significant people—a view that was not influenced by negative judgments from other people.[21]

(Continued from previous conversation)

THERAPIST: *When and from whom did you acquire such ability, knowledge, quality, or belief?*
PETER: *I learned this from my mother, who had a hard life after my father passed away when I was only ten. She was "determined" to "stand on her feet," and to raise the three of us all by herself, holding on to these values and beliefs. Also, I know that my family needs me, so I have to stand on my feet and take up my responsibilities as a husband and a father.*
THERAPIST: *If she [your mother] knew that you have been holding onto these beliefs during these challenging years, that they have helped you in maintaining a distance from [the] stroke and cherishing your family, what would she say?*
PETER: *I think she would feel very proud of me [in deep thought with tears].*

In outsider witness practice, narrative therapists invite an audience, which can include family, friends, or community members, to witness, acknowledge, and give feedback on the alternative stories and identity of the participants through the practice of telling and retelling.[22] These conversations with outsider witnesses thicken the participants' stories of coping and their preferred identity. Additionally, participants' testimonies can impress on and resonate with the audience members and can contribute to their resilience as well. At this point, the participants' senses of capability and worthiness are enhanced.[23]

Outsider individuals who faced similar physical conditions were invited to join as members of the reflecting team or to serve as witnesses. Following is an example of outsider witnessing:

THERAPIST: *Tom, what do you think about Joe's story? What expressions or images resonate with you?*

TOM/WITNESS: *The expression of "I'll always stand by you" and experiences of Joe and his wife resonated with me.*

THERAPIST: *Why did their experiences draw your attention?*

TOM/WITNESS: *I learned from their loving care and mutual support as a couple and the way they use their life wisdom to tackle the experience with illness. Now, I understand my wife's complaints are actually utterances of love, and I'm grateful that I am not walking alone. . . . I feel that I am treasured by my family and friends, who have been walking with me and supporting me all along.*

At the same time, as participants renamed the problem, their perspective on the stroke changes and its influence was evident. Examples of this shift in perspective include the following: from a "Tsunami" (unable to predict and control) to "Red Rain" (able to control when it occurs again) and from a "Stormy" station (the devastating impact of stroke) to a "Lucky Me" station (appreciation of self and others). Participants also recognized their preferred identities and rediscovered their values and beliefs—for instance, one member changed his self-description from being a "Useless" person (a problem-saturated identity of having no abilities and being a burden to others) to a person filled with "Gratitude" (a person who is valued by their spouse and respected by their children; a person who uses one's life experience to help others), from being a "Hopeless" person (with no sense of future) to a person filled with "Hope[s] and dreams."

STAGE 3B: CELEBRATING THE OPENING OF THE NEW TRAIN JOURNEY
The stroke survivors next constructed their "Future Life Station,"—that is, the beginning of their preferred ways of living. Participants were asked landscapes-of-action and landscapes-of-identity questions complete Step 5, Planning for a Future Life with Stroke. Examples questions are as follows: "What station do you want to create for your new journey with Stroke?"

and "Why is such a station so important to you and how can you reach that station?" Following are example answers from the group:

THERAPIST: *We are now planning for a future life journey. What station do you want to build in your new journey with a stroke?*
JOHN (PARTICIPANT): *A station of "health."*
THERAPIST: *A station of "health." What kind of health do you want?*
JOHN: *All kinds of health — social, psychological, and spiritual. However, the most important is physical health.*
THERAPIST: *What do you need to do to reach that station of "health"?*
JOHN: *I need to stop smoking and drinking, and eat healthily* [landscape of action].
THERAPIST: *Why do you need to be healthy? Why is such a station important to you?*
JOHN: *I want to regain my freedom, to have a wonderful life, and to spend more time with my wife and my family.*
THERAPIST: *I see that being a good husband and a good father* [landscape of identity] *is important in your life.*

Other examples of future life stations included hope, prudence, kindness, courage, and faith. Once all participants had individually created their new stations with stroke, the therapist invited the group to name their new journey with stroke collectively. Examples of the new life journey included the "Changing for the Better" rail line, "Silver Lining" rail line, and "Striving for Good Lives" rail line.

At the end of the group therapy, participants completed Step 6, "Celebrating the Unlocking of a New Journey." This definitional ceremony provided the context in which to celebrate significant steps along this journey and the participants' successful transition from a problem-saturated story to an alternative storyline.[24] Under the witness of the therapist, group members, and outsider audiences, the group navigated through their struggles and moved beyond their feelings of despair. They pulled a "life carriage" together, passed through the "tunnel of despair," and embarked on a new journey along the "Resilience" rail line.

The therapist introduced the opening of the new railway line by saying:

We would like to have a grand opening for our new train journey, to witness the start of the "Breakthrough and Rekindling the Light of Life" railway line beginning today.

Then, the therapist invited participants to cut a ribbon and start the opening ceremony as a group.

Throughout these therapeutic conversations, therapists may collect materials in any forms, such as letters, certificates, videotapes, pictures, or other documents. These materials not only contribute to the thickening of alternative stories but also can be referred to as therapeutic documents.[25]

PROJECT OUTCOMES

According to the demographic information and clinical characteristics of the sample participants at baseline, of the 192 original participants, 33 (17.19 percent) dropped out throughout the data collection time. More than half of the participants in the intervention group (61.46 percent) and the treatment as usual (TAU) group (62.50 percent) were men. The mean age of the stroke survivors in the intervention and TAU groups were $M = 72.49$ (SD: 7.27) and $M = 72.84$ (SD: 7.82), respectively. The majority of participants suffered an ischemic stroke (intervention: 83.72 percent, TAU: 81.82 percent). Initial Mini-Mental State Examination (MMSE) scores were similar in the two groups (intervention: 26.11 percent; TAU: 26.24 percent). We did not observe any other significant differences between the intervention and the TAU group for all clinical characteristics and selected demographic information. We did not observe any significant differences in the selected outcome variables at baseline between the intervention and TAU groups; thus, both groups were deemed comparable at baseline.

Repeated analysis of variance (ANOVA) measures were completed to compare the patterns of outcome change over time between the two groups. In the intervention group, significant time effects were demonstrated across all seven outcome measures: self-esteem, sense of mastery, hope, meaning of life, depression, life satisfaction, and stroke knowledge. For the control group, however, a significant time effect was found only in the meaning in life ($F (3, 246) = 3.28$, $p = 0.02$), hope ($F (3, 237) = 3.15$, $p = 0.03$), self-esteem ($F (3, 243) = 2.70$, $p = 0.49$), and stroke knowledge ($F (3, 234) = 43.35$, $p < 0.001$). We further investigated the noted change patterns over time in their mean plots, which suggested that the patterns of change over time in the outcome measures across intervention and the TAU groups were statistically different. Furthermore, many of these positive effects were sustained four-months postintervention, in the intervention group. Pairwise comparisons revealed that hope, meaning in life, self-esteem, and stroke knowledge had significant changes between T_0 and T_1, T_0 and T_2, and T_0 and T_3.

To further delineate intervention effectiveness, we conducted a regression of change between (1) T_1 and T_0, (2) T_2 and T_0, and (3) T_3 and T_0. These analyses indicated a delineated pattern: NT showed a higher improvement in most outcome scores over the conventional psychoeducation intervention. Results further indicated that the intervention group significantly improved in mastery ($R^2 = 0.04$, F $(1, 174) = 7.12$, $p = 0.05$), hope ($R^2 = 0.04$, F $(1, 176) = 7.24$, $p = 0.05$), meaning of life ($R^2 = 0.04$, F $(1, 172) = 7.04$, $p = 0.01$) and life satisfaction ($R^2 = 0.04$, F $(1, 178) = 6.72$, $p = 0.05$), at postintervention versus baseline. Improvement of self-esteem was marginally significant between interim and baseline in the intervention group $R^2 = 0.02$, F $(1, 179) = 3.60$, $p = 0.06$. Regarding stroke knowledge, a negative mean difference, although insignificant, seemed understandable, suggesting that the relative effects of NT and the psychoeducation group were similar.

The results of these analyses supported our contention that NT is beneficial in reconnecting a person's sense of mastery, enhancing self-esteem, and reconstructing the meaning of life with hope (i.e., ascribing more positive meaning to a critical life event) while also having other positive influences on depression and satisfaction of life.

At the beginning of this chapter, we presented Ms. Yeung's story as a case illustration. In our conversation with her, we invited her to name her pain by using the Train-of-Life metaphor. In unfolding her experience with pain, Ms. Yeung described the onset of her pain as a "burden" that had unconsciously and gradually worsened over time, limiting her mobility and restraining her abilities. By contextualizing her pain in the Life Train metaphor, she recognized that it had left her feeling trapped in a station of life she named "Harsh." After naming the pain and the life stations, we invited Ms. Yeung to reflect on the illness's impact on her life and her dialogue with the illness.

She feels that this "heavy burden" placed additional obstacles in her life. Although she was proud of her life after quitting gymnastics, she still experienced the feeling of being a victim of chronic pain. Holding the belief that chronic pain was problem-saturated, she felt helpless to fight it and that life had been unfair. This internalized belief of being the "burden," led her to give up trying to reach on higher achievements after she had to stop elite gymnastics. Since then, she described her life as becoming cold and depressed, and she no longer had the energy to move on.

Through scaffolding and an externalizing dialogue, Ms. Yeung learned to separate herself from that burden and to take control of her life. After having a direct conversation with the "burden," she recognized that chronic pain had become a part of her identity like an "invisible demon." At this point in her treatment, she became determined to move on from this "harsh" life station and to distance herself from this "burden."

Having named and deconstructed the effects of the problem, the next step was to coconstruct alternative storylines through reauthoring conversations using the train journey metaphor.[26] To reauthor the story, we invited Ms. Yeung to discover the "unique outcomes" during her illness. Despite the significant impact of living with this dreadful "demon" (i.e., a sense of failure as a result of limitations from chronic pain), she found that engaging in activities and learning new things helped to mitigate the "demon," which lessened the pain. Her curiosity and determination eventually turned the "invisible demon" into a "friend," enabling her to persevere through difficult times.

Ms. Yeung's deeply ingrained positive belief that "there are many solutions to every problem" played a crucial role in combating the "invisible demon" of chronic pain. Through a narrative reauthoring dialogue and good adherence to medication, her pain no longer was a central force in her life. She has since named her life carriage as "hopeful," drawing on curiosity, determination, and perseverance as the fuel for her future life journey. Rediscovering values behind the unique outcomes of her chronic pain that helped her conquer it, Ms. Yeung has a newly constructed life story and can now master her life and carry on with the power of hope. At the end of this conversation, Ms. Yeung happily described her growth of moving from the "Harsh" life station to the "Gratification" life station. In revisiting all her narratives, she identified continuous trials that testified to her faith and made her grow stronger.

Similarly, we can find the story of Mr. Huang and his wife Ms. Feng and their growth after completing the program.

MR. FENG AND MS. HUANG'S STORY   Couples who have been married for several years may not see each other's sincere love in their lives. In adversity, one partner will persevere, endure and understand, and give quietly to the other, while the other partner, in facing "his or her own difficulties," will freely vent his or her unhappy feelings. When they do feel the "loving care," however, this scolding will disappear, gratitude can be reversed, and mutual love will be restored. Following is the story between Mr. Feng and Ms. Huang (aka Mrs. Feng):

When he came home from [the hospital after] his stroke, he needed my close attention because of his mobility problems, which made me get very angry so easily. I got so angry," said Ms. Huang, who once thought about divorce. "I really wanted to jump to my death, but when I thought of my son and daughter and his dedication to the family, I stopped." Ms. Huang said.

"I can't volunteer, I can't sing Cantonese songs at the senior center to entertain the elderly, I feel stressed and have no fun in life." While suffering from back pain, she has been able to endure the scolding from her husband. She has not given up on her husband.

"Stroke is a devil, a witch, it makes me lose my freedom, I have to quit talking, and it makes me lose my temper." said Mr. Feng, her seventy-year-old partner. At this time, the couple's relationship was also in the dark, with constant bickering and conflict.

"Fortunately, we joined a support group which allowed my wife to vent her frustrations and receive more support from people other than her children; she also learned how to help me in testing my blood sugar levels. Moreover, I met a lot of positive people who are in the same boat, which made me start to appreciate the hard work and care of my family, especially my wife. My wife takes me to acupuncture, and my children worry about me. Therefore, I must take my medication on time, listen to the doctor, and exercise hard for my own good and for my wife's good, so that she could have a moment of freedom again. Also, I had a temper tantrum that hurt my wife and made me feel bad. After the stroke, I felt my wife's love for me, so I have to get rid of this demon and cannot have another stroke."

Since then, with the support of his wife, he started going out for walks every day after dinner. "After the stroke, I have to go out with my wife. After the stroke, I want to live a happier and better life with my wife, experiencing more colorful moments and traveling more together, like a rainbow after the rain. I hope we can work together until the end and be healthy all the way."

CONCLUSION

In NT, we have found that the Train-of-Life metaphoric framework is particularly useful for stroke survivors and chronic pain patients. By encouraging individuals to view their experiences as part of a life journey, this metaphor enables them to deconstruct their illness experience by naming and renaming different "life stations," gaining a broader perspective about their lives. On this voyage of self-discovery, they are able to deconstruct problem-saturated identities, reauthor a preferred identity, and regain their sense of agency. Moreover, we have emphasized the vital role of language and narrative in the therapeutic alliance. This is particularly important when helping individuals externalize their struggles. Therefore, it is crucial for practitioners to apply language- and narrative-based principles in counseling and psychotherapy. Individuals who have experienced a sudden loss of body control as a result of chronic pain or stroke often struggle with their self-esteem, especially when they are unable to fulfil their normal daily roles in the family or workplace. With a deeper understanding of these challenges, practitioners can provide effective support and guidance, empowering individuals to continue their life journey with joy and freedom, free from the unwanted limitations imposed by their illness.

NOTES

1. Esther Oi-Wah Chow, "Narrative Therapy and Evaluated Intervention to Improve Stroke Survivors' Social and Emotional Adaptation," *Clinical Rehabilitation* 29, no. 4 (2015): 315–26, https://doi.org/10.1177/0269215514544039.
2. Esther Oi-Wah Chow, "Narrative Group Intervention to Reconstruct Meaning of Life Among Stroke Survivors: A Randomized Clinical Trial Study," *Neuropsychiatry* 8, no. 4 (2018): 1216–26, https://doi.org/10.4172/Neuropsychiatry.1000450.
3. Chow, "Narrative Group Intervention to Reconstruct Meaning."
4. Karla Krogsrud Miley, Michael O'Melia, and Brenda DuBois, *Generalist Social Work Practice: An Empowering Approach*, 7th ed. (Boston: Pearson, 2013).
5. Michael White, "The Externalizing of the Problem and the Re-Authoring of Lives and Relationships," *Dulwich Centre Newsletter* (Summer 1989).
6. Maggie Carey and Shona Russell, *Narrative Therapy: Responding to Your Questions* (Adelaide, SA: Dulwich Centre, 2004).
7. Ruthellen Josselson, "Narrative Research and the Challenge of Accumulating Knowledge," *Narrative Inquiry* 16, no. 1 (2006): 3–10.
8. Esther Oi-Wah Chow, "Responding to Lives After Stroke: Narrative Therapy with Stroke Survivors and Caregivers," *International Journal of Reminiscence and Life Review* (10th Biennial Conference, New Orleans, LA, 2013).
9. Chow, "Narrative Therapy and Evaluated Intervention."
10. Yvonne Sliep, "A Narrative Theatre Approach to Working with Communities Affected by Trauma, Conflict and War," *International Journal of Narrative Therapy and Community Work* 2005, no. 2 (2005): 47–52.
11. Carey and Russell, *Narrative Therapy*; and Michael Kingsley White, *Maps of Narrative Practice* (New York: Norton, 2007).

12. David Denborough, *Collective Narrative Practice* (Adelaide, SA: Dulwich Centre, 2008).
13. White, "The Externalizing of the Problem."
14. Carey and Russell, *Narrative Therapy.*
15. Edward M. Bruner, *The Anthropology of Experience* (Urbana: University of Illinois Press, 1986); and White, *Maps of Narrative Practice.*
16. Denborough, *Collective Narrative Practice.*
17. White, "The Externalizing of the Problem."
18. Josselson, "Narrative Research and the Challenge of Accumulating Knowledge."
19. Carey and Russell, *Narrative Therapy.*
20. White, "The Externalizing of the Problem"; and White, *Maps of Narrative Practice.*
21. Maggie Carey and Shona Russell, "Externalising: Commonly Asked Questions," *International Journal of Narrative Therapy and Community Work* 2 (2002): 76–84.
22. Carey and Russell, *Narrative Therapy.*
23. G. W. Burns, *Healing with Stories in Your Casebook Collection for Using Therapeutic Metaphors* (Hoboken, NJ: Wiley, 2007); Denborough, *Collective Narrative Practice*; and David Denborough, *Kite of Life: From Intergenerational Conflict to Intergenerational Alliance* (Adelaide, SA: Dulwich Centre, 2010).
24. Josselson, "Narrative Research and the Challenge of Accumulating Knowledge.
25. Josselson, "Narrative Research and the Challenge of Accumulating Knowledge."
26. Carey and Russell, *Narrative Therapy*; and White, *Maps of Narrative Practice.*

14

UNIFYING NARRATIVES

Building Inclusive Community Through Collective Practice

TRADITIONAL CLINICAL PRACTICE of narrative therapy (NT) has been one on one or in groups (e.g., family members). In recent years, however, the growing trend has been toward the use of NT on a collective level (i.e., groups and communities) to address life challenges, specifically for people experiencing stigma and trauma. Research on the effects of NT at the collective level is still developing. Limited studies have shown that this relatively novel use of NT is beneficial for chronically ill survivors, community-dwelling older adults, mental health professionals, and society at large. This chapter summarizes some of the existing research on the impacts of collective narrative practice among different stakeholders (i.e., chronically ill survivors and their caregivers, and older and younger learners) and also presents some recent studies.[1] These studies have included applications of "narra-drama" and intergenerational Playback Theater performances to document their effects on rediscovering life wisdom and coping strength in middle-age and older people living with chronic illnesses, such as stroke and chronic pain.[2] This chapter also discusses the use of Playback Theater to facilitate cross-generational understanding and exchanges through collective narrative practice in Hong Kong.

INDIVIDUAL AND GROUP NARRATIVE PRACTICE

Over the past two decades, the outcomes of NT used on individuals who suffer from physical and psychological illnesses and their family or informal caregivers have been widely discussed (chapter 2). Examples of targeted populations in the existing studies include families living with acquired brain injury,[3] people with chronic pain,[4] stroke survivors,[5] people with trauma,[6] and primary caregivers of people with schizophrenia.[7] A number of studies have examined the effects of both NT and drama therapy on people who have substance use issues.[8] Individual and group therapies have also been applied to people who live with abusive partners, legal offenders, and chronically homeless people.[9] As mentioned in chapters 4 and 11 to 13, externalizing conversation skills can be used to separate personal problems from a person's problem-saturated identity through group practice, rediscover inner strengths, facilitate meaning-making, and create alternative narratives of life events.[10] All of these skills can help individuals rediscover and reconstruct their preferred identities as they begin to live a new life. Because our social structures have embedded misunderstandings of and bias toward stigmatized groups, other levels of intervention have to be in place to allow their voices be heard. Providing interactive platforms for different stakeholders through drama can be a means to bridge and cultivate understanding and positive changes.

WHAT IS COLLECTIVE NARRATIVE PRACTICE?

The rationale underpinning the collective narrative practice lies in postmodernism and social constructionism, which challenge the dominant and privileged narratives and question the power involved in the story construction process.[11] These practices suggest the redistribution of power between the therapist/practitioner and the client/individual.[12] According to postmodernism and social constructionism, "no fixed truth" and "no master narrative" will totalize the experiences of different people.[13] In clinical practice, postmodernist therapists/practitioners are aware of the power imbalance between the therapists/practitioners and the clients/people in the therapeutic process, and they seek to ensure the active participation of the people who consult social workers/practitioners or counselors so that their voices and beliefs can be heard through a collective process of therapeutic inquiry.[14] Practitioners favor stories that are derived from individual lived experiences and suggest that the therapist and the person work together to coconstruct preferred life narratives, with the therapy role supporting the narrative flow of these people to honor individual stories and strengths.[15]

Following the underlying principle of postmodernism and social constructionism, collective narrative practice goes beyond the group setting, and links individuals with similar experiences to give voice to parts of society that have been marginalized or historically seen as disadvantaged. The goal is to reduce stigmatization by recreating narratives and bringing them back to society's center.[16] By mobilizing societal groups with shared concerns, skills, knowledge bases, and abilities,[17] their voices and contributions can collectively bring about societal change, inspire hope, enhance societal understanding, and rectify societal misconceptions.[18] Collective narrative practice can be used to facilitate "narrative justice."[19] According to David Denborough, when trauma or life challenges are encountered by the people who seek therapeutic help, this process involves a form of social injustice that cannot be manifested in the existing justice system alone. The process of enabling these people to regain justice through narrative practices allows for deeper healing at the individual, community, and societal levels.[20] Given that the importance of bringing justice back to these people has often been neglected in traditional psychotherapeutic settings, Denborough has proposed the following three-stage framework of facilitating "narrative justice" through a collective narrative practice: (1) acknowledging multiple injustice and effects; (2) acknowledging the shared ideals and values that have survived through the injustice; and (3) convening forums of narrative justice to enable the contributions of the "survivors" of the injustice, thereby honoring their experiences and promoting their ability to seek justice collectively. This three-stage framework is elaborated in a later part of this chapter.

EXAMPLES OF COLLECTIVE NARRATIVE PRACTICES IN OTHER COUNTRIES

Only limited studies have discussed the impact and benefits of using collective narrative practice, and studies to date have usually been qualitative. This may be partly because collective narrative practice is presented as a practice, or an event, despite the fact that it has been developed and widely used in many places globally, and has involved collaboration and support from various stakeholders in society. The goals of collective narrative practice can be achieved through different mediums, including drawing, drama,[21] poems and letter writing,[22] and other approaches. In this section, we introduce the use of collective narrative practice in theater performances and therapeutic documents.[23]

The first example is Playback Theater. Playback Ψ, the first Playback Theater team in Greece, was formed by a group of professional performers and psychotherapists in 2004.[24] Playback Theater is an approach in which the audience shares their personal stories, and the playback players and performers enact the stories in an improvisational manner immediately after they hear these stories.[25] A Playback Theater performance provides a platform for a combination of different stories that are shared by the audience. The significance of the story and the dialectic process are created through the connection among the different storytellers.[26] This process provides an opportunity for reflection from different perspectives for the storytellers, players and performers, and the audience. Playback Ψ has used Playback Theater as a tool to increase understanding and reduce the societal stigma associated with individuals with mental illnesses, their families, and mental health professionals since 2004. With the trust and support of many people, the Playback Ψ performance team has successfully staged around five hundred performances with a wide platform of styles and audiences, including in group homes, day centers and hospitals, and mental health seminars, as well as at international festivals like the World Playback Week in London in 2012, which included not only patients and mental health professionals but also the general public. Playback Ψ is a rare example of conducting a long-running collective narrative practice established nationwide, a number of collective narrative practice projects or programs have been implemented on a smaller scale in different countries.

Programs using drama and theater as aids also have been adapted to other contexts to develop mutual understanding. In Memphis, Tennessee, in the United States, a program called "Performing the Peace" brought together police officers and ex-offenders to learn about and perform each other's life experiences.[27] Although mostly done in a closed setting, this program has also been performed before a general audience. Similarly, in the United Kingdom, a minimum-security forensic mental health service, under the Forensic Directorate of the Mental Health National Health Service Trust, organized a thirteen-week pilot project collective narrative called the "Knowledge Group," which enrolled a small group of its service users who were preparing for discharge.[28] The group made a booklet about their life experiences that included the phases of their life before offending, living in the ward, preparing for discharge, and their hopes for the future. This project attracted the interest of involved stakeholders, and the closing ceremony of the program included other service users as well as mental health and welfare professionals who took turns as both audience and players and performers to discuss how the "Knowledge Group" affected them.

SUMMARY OF FINDINGS

Current findings indicate that collective narrative practices are beneficial to individuals, groups, and society. At the individual and group level, these narrative practices, such Playback Theater, facilitate meaning-making by recognizing and validating personal strengths and abilities openly on the stage; which provides a cathartic outlet for societal misunderstandings, biases, stereotypes, and labels.[29] In addition, these practices give society's disadvantaged groups the opportunity to refute these misconceptions with diverse stakeholders within society.[30] Moreover, collective narrative practices give them an opportunity to be seen in an alternative role as "the expert" or "the educator" of their own lives and struggles, rather than just patients and aid recipients.[31] In this expert role, they can transfer knowledge gained from their experiences to their audiences at large, which places them in a special social role to educate the public and give back to society.[32]

At the collective level, narrative practices could be a tool for social education and cultural reform. When the general public engages in narrative practices, they gain firsthand, authentic, positive insight from people who have been regarded as marginalized.[33] For instance, Playback Ψ audiences not only found the storytellers entertaining but also felt comfortable approaching the patients after the performance to express appreciation for the shared narratives and their active resistance to stigma.[34] After participating in "Performing the Peace," both police officers and ex-offenders showed significant allophilia scale improvements, which indicated that attitudes toward each other had improved.[35] Police-community relations also improved as the public audience witnessed the sharing of narratives between police and ex-offenders. Concrete measures confirmed decreased mutual distrust and hostility between police and the public.[36]

COLLECTIVE NARRATIVE PRACTICE IN HONG KONG: SELECTED EVIDENCE

BACKGROUND OF PROJECT 1: REKINDLING THE GLORY OF LIFE THROUGH NARRA-DRAMA

Although the positive impacts of collective narrative practice have been studied and are found in various Western countries, research in this area remains lacking in Eastern countries. A glaring oversight in collective narrative practices is that even when it is used, it is seldom applied in work with older adults who are encountering aging-related challenges (such as chronic physical health issues and caregiver burden), despite the fact that previous research has demonstrated the effectiveness of both one-on-one and group narrative practices in these populations.[37] It is very likely that such populations could benefit from collective narrative practices, because these individuals also lack a voice within the societal power structure, having been marginalized, and thus facing the risk of negative labeling and stigmatization,[38] resulting in low social participation.[39]

Since 2015, I have, along with my coworkers, been using narra-drama to give a voice to older adults and their families in Hong Kong. I hope to achieve narrative justice, social education, and wisdom transfer as well as to facilitate individual and structural changes. The following narra-drama programs have been conducted to date:

2016: "Rekindling the Glory of Life Through Narra-drama" (a CADENZA initiative with stroke survivors and caregivers)

2019: "Your Story, My Story, Our Stories: Embracing Diversity Through Playback Theater" (international undergraduate students)

2020 to 2021: "Intergenerational Solidarity: Narrative Approach Playback Theater Project" (undergraduate students serving older adults)

2022: "We Playback . . . to Move Forward" (online, a student-initiated project about online learning during the COVID-19 pandemic)

2022: Lifelong learning at CityU: Intergenerational Exchanges, Mentorship and Solidarity (university students and older learners from the Elder Academy)

In 2016, with a funding grant supported by the Hong Kong Jockey Club Charities Trust, I had the privilege to work with stroke survivors and their caregivers to launch "Rekindling the Glory of Life Through Narra-drama." Participants were invited to join this collective narrative practice designed for the older adults with strokes and their support networks (including families, students, and health professionals). After completing work with their respective NT groups, participants were invited to a reunion six months later. We also performed the narra-drama performance in front of the general public, including new stroke survivors and their caregivers as participants.

In our practice, we invited older adults with strokes and their caregivers, after they had completed NT group practice, to share their personal stories in conquering the challenges brought about by the strokes. These stories were made into a collective declaration and a song, which were then integrated into a play. After ten sessions of preparation, the participants were invited to go on stage and perform their play, giving voice not only to their own story but also to other people who had similar experiences. We adopted the three-stage framework proposed by Denborough, and our collective narrative practice was introduced through the following three steps: (1) acknowledging the injustice faced by the person, (2) acknowledging shared ideals and values, and (3) convening forums of narrative justice.[40] The following section presents our observations and findings from "Rekindling the Glory of Life Through Narra-drama," with the application of Denborough's narrative framework.

STAGE 1. ACKNOWLEDGING THE INJUSTICE FACED BY THE INDIVIDUALS: DECONSTRUCTING PROBLEM-SATURATED LIFE STORIES

As suggested by Denborough, enabling people to express the effects of injustice in their own words allows their experiences to be named, understood, and acknowledged in ways that align with their local cultures.[41] As such, the therapist or practitioner may provide a safe context that allows individuals to comfortably voice their challenges with and experiences of injustice. To acknowledge the injustice and challenges faced by these people, it is important to distance the "problem" from the person. This can be achieved by "externalizing conversations."[42] Through these externalizing conversation, we invited the older adults to name the problem (i.e., strokes), by asking questions like "How do you describe strokes?" and "What is the stroke like?" Some older adults imagined their strokes to be a big *thief* or a *tsunami* that they faced in their life journey. We then asked them about the effects of the strokes, such as how strokes have influenced their lives. They stated that the strokes had "taken away their mobility" like a thief, and "wiped out all the things" they treasured in their lives, just like a tsunami. Despite these challenges, however, they believed that this was not the endpoint of their lives. In our narra-drama setting, the older adults and their caregivers visualized the strokes as a "thief" and "tsunami" and enacted them on the stage through body language and colored clothes.

> I have met a "big thief" in my life, who wanted to take away mobility from me; I have met a "tsunami" in my life, which wiped out all the things I like. However, I truly believe that this is not the endpoint of my life.
>
> —MR. NG, PERFORMER, "REKINDLING THE GLORY OF LIFE THROUGH NARRA-DRAMA"

Through the performance, the older adults and their caregivers' resilient attitudes toward the challenges were presented to the audience. Through such a collective practice, these individuals are no longer portrayed simply as "people who have problems" but instead as people who are "actively facing and conquering these problems." This process was effective in deconstructing the problem-saturated life stories and providing opportunities to construct a new life story for themself and their audience.

STAGE 2. ACKNOWLEDGING SHARED IDEALS AND VALUES: REAUTHORING HOPEFUL LIFE STORIES The second stage of facilitating "narrative justice" acknowledges shared ideals and values as a way to discover the personal resources that have helped these individual face their life challenges. To achieve this, individuals are invited to join a group sharing session. In the session, they rediscover the "unique outcomes" and reauthor alternative life storylines for themselves, which allows them to recall the personal resources they possess in conquering the challenges. This practice facilitated the coconstruction of alternative personal life stories with strengths, and reconnection with preferred identities.[43] Through this sharing process, the older adults and their caregivers were able to rejuvenate their values and resources (e.g., life wisdom, mutual support), which helped them to endure the difficulties. Following is a testimony by one of the participants:

> We live with strokes through the journey of "Happy and Healthy" along the railway line of "Happiness and Health." During this period, we shared the hardship, hard work, life wisdom, ability, resilience, and support of family members and medical staff, and the joy of overcoming it (stroke). Then, we let go of our heavy hearts, live[d] anew, and regain[ed] our smiles. During the period, we found that the sentiments of our groupmates/team members were filled with selfless love. Everyone overcame challenges during the journey in living with adversity of stroke and found a beautiful rainbow with mutual support.[44]

STAGE 3. CONVENING FORUMS OF NARRATIVE JUSTICE In the third stage of facilitating "narrative justice," Denborough states the importance of creating a platform to connect people with similar experiences together to strengthen their new life stories.[45] Through these "enabling contributions," the pain and injustices of individuals are "transformed" into a driving force to pursue collective justice for a wider group of people who share similar life challenges. This empowers individuals to advocate for social change and promotes a sense of agency.

The concept of "enabling contributions"[46] is based on the idea that the individuals are the "experts" of their own life stories and are capable of assisting others with the wisdom gained from their experiences.[47] By engaging in outsider witness practice in which they shared their valuable life experiences with the audience, participants' core values were recognized, and they found reassurance in one another. Players and performers were also able to understand the positive effects of their shared experiences on others and to reflect on their newly written stories.[48] As Denborough has suggested, enabling contribution enhances older adults' and their caregivers' self-confidence, agency, and self-worth.[49] Recognizing they can also contribute to others' lives helped the older adults and caregivers make sense of their own lives in a hopeful way, thereby strengthening their reconstructed life narratives.[50]

In our collective narrative practice, we engaged the older adults and their caregivers in sharing their lived experiences of chronic illnesses, struggles, and regaining mastery in life activities after stroke by singing the "Song of Life," which they composed in the narra-drama theater performance.[51] In this theatrical setting, the stroke survivors and caregivers performed a series of plays depicting physical changes to their bodies, altered daily activities poststroke, rehabilitation challenges, and caregiving while juggling family and work. Their experiences of living with strokes were also made into a collaboratively written theme song by the participants with the support of Mr. Ho Pak Chuen, the conductor, and the Life Education Project, Stewards of Hong Kong.[52] In the "Song of Life," the older adults and caregivers honored what their lives have brought, expressed their hopes for the future, and shared their desire to cherish everything and move forward despite life challenges.

THE SONG OF LIFE

Life is like running water,
Rugged and endless,
Life is like ripples,
It started from a droplet,
Gradually spread its energy.
Life is like a shooting star,
It's short but it brings hope to people.
Wishing for blissfulness and happiness,
Eternal glory, brightening the world,
Life is ever-changing,
But take things calmly, and treasure all we have at present,
Life inspires life,
Supporting one another,
To move forward bravely.

Their hopes revealed a sense of collective agency, renewed social roles, an appreciation of life challenges, the impact of mutual understanding and care, and their expectations for the future. These hopes demonstrated that the participants were ready to "move forward" despite the challenges they had faced in their lives.[53] Following is some of the feedback from participants after taking part in "Rekindling the Glory of Life Through Narra-drama":

I never thought that my recovery experience could give strength and encouragement to other persons and their caregivers who are trapped by stroke. As a patient, we just stayed at home to follow our medical regime, to take care of ourselves. Now, I learnt I have to reach out as I have an important social role to encourage my peers individually, reciprocally, and collectively that we can turn a new page of our life together.

—MR. LAI, A PERFORMER WHO HAD A STROKE THREE YEARS AGO, VOICING HIS TRANSFORMATIVE EXPERIENCE AFTER JOINING THE NARRA-DRAMA PERFORMANCE

I hope the government will include psychosocial support to both stroke survivors and their family members as part of rehabilitation. The stroke survivors are able to support each other, so that everyone will treasure the people around us more and appreciate the time spent with family more after our performance tonight.

—MRS. YIK, PERFORMER AND SPOUSAL CAREGIVER

The program director also linked the survivors' and caregivers' skills and knowledge, hopes, and dreams, with the audience, using a definitional ceremony practice, through a dialogue between the performers and the audience. We were able to connect and share the participants' feelings, experiences, inspiration, and demands for better care in living with stroke. The audience also benefited from the experience, as they related to the stories and developed a better understanding of the recovery experience from the performers:

What impressed me the most is the idea of "life inspires life." My husband is a stroke patient. I often said that after he got the stroke, his caregiver has become a "person with depression" (laughed wryly). Every time I join (these activities here), I am touched by their family members who are very active and positive, which gives me a sense of hope that it will get better. This motivates me.

—MS. HUNG, AUDIENCE MEMBER, "REKINDLING THE GLORY OF LIFE"

I am very touched by the strengths of mutual care among patients and carers supporting each other, especially during the rehabilitation. Patients' and carers'

support network is definitely an important source of support when they are dealing with the hardships of their lives. We fully acknowledge the precious recovery experience of the stroke survivors and their caregivers, that they have a definite social role as peer models to the new stroke victims and their caregivers. . . . Appropriate psychosocial support for both stroke survivors and their family members as part of rehabilitation provides additional coping strengths to the patients and the rehabilitation team.

—DR. CHAN, INVITED PHYSICIAN AND AUDIENCE MEMBER,
"REKINDLING THE GLORY OF LIFE"

Narra-drama enables stakeholders to voice their struggles and share knowledge, skills, and insight through an interactive applied theater performance with the audience. This practice, however, is more time consuming than other therapeutic interventions because it requires obtaining consent, generating descriptive narratives with participants, transforming these narratives into dramatic scenes, training participants, and securing funding. Alternative practices have been explored.

LIFELONG LEARNING AT CITYU PROJECT 2: INTERGENERATIONAL EXCHANGES, MENTORSHIP, AND SOLIDARITY THROUGH PLAYBACK THEATER

Although young people and older adults have respective developmental needs and interests, only a limited number of mutual platforms are available for both generations to communicate and exchange ideas with each other. In supporting the lifelong learning initiative of the Hong Kong government, the City University of Hong Kong launched an Elder Academy in 2008, in which older adults, aged sixty and above, could register to audit courses across disciplines offered by different undergraduate studies. To promote cross-generational interactions and exchanges, we adopted a Playback training model to facilitate the cross-generational communication between older and younger learners to enrich mutual understanding and respect. We formed an intergenerational Playback team with an open theater performance to create a collaborative learning experience between younger and older peers.

Drawing on Yotis et al.'s use of Playback Theater to facilitate mutual understanding and reduce the stigmatization of people with mental health issues, we initiated the "Intergenerational Solidarity: Narrative Approach x Playback Theater Project" (2021) and "Lifelong Learning at CityU: Intergenerational Exchanges, Mentorship, and Solidarity" (2022).[54] We invited university students from the social and behavioral sciences programs at the City University of Hong Kong to enact the stories of older adults in a Playback Theater. Under professional guidance, older adults shared their life challenges, recovery experiences, and life wisdom with the university students to form the basis for the drama practice. Students then improvised stories with both narratives and body language during training sessions.

Following are some testimonials from the participants:

"Games" are the best way to learn. In the training for theater practices, I had several experiences where my "scenarios" and "inner feelings" were intertwined. This training breaks the traditional learning pattern with a new highly-effective practical mode of "doing more, thinking less." I also deeply appreciated that the university provided us with this opportunity to rediscover our core values, share with the younger generation, with hopes that we can transfer our life wisdom and make contributions from the "older adults" in today's Hong Kong society.

—MR. YUI, ELDER PROGRAM PARTICIPANT

It's amazing how in such a short time we've developed a rapport and under-standing of each other. Joining this intergenerational program is indeed beyond classroom experiences. . . . The life experiences and perspectives that we shared here have transported the young people and have been really profound and insightful. This intergenerational playback has been so meaningful by bringing all of us together. We have learned a lot from our elder peers. This encouraged my curiosity to find more opportunities to talk with older persons, including my grandparents.

—MS. YUEN, STUDENT PROGRAM PARTICIPANT

Indeed, the older learner peers are our life mentors who always remind us to dare to adventure and step out of our comfort zone. This spirit is applicable not only in theater, but also in the journey of life. . . . It was a great and life transforming experience for me.

—MS. KAN, STUDENT PROGRAM PARTICIPANT

Other than auditing university courses, I am so privileged to join this Play-back training program, to interact and collaborate with young people in greater depth. This provides us with a better understanding of the young generation. During rehearsals, we gained insights into their thinking, vitality, lifestyles and daily experiences, which deepens our mutual understanding.

—MR. WONG, ELDER PROGRAM PARTICIPANT

As a result of this program, both students and older adults benefited from the Playback project, which served as collective practice in promoting intergenerational interactions and exchanges. In this program, participants reported that the use of drama was a challenging yet creative means that helped them improve self-confidence, communication skills, brain function, language and physical expression, listening skills, public speaking, and patience in general. For the older participants, in particular, the activities provided a space for light physical exercise. Moreover, it promoted values and attitudes of respecting others, art inheritance, striving for excellence, and daring to take risks. Both older and student participants agreed that these experiences bridged intergenerational communication and solidarity.

Playback Theater has also been a useful tool in enhancing cross-generational communication through mutual storytelling, interaction, and teamwork nature. As mentioned earlier, participants gained a better understanding of the other generation during the program, forming new friendships across age-groups. As the participants enacted the stories of each other's lives, they gained insight into other individuals' experiences, values, and life wisdom, growing in respect for each other. Such a process highlighted the commonalities between youth and elders, reducing stereotypes and facilitating intergenerational bonding. Therefore, by collaboratively creating and performing stories, the practice of narra-drama helped form intergenerational relationships and developed understanding in a meaningful way.

At a societal level, not only can narra-drama programs bridge the gap between younger and older participants but also created connections between the older generation and the public. During an end-of-semester ceremony, this intergenerational Playback Theater team performed in front of an audience, which included other university students, members of the Elderly Academy, and government funders. This performance created a platform on which to demonstrate intergenerational solidarity and allowed the older adults to share their life wisdom and be acknowledged by youth and the general public. By improvising the life stories of the older adults, youth participants honored and voiced the underlying stigmas and enduring beliefs of the elders, which enabled the audience to witness mutual growth and development for this intergenerational Playback Theater team. Furthermore, this performance raised public awareness of social support, care, and welfare of older adults and advocated for a more inclusive community.

CROSS-CULTURAL COMMUNICATION

In addition to bridging different generations, the Playback Theater is also applicable to facilitate cross-cultural understanding. Before conducting cross-generational projects, we applied this technique in student groups with diverse cultural backgrounds, and the initial results were positive. This student-initiated project was called "Your Story, My Story, Our Stories: Embracing Diversity Through Playback Theater" (2019) and was developed to give voice to international students who struggled to adapt to university life in Hong Kong. A similar project was "We Playback . . . to Move Forward" (2022), which connected students from different cultures through a virtual Playback Theater performance on a video conference platform during the COVID-19 pandemic. We were delighted to have obtained positive feedback from the participants. In the "We Playback . . . to Move Forward" project, participants reported that the program gave them the opportunity to share their feelings and to connect with others while feeling safe and respected. In addition, among the thirty respondents, 90 percent reported learning more about how to interact with people from different cultural backgrounds through the training program. Participants also said that Playback Theater was a helpful tool for building harmony among people of diverse cultural backgrounds on campus.

CONCLUSION

Research on collective narrative practice is still emerging, but studies to date have demonstrated its value and positive impact. Several platforms have been shown to be effective in positive health outcomes, including my own and other research using narra-drama and other narrative practices to give voice to older adults with chronic illnesses (e.g., stroke, chronic pain, dementia) and their caregivers. In addition to narra-drama, we borrowed the experiences of previous research at the collective level to launch Playback Theater projects and to facilitate cross-generational communications. As a result, these adaptations empowered older adults in Hong Kong by facilitating the reconstruction of hopeful life stories, fostering intergenerational exchanges with youth, and creating greater public awareness of older adults' struggles. To optimize these interventions, further research is needed to explore the possibility of expanding applications to new groups. We believe that through the flexible use of various mediums, the voices of historically marginalized groups of people can be conveyed and heard by society. Hopefully, with more research and practice, the potential of collective narrative practice can be harnessed to promote a more empathetic and inclusive society with love, care, and respect.

NOTES

1. Esther Oi-Wah Chow, *Narrating Faith. Love. Hope: A Practical Manual on Narrative Therapy* (敘出信。愛。望: 敘事治療實務手冊), 2nd ed. (Hong Kong: City University of Hong Kong, 2016); and Esther Oi-Wah Chow, *I Have a Story with Chronic Pain: Narrative Practice in Application* (「我和疼痛有個故事」敘事治療小組實踐): A Report (Hong Kong: Neighbourhood Advice-Action Council, 2018).

2. Esther Oi-Wah Chow and Andrew Yiu Tsang, *Low Applications of Interactive Pedagogical Learning Model in Promoting Intergenerational Communication to Enhance Teaching and Learning* (Hong Kong: City University of Hong Kong, 2021–2023).

3. Franca Butera-Prinzi, Nella Charles, and Karen Story, "Narrative Family Therapy and Group Work for Families Living with Acquired Brain Injury," *Australian and New Zealand Journal of Family Therapy* 35, no. 1 (2014): 81–99, https://doi.org/https://doi.org/10.1002/anzf.1046.

4. Laurel Phillips, "A Narrative Therapy Approach to Dealing with Chronic Pain," *International Journal of Narrative Therapy and Community Work* (2017): 21–30, https://doi.org/10.3316/informit.768720305988235; and Esther Oi-Wah Chow, "Narrative Group Intervention to Reconstruct Meaning of Life Among Stroke Survivors: A Randomized Clinical Trial Study," *Neuropsychiatry* 8, no. 4 (2018): 1216–26, https://doi.org/10.4172/Neuropsychiatry.1000450.

5. Esther Oi-Wah Chow, "Narrative Therapy an Evaluated Intervention to Improve Stroke Survivors' Social and Emotional Adaptation," *Clinical Rehabilitation* 29, no. 4 (2015): 315–26, https://doi.org/10.1177/0269215514544039; and Chow, "Narrative Group Intervention to Reconstruct Meaning of Life."

6. Emily Pia, "Narrative Therapy and Peacebuilding," *Journal of Intervention and Statebuilding* 7, no. 4 (2013): 476–91, https://doi.org/10.1080/17502977.2012.727538.

7. De-Hui Ruth Zhou et al., "An Unexpected Visitor and a Sword Play: A Randomized Controlled Trial of Collective Narrative Therapy Groups for Primary Carers of People with Schizophrenia," *Journal of Mental Health* (2020): 1–12, https://doi.org/10.1080/09638237.2020.1793123.

8. Gregory Clark et al., *The Son Also Rises: Surnames and the History of Social Mobility*, The Princeton Economic History of the Western World (Princeton,

NJ: Princeton University Press, 2014); and Jozsef Szabo, Szilvia Toth, and Annamaria Karamanne Pakai, "Narrative Group Therapy for Alcohol Dependent Patients," *International Journal of Mental Health and Addiction* 12, no. 4 (2014): 470–76, https://doi.org/10.1007/s11469-014-9478-1.

9. Tod Augusta-Scott and Juergen Dankwort, "Partner Abuse Group Intervention: Lessons from Education and Narrative Therapy Approaches," *Journal of Interpersonal Violence* 17, no. 7 (2002): 783–805, https://doi.org/10.1177/088626050 2017007006; Gwen Adshead, "The Life Sentence: Using a Narrative Approach in Group Psychotherapy with Offenders," *Group Analysis* 44, no. 2 (2011): 175–95, https://doi.org/10.1177/0533316411400969; and Barbara Baumgartner and Brian Williams, "Becoming an Insider: Narrative Therapy Groups Alongside People Overcoming Homelessness," *Journal of Systemic Therapies* 33, no. 4 (2014): 1–14, https://doi.org/10.1521/jsyt.2014.33.4.1.

10. Suet Lin Hung, "Collective Narrative Practice with Rape Victims in the Chinese Society of Hong Kong," *International Journal of Narrative Therapy and Community Work* 1 (2011): 14–31, https://doi.org/10.3316 /informit.870589297245238.

11. Robert E. Doan, "Narrative Therapy, Postmodernism, Social Constructionism, and Constructivism: Discussion and Distinctions," *Transactional Analysis Journal* 27, no. 2 (1997): 128–33, https://doi.org/10.1177/036215379702700208.

12. Kathy Weingarten, "The Small and the Ordinary: The Daily Practice of a Postmodern Narrative Therapy," *Family Process* 37, no. 1 (1998): 3–15, https://doi.org/10.1111/j.1545-5300.1998.00003.x.

13. Doan, "Narrative Therapy, Postmodernism, Social Constructionism, and Constructivism"; and Weingarten, "The Small and the Ordinary."

14. Doan, "Narrative Therapy, Postmodernism, Social Constructionism, and Constructivism"; and Weingarten, "The Small and the Ordinary."

15. Weingarten, "The Small and the Ordinary."

16. Hung, "Collective Narrative Practice with Rape Victims"; and L. Yotis et al., "Using Playback Theatre to Address the Stigma of Mental Disorders," *Arts in Psychotherapy* 55 (2017): 80–84, https://doi.org/10.1016/j.aip.2017.04.009.

17. Grant Lesley, "Bringing Together Women Like You and Me: Collective Narrative Practice with Women and Trauma," *International Journal of Narrative Therapy and Community Work* 1 (2022): 1–8, https://doi.org/10.3316/informit .429037128627631; and Hung, "Collective Narrative Practice with Rape Victims."

18. Catherine Gardner-Elahi and Sannam Zamiri, "Collective Narrative Practice in Forensic Mental Health," *Journal of Forensic Practice* 17, no. 3 (2015): 204–18, https://doi.org/10.1108/JFP-10-2014-0034; and Jamison S. Bottomley et al., "Mental Health Symptomatology and Exposure to Non-Fatal Suicidal Behavior: Factors That Predict Vulnerability and Resilience Among College Students," *Archives of Suicide Research* 22, no. 4 (2018): 596–614, https://doi .org/10.1080/13811118.2017.1387632.

19. David Denborough, "Healing and Justice Together: Searching for Narrative Justice," *International Journal of Narrative Therapy and Community Work* 3 (2013): 15, https://doi.org/10.3316/informit.697583733979367.
20. Denborough, "Healing and Justice Together."
21. David Denborough, *Collective Narrative Practice* (Adelaide, SA: Dulwich Centre, 2008); and Esther Oi-Wah Chow and Sai-Fu Fung, "Narrative Group Intervention to Rediscover Life Wisdom Among Hong Kong Chinese Older Adults: A Single-Blind Randomized Waitlist-Controlled Trial," *Innovation in Aging* 5, no. 3 (2021): igab027, https://doi.org/10.1093/geroni/igab027.
22. Lesley, "Bringing Together Women Like You and Me"; and Hung, "Collective Narrative Practice with Rape Victims."
23. Melissa A. Smigelsky and Robert A. Neimeyer, "Performative Retelling: Healing Community Stories of Loss Through Playback Theatre," *Death Studies* 42, no. 1 (2018): 26–34, https://doi.org/10.1080/07481187.2017.1370414; Yotis et al., "Using Playback Theatre"; and Gardner-Elahi and Zamiri, "Collective Narrative Practice in Forensic Mental Health."
24. Yotis et al., "Using Playback Theatre"
25. Ben Rivers, "Narrative Power: Playback Theatre as Cultural Resistance in Occupied Palestine," *Research in Drama Education* 20, no. 2 (2015): 155–72, https://doi.org/10.1080/13569783.2015.1022144.
26. Rivers, "Narrative Power."
27. Smigelsky and Neimeyer, "Performative Retelling."
28. Gardner-Elahi and Zamiri, "Collective Narrative Practice in Forensic Mental Health."
29. Smigelsky and Neimeyer, "Performative Retelling"; and Gardner-Elahi and Zamiri, "Collective Narrative Practice in Forensic Mental Health."
30. Yotis et al., "Using Playback Theatre."
31. Chow, *Narrating Faith. Love. Hope.*
32. Denborough, *Collective Narrative Practice*; and Gardner-Elahi and Zamiri, "Collective Narrative Practice in Forensic Mental Health."
33. Chow, *Narrating Faith. Love. Hope.*
34. Yotis et al., "Using Playback Theatre."
35. Smigelsky and Neimeyer, "Performative Retelling."
36. Smigelsky and Neimeyer, "Performative Retelling."
37. Chow, "Narrative Therapy an Evaluated Intervention": Esther Oi-Wah Chow and Doris Yuen Hung Fok, "Recipe of Life: A Relational Narrative Approach in Therapy with Persons Living with Chronic Pain," *Research on Social Work Practice* 30, no. 3 (2020): 320–29, https://doi.org/10.1177/1049731519870867; and Doris S. F. Yu et al., "Effects of Strength-Based Intervention on Health Outcomes of Family Caregivers of Persons with Dementia: A Study Protocol," *Journal of Advanced Nursing* 76, no. 10 (2020): 2737–46, https://doi.org/10.1111/jan.14470.

38. Cui Yu Deng et al., "Factors Associated with Stigma in Community-Dwelling Stroke Survivors in China: A Cross-Sectional Study," *Journal of the Neurological Sciences* 407 (2018): 1–6, https://doi.org/10.1016/j.jns.2019.116459; Fred Stephen Sarfo et al., "Stroke-Related Stigma Among West Africans: Patterns and Predictors," *Journal of the Neurological Sciences* 375 (2016): 270–74, https://doi.org/10.1016/j.jns.2017.02.018.

39. Qi Lu et al., "The Effect of Stigma on Social Participation in Community-Dwelling Chinese Patients with Stroke Sequelae: A Cross-Sectional Study," *Clinical Rehabilitation* 36, no. 3 (2022): 407–14, https://doi.org/10.1177/02692155211050558.

40. Denborough, "Healing and Justice Together."

41. Denborough, "Healing and Justice Together."

42. See chapters 3 and 11 for the four principal steps of externalizing conversation: (1) naming the problem, (2) mapping the effects of the problem, (3) evaluating the effects of the problem, and (4) justifying the evaluation.

43. Geoffrey Cowley and Karen Springen, "Rewriting Life Stories: Mind: Instead of Looking for Flaws in People's Psyches, 'Narrative Therapy' Works at Nurturing Their Forgotten Strengths," *Newsweek* 125, no. 16 (1995): 70–74; and Chow, *Narrating Faith. Love. Hope.*

44. Chow, *Narrating Faith. Love. Hope.*

45. Denborough, "Healing and Justice Together."

46. Denborough, *Collective Narrative Practice*; and Denborough, "Healing and Justice Together."

47. Chow, *Narrating Faith. Love. Hope.*

48. Lesley, "Bringing Together Women Like You and Me."

49. Denborough, *Collective Narrative Practice.*

50. Denborough, *Collective Narrative Practice*; and Lesley, "Bringing Together Women Like You and Me."

51. Lesley, "Bringing Together Women Like You and Me."

52. Chow, *Narrating Faith. Love. Hope.*

53. Lesley, "Bringing Together Women Like You and Me."

54. L. Yotis et al., "Using Playback Theatre."

15

UNLEASHING THE POWER OF COLLECTIVE NARRATIVES

Narrative Therapy in Group and Community Practice

THE GLOBAL POPULATION is aging rapidly, which has necessitated evidence-based psychosocial interventions tailored to older adults across diverse cultural settings. Although most research to date has focused on Western populations, emerging evidence suggests that narrative therapy (NT) may confer similar benefits to Eastern seniors. Older adults are often vulnerable because of chronic illness and lack of social support. What can we do to improve the lives of these seniors who were once the driving force of our society? Therefore, in this chapter, we focus on mental support that we can provide as social workers by sharing the what and how of the NT psychological intervention. NT originated in Australia and New Zealand through the work of Michael White and David Epston to help individuals and couples for a certain period.[1] This approach, however, has been rarely adapted to the Eastern context. Chapters 11 through 14 have highlighted empirical studies and methods that show the promise of NT in providing older adults with a sense of meaning, community, and emotional support through group and collective practice.

GROUP PRACTICE AND SOCIAL CONSTRUCTIONISM

Based on social constructionism, psychological interventions aim to assist marginalized individuals to deconstruct negative beliefs and reconstruct preferred identities (chapters 2 and 3).[2] Just like authors and editors proofreading their books, this process allows the individuals to examine and review their experiences, recreating their identity and life narrative. To achieve this narrative change, therapists use core conversational tools from NT as a guide (chapter 4). Externalizing conversations help individuals

separate their identity from the problem by viewing the problem as external, thus reducing self-guilt and blame.[3] Reauthoring conversations allow
individuals to rediscover unique outcomes and strengths by exploring the
landscapes of action and identity from their past life experiences. Re-membering conversations reconnect participants to significant figures who have
supporting their preferred story. Outsider witness practices and therapeutic
documents further validate the alternative narrative. Together, by rejuve-
nating life values and wisdom, this process empowers individuals to regain
a sense of power and self-agency, which are crucial qualities for living a
fulfilling and prosperous life.

In this part of the book, we provided concrete examples of applying these
methods to collective settings. We discussed the use of metaphoric frameworks and empathetic questioning to elicit individuals' perspectives and to
facilitate their own meaning-making. We offered step-by-step techniques
and sample questions as a road map for structuring productive narrative
conversations to help individuals rewrite their stories in line with their values and preferred identities.

METAPHORIC FRAMEWORKS

We also introduced the use of metaphoric frameworks in narrative practices
among older adults in Hong Kong. Troubled by chronic illnesses, such as
pain and stroke, older individuals, especially in Eastern cultures, may lack
the relevant health information and strategy to articulate or express their
feelings. Metaphoric frameworks provide an accessible way for these adults
to externalize their thoughts, emotions, concerns, and coping strengths.
The three tested metaphoric frameworks, Tree-of-Life, Recipe-of-Life, and
Train-of-Life interventions, can be applied to empower individuals to view
their lives with a fresh and imaginative perspective, creating space for them
to form alternative narratives apart from problem-saturated ones. Initial
data has indicated uniformly positive outcomes from these three methods, including rediscovering one's values and beliefs, regaining a sense of
agency, and cherishing life with hope.

TREE OF LIFE

The Tree-of-Life intervention guides individuals through a collective
rediscovery journey with the metaphor of a tree as life.[4] As participants

symbolically map their lives onto the parts of a tree, individuals have the opportunity to share the uniqueness of their life experiences and wisdom. As they gather their trees to form a forest on a wall, this process further enhances the sense of connectivity and the "we-ness" within the group. With mutual support and understanding, participants are able to share their vulnerability and hardships candidly; later, they can celebrate their new life narrative together.

Promising results have been obtained from our research of groups in Hong Kong using the Tree-of-Life metaphor with older adults. Qualitative interviews revealed that participants gained insight into their abilities, reconnected with purpose and values, and increased hope and self-acceptance.[5] Quantitative data showed significantly improved wisdom, mastery, self-esteem, and well-being compared with controls.[6] The group process of acknowledging shared struggles while also recognizing members' strengths fostered mutual support. Overall, the Tree of Life shows promise as a culturally adaptable narrative practice for helping diverse older adults rediscover life wisdom.

RECIPE OF LIFE

The Recipe-of-Life metaphoric framework has been used in NT for older adults with chronic pain. Participants are guided to consider life's ingredients; reflect on their sources, methods, and rituals; and share their recipes with others.[7] This process externalizes and deconstructs the problem of chronic pain. Reauthoring dialogues support individuals in reclaiming and foregrounding their strengths, values, and preferred identities as core ingredients in their recipes. Moreover, reciprocally exchanging recipes enables the participants to contribute their accumulated life wisdom as a gift to others facing similar challenges.

Our study in Hong Kong found that this intervention increased self-efficacy and hope regarding pain, validated participants' values, and built a mutual support community.[8] Case examples highlighted individuals rediscovering their resilience despite challenges. The metaphor provides an empowering narrative approach for chronic pain and likely other health conditions as well. Using food and flavors as a metaphor also provides a universal context for narration. Therefore, further research is needed to adapt this approach to other cultures.

TRAIN OF LIFE

The Train-of-Life metaphor has been valuable as a recovery journey for stroke survivors and their caregivers. Life events are identified as stations along a railway line to facilitate perspective-taking. According to a random-ized controlled trial in Hong Kong, narrative groups using this metaphor significantly improved mastery, hope, life satisfaction, and other outcomes compared with controls.[9] Case studies have revealed rich processes of reconstructing agency and wisdom.

We provided a six-step plan for orienting participants to this metaphor, including externalizing stroke, identifying unique outcomes, coconstructing preferred identities, thickening alternative stories, and celebrating the new journey. What makes this approach unique is that the ongoing train jour-ney metaphor further promotes a sense of moving forward, thus empowering participants to envision their future with optimism and hope. Overall, the Train of Life shows promise as a creative narrative approach to empowering chronically ill patients. Imagining life as a journey can help people decon-struct limiting narratives and rediscover purpose and meaning. Evidence indi-cates a capacity to strengthen self-esteem, relationships, and quality of life.[10]

In this book, we documented three empirical metaphoric frameworks that have been developed in the Hong Kong context. Many other metaphors, however, have been adopted in other studies—for example, the narrative house,[11] team of life,[12] kite of life,[13] and suitcase of life,[14] just to name a few. In addition, the Recipe-of-Life metaphor was adapted from a Western research study with children and was tailored to older adults living with chronic pain in Hong Kong. Hence, drawing on these studies that employ metaphors as a tool and guide, we observed the infinite possibilities and com-binations of metaphoric frameworks and therapy users. In future research, narrative practitioners will continue to explore the potential of metaphoric frameworks and its applications. Other metaphors should be explored in different cultural contexts to benefit a wider range of populations.

COLLECTIVE NARRATIVE PRACTICE

In addition to group work, collective narrative practice also provides a channel to renew the societal levels of practice. By participating at the com-munity and collective level, marginalized groups can voice their struggles and share their stories with a wider public. This practice can enhance the public's understanding and reshape the public's view of these individuals, enabling them to regain power and respect from the society. Ultimately, we hope this practice can help achieve social justice for these individuals from marginalized groups.[15]

We examined the emerging collective practice by adopting Playback Theater to bring groups and communities together.[16] Theater, documentation, and other methods have helped marginalized groups reconstruct their social narrative. Studies have suggested that collective practices facilitate education, empowerment, and social justice by reducing stigma[17] and enabling new roles for participants as experts sharing knowledge.[18] Intergenerational theater has successfully forged cross-generational empathy. New evidence from research in Hong Kong groups using narra-drama theater as a bridge narrowed the gap between younger and older adults. Participants were given the opportunity to speak for themselves in the format of drama. Such a practice has proven to facilitate public education among the participants and the audience. Participants reported finding common ground and building relationships across age-groups. Although collective narrative practice research remains limited, initial findings point to its strong potential as a means of community building and social change. This chapter shed light on the possibilities of using collective narrative practice with different societal groups and provided a framework for acknowledging injustice, coconstructing solutions, and convening public forums to legitimize the wisdom of marginalized voices.

CHARACTERISTICS AND BENEFITS OF NT IN COLLECTIVE PRACTICE

GROWTH IN REDISCOVERING LIFE

NT helps individuals rediscover life values, wisdom, and meaning. Instead of focusing on what has affected the behaviors, the focus is on releasing the individual's intentional understanding of self, such as their beliefs, values, commitment, abilities, skills, and problem-solving capacities from their narratives, which may have led to successful coping in the past.[19] According to NT, "the problem is the problem, not the people," and the practice is devoted to rescuing the individual's life wisdom, as well as valuable local knowledge, to deconstruct the social image afflicted by negative life challenges.[20] NT relies on the person's strengths, values, and beliefs, rather than focusing solely on their symptoms or problems, which is consistent with the values and beliefs of social work practice. The practitioner acts as an ally along with group participants instead of as a hierarchical expert, embodying a respectful, curious, nonblaming attitude in working together with the individuals and participants, while witnessing and acknowledging they are indeed the "expert" of their lives.

MUTUAL AID AS A COMMUNITY

Collective narrative practice demonstrates the characteristics of mutual aid by working with groups collectively. As proposed by Lawrence Shulman, as individuals of similar backgrounds gather, they share the "all-in-the-same-boat" characteristic of mutual aid.[21] When people with similar experiences come to a group, participants are more comfortable to develop trust and vulnerability in the group with respect to each other's life experiences. They can then release and normalize negative thoughts and emotions, decreasing feelings of self-guilt and self-blame and establishing the basis for a shift in problem-saturated perspectives. Receiving feedback from one another, this practice allows participants to reembrace themselves for their values and wisdom. This process generates a sense of hope and supports the formation of a new identity for future prospects. By elevating them as they deal with the personal as well as social situations in which they are trapped, participants can break the cycle of a self-fulfilling prophecy.

GATHERING FOR SOCIAL JUSTICE

The transformational impact of all being the "in the same boat" can further cultivate the second characteristic of mutual aid—that is, "strength in numbers."[22] This belief provides both psychoemotional and social support to reduce the self-destructive inclinations of group members. When all of the members join together as a collective power, like in survivors' groups, they can gain courage from this shared solidarity. The collective power in a group invigorates phenomenal courage and promotes positive change not just individually but also across groups and even society. As narrative practice involves outsiders as witnesses, group members are empowered to voice their experiences, further educating the public about their lives, struggles, and needs.[23] This process can alleviate preexisting stereotypes and labels that have been imposed on the group by society. Furthermore, this practice reinforces the need for society to reflect on and enhance existing systems to better tackle the deep-seated difficulties of marginalized groups, eventually creating narrative social justice and a more inclusive society.

SHARING PUBLIC OPINION

Collective interventions can play a crucial role in shaping public opinion by raising awareness, reframing and challenging dominant narratives, and mobilizing support to address social concerns with specific causes. The following sections demonstrate how these interventions can contribute to setting social agendas and shaping public opinion.

VISIBILITY AND AWARENESS

Collective interventions, such as public education, direct conversation, protests, rallies, and demonstrations, draw attention to social issues that might otherwise be overlooked or marginalized. By bringing these concerns and issues into the public sphere, they increase visibility and generate awareness among the broader population. Through media coverage and social media sharing, collective interventions amplify the voices of marginalized groups, illustrate that they are not alone, and shed light on their experiences, concerns, strengths, hopes, and dreams, thereby influencing public opinion by exposing people to perspectives they may not have encountered otherwise.

FRAMING THE NARRATIVE AND SHIFTING SOCIAL NORMS

Collective interventions often involve framing the narrative around a particular issue or cause. Activists and organizers use various communication strategies, such as stories, drama, slogans, speeches, and public service announcements, to shape the narrative and define the terms of the discussion. By providing alternative viewpoints and challenging existing narratives, collective interventions can shift public opinion and reduce bias by offering new perspectives, highlighting impartialities, and reframing the way people and society at large thinks about a particular issue.[24]

MOBILIZING SUPPORT

Collective interventions mobilize individuals and communities to act and increase involvement to support a cause. These interventions provide opportunities for people to join together, share their stories, and collectively demand change. By fostering a sense of solidarity and empowerment, these interventions also encourage individuals to engage with the issue, enlighten themselves, enrich their civic roles, and advocate for what they need. This mobilization of support can set an agenda to address concerns and influence public opinion by expanding the reach of a movement, thus creating a broader base of support and demonstrating the significance of the issue to the wider population.

MEDIA INFLUENCE

Collective interventions often attract media attention, which can significantly affect public agenda and opinion. Media plays an important role in the communication between the government officials and citizens.[25] Mass media, such as newspapers and television, set the agenda for media coverage, which can help disseminate the message, images, and goals of the movement to a wider audience. Note, however, that media coverage can also be biased or distorted, which may influence public opinion in different ways depending on the presentation and framing of the collective intervention.

In the age of Web 2.0,[26] in which multidirectional interactions have become the norm for online media ecosystem, we have begun to explore the potential of the new media (i.e., social media) as a tool of communication. In recent years, cohesive and interactive communities have emerged on social media. For example, the "youth cancer hk"[27] and "we are all mental"[28] on Instagram are some of the online community models that are not only confined to the social media platform but also have expanded to face-to-face meetings among members. These accounts create a new channel for interactions among social workers and community members, which strengthens community bonds. Moreover, these platforms provide informative content, such as facts of a certain cancers[29] and specific topics on mental health,[30] which help educate the general public about the challenges faced by these communities. In fact, collective NT practices have been using Instagram, including the "narrative_playback_theatre_tribe" (拿破輪劇團) in Hong Kong.[31] The tribe has posted photos and video footage of their rehearsals and also has promoted their drama training courses on Instagram. These community models shed light on the possibility for NT to incorporate new venues in maximizing service and impact. By providing related information and community updates on social media, these platforms could also expand and act as hubs for narrative reconstruction, outsider witness, and social justice.

Shaping public opinion is a complex process influenced by multiple factors, and collective interventions are just one aspect. By raising awareness, framing narratives, mobilizing support, challenging norms, and influencing media coverage, collective interventions can have a substantial impact on reactivating social agendas, shaping public opinion, and driving social change.

CONCLUSION

We have to face challenges and changes every day in society. It is inevitable that people's reactions and the voices around us will have an impact on our way of living. Some people develop self-knowledge and tools to help them navigate through negative connotations, whereas other people are greatly affected and entrapped by their difficulties. Without interventions of self-help or mutual aid, these individuals may externalize their problems. They need to understand that they are the protagonist/hero trapped in a difficult story and find space to rediscover their purpose in life away from these problem-saturated narratives.

Social constructionism suggests that people internalize their values and norms through socialization, both communally and culturally, throughout their lifespan; however, with the rapid changes in our dynamic society, the values, norms, and beliefs that we acquire from our social contexts may not reflect reality and can be limited in many ways. Because reality is socially constructed, it can also be explored, questioned, and reconstructed to allow for new perspectives to develop that are more conducive to the well-being of the individuals and the society.

From the clinical level, therapists help individuals in the process of telling and retelling their narratives, creating alternative stories that align with their preferred identity. Helping people to navigate their egos depends significantly on the way they see themselves and this world. Just like filters of a camera, one can select a gloomy filter to see a cloudy gray sky or a highly saturated filter to see a bright blue sky. Of course, a person's life narrative is far more complicated. It consists of a series of intertwined moments that progress with endless possibilities of encounters. Yet, the logic is similar. It depends on how you define these moments and encounters in your life.

By using a storytelling approach, people can begin to separate themselves from their experiences, especially negative ones. People gain a sense of agency as they speak of their stories, being the narrator of their lives.

Despite the fact that life encounters are not something that we as humans can control (i.e., the events), we can control how the protagonist reacts to them. To reauthor their stories, individuals have to first deconstruct their beliefs and views toward the "protagonist." As they listen to the person's narration, peers and the therapist can provide feedback to help the individual break down harmful misconceptions and myths they have created for themselves. In this way, more space is cleared for reinterpretation and imagination. The next step is to select healthier thoughts and support for the person to rebuild their conceptions and beliefs through coconstruction. The person has the chance to review their life journey, uncovering the treasures hidden in their past, to rediscover and reconnect to their life wisdom and core values.[32] These values are vital for the person to reconstruct their narrative, or even their living mechanism. At the end of the narrative practice, we celebrate the individual's conquest over adversity and recognize this as a happy resolution to enable them to embark on a new adventure.

This process is not only about rewriting one's story but also about the whole story of society. As we rewrite the stories of groups of individuals, it is probably time for society to change its narrative about marginalized groups. We have to ensure that the voices of these groups of people are heard by more people—remembering and reminding all of us that at one point we have been or will be part of a marginalized group. Moreover, these groups and the witnesses supporting them can share these new narratives by reaching out to those who are in need and giving back to the society from which they have received care. Eventually, we believe that these new narratives will bring continuing changes to society, rewriting our society into a more inclusive and empowering one.

NOTES

1. Michael White and David Epston, *Narrative Means to Therapeutic Ends* (New York: Norton, 1990).
2. R. G. Smith, "Structuralism/Structuralist Geography," in *International Encyclopedia of Human Geography* (Oxford: Elsevier, 2009), 30–38.
3. Michael White, *Map of Narrative Therapy* (Adelaide, SA: Dulwich Centre, 2007).
4. Ncazelo Ncube, "The Tree of Life Project: Using Narrative Ideas in Work with Vulnerable Children in Southern Africa," *International Journal of Narrative Therapy and Community Work* 1 (2006): 3–16, https://doi.org/https://search.informit.org/doi/10.3316/informit.197106237773394.

5. Chow Oi-Wah Esther, "Rediscovery of Older Adults' Life Wisdom: Application of Narrative Therapy Using a Tree-of-Life Metaphor," *Innovation in Aging* 4, Suppl. 1 (December 1, 2020): 835–35, https://doi.org/10.1093/geroni/igaa057.3059.

6. Esther Oi-Wah Chow and Chau-Kiu Cheung, "Contribution of Wisdom to Chinese Elders' Wellbeing," *Innovation in Aging* 1, Suppl. 1 (June 30, 2017): 605, https://doi.org/10.1093/geroni/igx004.2117.

7. Natale Rudland Wood, "Recipes for Life," *International Journal of Narrative Therapy and Community Work* 2 (2012): 34–43.

8. Esther Oi-Wah Chow and Doris Yuen Hung Fok, "Recipe of Life: A Relational Narrative Approach in Therapy with Persons Living with Chronic Pain," *Research on Social Work Practice* 30, no. 3 (August 25, 2019): 320–29, https://doi.org/10.1177/1049731519870867.

9. Esther Oi-Wah Chow, "Narrative Group Intervention to Reconstruct Meaning of Life Among Stroke Survivors: A Randomized Clinical Trial Study," *Neuropsychiatry* 8, no. 4 (2018): 1216–26, https://doi.org/10.4172/neuropsychiatry.1000450.

10. Chow, "Narrative Group Intervention to Reconstruct Meaning of Life."

11. Rene Van Wyk, "Narrative House: A Metaphor for Narrative Therapy: Tribute to Michael White" (2008).

12. David Denborough, "The Team of Life with Young Men from Refugee Backgrounds," *International Journal of Narrative Therapy and Community Work* 2 (2012): 44–53.

13. David Denborough, *Kite of Life: From Intergenerational Conflict to Intergenerational Alliance* (Adelaide, SA: Dulwich Centre, 2010).

14. Glynis Clacherty, "The Suitcase Project: Working with Unaccompanied Child Refugees in New Ways," in *Healing and Change in the City of Gold* (Cham: Springer International, 2014), 13–30, http://dx.doi.org/10.1007/978-3-319-08768-9_2.

15. David Denborough, "Healing and Justice Together: Searching for Narrative Justice," *International Journal of Narrative Therapy and Community Work* 3 (2013): 13–17, https://doi.org/10.3316/informit.697583733979367.

16. Yotis et al., "Using Playback Theatre to Address the Stigma of Mental Disorders," *Arts in Psychotherapy* 55 (September 2017): 80–84, https://doi.org/10.1016/j.aip.2017.04.009.

17. Melissa A. Smigelsky, and Robert A. Neimeyer, "Performative Retelling: Healing Community Stories of Loss Through Playback Theatre," *Death Studies* 42, no. 1 (January 2, 2018): 26–34, https://doi.org/10.1080/07481187.2017.1370414.

18. Catherine Gardner-Elahi and Sannam Zamiri, "Collective Narrative Practice in Forensic Mental Health," *Journal of Forensic Practice* 17, no. 3 (August 10, 2015): 204–18, https://doi.org/10.1108/jfp-10-2014-0034.

19. Geoffrey Cowley and Karen Springen, "Rewriting Life Stories: Mind: Instead of Looking for Flaws in People's Psyches, 'Narrative Therapy' Works at Nurturing Their Forgotten Strengths," *Newsweek* 125, no. 16 (1995): 70–74; Esther Oi-Wah Chow, *Narrating Faith. Love. Hope: A Practical Manual on Narrative Therapy* (敍出信。愛。望: 敍事治療實務手冊), 2nd ed. (Hong Kong: City University of Hong Kong, 2016).

20. Michael White, "The Externalizing of the Problem and the Re-authoring of Lives and Relationships," *Dulwich Centre Newsletter* (Summer 1989).

21. Lawrence Shulman, *Dynamics and Skills of Group Counseling* (Belmont, CA: Cengage Learning, 2010): 27.

22. Lawrence Shulman, *Dynamics and Skills*, 27.

23. Chow, *Narrating Faith. Love. Hope*, 30.

24. Esther Oi-Wah Chow, "Narrative Therapy an Evaluated Intervention to Improve Stroke Survivors' Social and Emotional Adaptation," *Clinical Rehabilitation* 29, no. 4 (August 20, 2014): 315–26, https://doi.org/10.1177/0269215514544039.

25. Jesper Strömbäck, "Four Phases of Mediatization: An Analysis of the Mediatization of Politics," *International Journal of Press/Politics* 13, no. 3 (July 2008): 228–46, https://doi.org/10.1177/1940161208319097.

26. José Van Dijck and David Nieborg, "Wikinomics and Its Discontents: A Critical Analysis of Web 2.0 Business Manifestos," *New Media and Society* 11, no. 5 (July 21, 2009): 855–74, https://doi.org/10.1177/1461444809105356.

27. 青春頌 | 青少年癌症 · 認識 · 同行 · 改變 (@youthcancerhk), Instagram Photos and Videos, accessed September 14, 2023, https://www.instagram.com /youthcancerhk/.

28. Support Community (@_were_all_mental), Instagram Photos and Videos, accessed September 14, 2023, https://www.instagram.com/_were_all_mental/.

29. 什麼是睪丸癌？, 青春頌 | 青少年癌症 · 認識 · 同行 · 改變 (@youthcancerhk), Instagram Photos and Videos, May 20, 2023, https://www.instagram.com/p/ Csd9uICBxhW/?img_index=1.

30. "This Weeks Mental Meetup Topic Is Anxiety," Support Community (@_ were_all_mental), Instagram Photos and Videos, August 28, 2023, https://www .instagram.com/p/Cwd3I5LtBsQ/?utm_source=ig_web_copy_link&igshid =MzRlODBiNWFlZA==.

31. 拿破輪劇團🎭 (@narrative_playback_theatre), Instagram Photos and Videos, accessed September 14, 2023, https://www.instagram.com/narrative_playback _theatre/.

32. White, "The Externalizing of the Problem."

CONCLUSION

16

EVOKING NARRATIVES IN TELETHERAPY'S DIGITAL REALM

Teletherapy levels the playing field. It makes the therapist seem more human.

— MICHAEL, CLIENT, EIGHTY-TWO YEARS OLD

Mary's face appears on the screen. I have never met her in person, but suddenly I am in her living room, and she is in mine. She takes the oxygen cannula out of her nose and rolls a cigarette. I am aghast and want to pull the cigarette away from her before she sets the house on fire. I can't help but wonder what I would have done, had I actually been sitting across from her. I can almost smell the smoke, and it is making me feel ill.

Mary and I have now been working together for almost a year. We have built a foundation of shared stories filled with both pain and joy, which has developed into a strong therapeutic alliance. I have other therapists as supports, and it has been a struggle to build rapport in a new way for those of us who had to switch their entire practice to telemedicine (telehealth).

Doing some self-education on the inception of telehealth, I was surprised to learn that the first documented discussion of phone-based medical appointments appeared in the *Lancet* in 1879 (the first phone was only just invented in 1876).[1] As early as 1925, *Science and Invention* foresaw the advent of video-based telehealth encounters. Before the COVID-19 pandemic, less than 10 percent of the U.S. population used telehealth for clinical encounters, and only 18 percent of physicians provided virtual services. The strongest barrier to the use of telehealth services in the past has been insurance parity state by state, but as a result of the granting of emergency coverage during the pandemic, telehealth was able play a critical role in the field of mental health treatment.

IMPACT ON LONELINESS

The pandemic has changed the way in which many of us practice, which enabled us to keep practicing during the pandemic. It is hard for me to conceive of how alienated those needing help during the 1918–1919 influenza pandemic (the so-called Spanish flu) must have felt. History shows in pictures how health professionals were the only ones in physical contact with their patients, risking and sometimes giving their lives to help others; the sufferers' loneliness was well-documented. Noah Y. Kim writes that:

> Because of the isolated nature of quarantine, the 1918 pandemic was suffered largely in private. Unable to lean on their friends and neighbors for support, people experienced the crisis alone in houses with shuttered windows. . . . Despite many similarities to the present moment, lockdown in 1918 was nevertheless a much lonelier experience than it is today. Lacking the many communication technologies that have allowed us to stay in contact with friends and family, early-20th-century Americans also struggled with the sudden loss of strong community ties, an experience that, to many, even outweighed the fear of a deadly and contagious disease.[2]

In today's technological world we can now, virtually, stay connected with previous clients and form new therapeutic alliances with beginning clients. Through case examples, this chapter focuses on the successful role of therapeutic narrative through the challenge of offering telehealth services to an aging population.

The pandemic has had a profound effect on perspective and reframing of one's life course for older adults. Compounding this is the decreased autonomy for some of those older adults, sending their life course on a new trajectory. Despite the enormous toll taken by the pandemic on the population of older adults worldwide, however, a survey conducted by the Centers for Disease Control and Prevention in August 2020, showed that older adults demonstrated a lower incidence of depression, anxiety, and stress-related disorders compared with younger adults during this time frame.[3] Providing support to older adults as caregivers for themselves and their younger cohorts is more crucial than ever to societal welfare.

IS TELEHEALTH TECHNOLOGY LEAVING
OLDER ADULTS BEHIND?

Florence has been a caregiver all her life. Her mother had a breakdown when Florence was a young teenager, and Florence had to take care of her younger sister. Florence is now in her eighties and, once again, she has become a caregiver, at a time of her life when she should be the one receiving the care. When the pandemic began to escalate, Florence's son moved in with her. He suffers from severe obsessive compulsive disorder and emotional regulation difficulties, and the pandemic exacerbated his symptoms. Under the guise of protecting his mother, he began to hover over her and monitor her every move. Florence tried her best to help him, but the pandemic made her a prisoner in her own home.

Diane faced a different challenge. Her husband, already in his early nineties, had needed care before the pandemic began. She had arranged for a home health aide, but when the pandemic hit, the aide went home and would not come back. Diane, who suffers from mobility problems, was trying to care for her husband alone, but she could not handle it by herself. She contacted an agency, which sent her a new aide. Diane liked the aide, but unfortunately the aide brought COVID-19 with her, and Diane's husband died in the hospital a few weeks later. She remembers his struggling for breath as the paramedics took him out on a stretcher. Diane was not allowed to visit him in the hospital, and her last image of him was when the nurses held up a phone and his face appeared on the screen.

These stories are only two in a vast sea of such narratives. The pandemic brought challenges to all caregivers, many of whom were already in challenging situations. Some 80 percent of all U.S. COVID-related deaths occurred in people over sixty-five years old, and disparities in access to health care, and other resources, have had a devastating impact on racial and ethnic minority and immigrant communities.[4] In an editorial on the impact of the pandemic on aging, Liat Ayalon et al. speak about the increase in ageism that has occurred since the pandemic began.[5] The concept of "stereotype embodiment," which is the internalization by older adults of the societal tendency to group all older adults together as frail and helpless, has been shown to have a negative impact on health. This phenomenon has worsened with the pandemic, as older adults have become more isolated, and have suffered the consequences on COVID-19. Even before the pandemic, inadequate attention was being paid to the mental health needs of older adults, with social isolation and disconnection directly correlated with worsened depression and anxiety.[6]

Multiple studies have shown that virtual therapy can be as effective as in-person treatment.[7] Telehealth provides many advantages for older adults, including accessibility and continuity of care.[8] Although issues of confidentiality and technology remain, the majority of my clients are pleased with the virtual care they are receiving. New obstacles within the auspice of virtual counseling include intuiting nuanced body language, physical spacing, audio delay inhibiting verbal cues, increased chance of distractions, and technological difficulties, among others. Using a narrative approach has become central to my virtual work with the elderly as it helps to minimize the obstacles in light of the person's story becoming the foundation of the work. Most of my current clients were seen in person before the shutdown, so even those I speak to only on the phone remain visually present in my mind. Interestingly, for some of these clients, the security of being in their own homes with the physical distance created by the screen, has enabled them to feel safer and externalize their issues to speak more openly about painful topics. One such person is Anna.

COUNTERING AGEIST BIAS

ANNA'S STORY: SIGHT UNSEEN

I have never seen Anna, yet we have developed a close therapeutic relationship through our phone calls for her weekly session. At ninety-two, she has been losing her vision. Even before meeting her, I knew I had some ageism to process—I was imagining her as a frail, white-haired old woman, but I had no proof of this. I reprocessed this through my years of experience as a geriatric social worker and recalled a "learning moment" of a client I had seen many years ago, whose intake sheet made her sound like a decrepit old woman. When I met her for the first time, however, she was dressed in a tennis outfit and carrying a racquet, having just come from her regular tennis game. I have to remember my own mother as well, who, at ninety-one, was still going to her office and playing tennis.

Anna was the daughter of Scandinavian immigrants. Her parents had a strong work ethic, but they showed little affection for Anna and her brother. Anna's brother was encouraged to pursue higher education, and he became a pioneer in the world of medical research. Anna, in contrast, was "just a girl" and was encouraged to get married and have children. She followed her parents' directive and dropped out of a prestigious university to marry and have a family. (She would later rebel, and go on to earn her doctorate in landscape architecture.)

From the start, Anna knew something was wrong in her marriage. Her husband excelled in his work as a teacher and became the principal of a high school, but at home he was abusive, criminally, to both Anna and her children. Anna, like many victims of abuse, could not perceive the seriousness of the abuse, trying herself "to make it right" for years. Eventually the truth came out, and her husband was arrested on several counts of child molestation. Shortly before he was to go to prison, he committed suicide. At that time, Anna was devastated to realize that he had molested their children as well as dozens of other children in the schools where he worked.

Anna started therapy at this late stage of her life, motivated by emotional distress and no longer wanting to be "an angry, bitter old woman." Anna's children refuse to talk about what happened, and this is painful for Anna, because she is ready to face the truth. Her children see her as a victim, but she does not want to characterize herself in that way because this creates a sense of powerlessness for her. She would rather be empowered as the narrator of her life without this being hijacked by her husband's actions. The most difficult part of this for her now is rumination of guilt: Could she somehow have seen what was going on earlier? Could she have protected others? She punctuates her reflections with the phrase: "I keep trying to make it right."

Her efforts to make it right included her desire to protect others and her false guilt for what her husband did. According to her rigid upbringing, the idea that she could do nothing would have been considered selfish. She said: "I was always on the bottom. Now I have to build my own totem pole."

We are continuing to build that totem pole together using narrative. Every week, Anna tells me another piece of her story, and I help her tease out the themes of strength and resilience, which have deconstructed her false guilt. Once, during a session, Anna accidentally pressed the FaceTime function on her phone. For a brief moment she appeared—stylishly coiffed and dressed. We said hello "face to face," but she did not want to continue on the screen; her vision makes it too stressful for her. We quickly went back to our audio conversation. This brief visual interaction, however, provided me with the understanding that her vision, although waning on the outside, was perhaps providing an opportunity to view things differently on the inside.

I have reminded her that the era in which this narrative took place is important; women were taught that they were supposed to "make things right." As I learned about her during our sessions and reflected on her virtual communication style, including repeated statements, I have been able to let her perspective shine through more than my imagining of her. Through narrative therapy, Anna is beginning to craft a new story in which she is finding her voice and learning how she can use the past to heal the present and future for herself, as well as allow her story to build up others.

THE OPPORTUNITY TO TRAVEL VIRTUALLY

DIANE'S STORY: STRANGERS ON THE SCREEN

Diane had once had voyages and trips around the world through her travel business, leading such an active social life that she never married. She was my first new referral after the pandemic shutdown began, seeking therapy after the loss of both her brother and sister. She was grieving and needed to talk. Ordinarily, I would have done a home visit with someone who is homebound such as Diane, who had become disabled by stenosis and COPD (chronic obstructive pulmonary disease). Now, she was alone in a small apartment, with only her cat for company, and was feeling isolated and depressed. At first, she addressed her losses, but after a while, she began to speak of other aspects of her life. I asked her questions about her travels, and she delighted in recounting her adventures. As we laughed over her tales together, our therapeutic bond grew, and we both looked forward to our weekly meetings. When I mentioned to Diane that I was writing material for a book on narrative therapy, she said excitedly: "I always wanted to be a case study." It has brought both Diane and me joy to see her words of travel to unknown destinations while her body remains still. I hope someday to meet Diane in the flesh, but for now, we share a spiritual connection as strong as any of the clients I was seeing before the shutdown.

WORKING WITH A HIGH-RISK CLIENT

SANDRA'S STORY: "IN WITH THE WRONG CROWD"

Sandra was considered to be a high-risk client, and her history of problems at first seemed just too daunting for me to help in a meaningful way. She had a litany common to many today: history of drug and alcohol abuse, a binge eating disorder, and several inpatient courses of treatment for the eating disorder, with limited success. Similar to substance use disorders, eating disorders tend to be treatment in refractory manner, leading to numerous admissions. The good news for Sandra, however, was that she had hope and was still seeking treatment, which encouraged me to try to help her. At first, the prospect of working with her only by phone did not seem like an option, as I had never before treated someone with this level of health acuity by phone only. I was mostly concerned about establishing trust only with voice cues and innuendos, when I have relied mainly on physical presence and visual cues to establish trust and to understand how substances and eating disorders are affecting a person. How could she build trust in me, without the possibility of actually seeing me?

Sandra, a single woman in her late sixties, lived with her beloved dog. Although her relationship with food has remained a constant issue, she has maintained substance sobriety for twenty-seven years, although during the pandemic, she began drinking episodically. She reports some passive sui-cidal ideation, thinking at times that the world would be better off without her, but said she would never do anything because of her dog, whom she said was her most trusted and valued friend since her breakup with her boyfriend. She denied any serious difficulties in childhood, but stated that her problems began when she went away to college and "got in with the wrong crowd." Sandra worked as an office assistant for a number of years, but for the past few years, she was unemployed, and now her finances were dwindling. She stated she did not binge or drink as much as she did in the past, but she did buy her dinners at a restaurant several nights a week, which was draining her financially. She would come home and eats ice cream and sweets, and afterward would be regretful and took laxatives. She knew this was not good for her health, but felt it was the only way to have some control in her life circumstances. Sandra was still reeling from the breakup of her relationship with a boyfriend, who became abusive. She blamed herself, saying: "How could I not have seen it coming!"

Self-blaming and low self-esteem were themes in Sandra's life and were the main focus of our work together. Surprisingly to me, working with her by phone was more helpful than I thought it would be and, in offering kind-ness and support, we have been exploring how her self-blame has served to exacerbate her self-sabotaging behaviors.

For those who struggle with substance use and eating disorders, seeing them in person is crucial from time to time to assess the physical ravages of their disorders. Fortunately, because things started opening up after the pandemic, I had an appointment recently in Sandra's neighborhood and asked if she would be willing to meet in person for her session. I wanted her to know that I would not pressure her to meet in person and that I would only do so if she felt comfortable. Sandra jumped at the opportunity and thanked me repeatedly for my offer. Upon seeing her, I was stunned to find that she was also anorexic, and I could not have known the degree of her body dysmorphia until I saw her in person. She was painfully thin, and her clothes hung off of her body. To gauge her perspective, I shared mine that I thought she was very thin. Sandra's response tipped me off to the extent of her struggle, saying, "Really? I like the way I look."

CAREGIVER SUPPORT

HENRY'S STORY: FIRST ON THE SCREEN, THEN IN PERSON

Henry and I first met on a video call during the pandemic, and we continued meeting virtually every week for more than a year, until the restrictions on face-to-face meetings were lifted, and I went back in person to the clinic where I worked. He reached out for counseling when he was feeling overwhelmed being a caregiver to a friend and the resulting tension in his marriage from this caregiving. He and his husband had an old friend who was ill, and Henry took it upon himself to be the caregiver. He went every day to see his friend, but the task of caring for his medical needs became too difficult for Henry to handle alone. His husband worked during the day and was unable to help out, except on weekends. Henry had trouble asking for time for himself at home as well, and this led to feelings of resentment toward his husband. Henry dreamed of getting away, and he thought suicide seemed like the only viable escape. He had been having increased suicidal thoughts, and his plan was to use helium to end his life. Thankfully, this plan was not well developed, and he was able to abandon this notion during our sessions.

Henry's weekly video sessions became a lifeline for him, and over time, he learned to establish boundaries for himself. He contacted an agency that helped him get services in place for his friend, and he was able to express more of his own needs when at home. When we eventually met in person, Henry said: "You exist!" And with affectionate humor he added: "You really are short." At first, the in-person meeting felt a bit awkward, but in the weeks that followed, our work together flowed as naturally as it had on the screen.

TELETHERAPY WITH GROUPS

"SHIFTING SANDS"

Teletherapy with groups poses significant challenges, but it can be used effectively in times of crisis to help ease distress. Before the pandemic, we had no inkling that group members would become constant video portraits, framed in individual boxes on a screen, rather than in person participants in a semicontrolled environment. In the three groups I am currently running, I feel at a disadvantage having not met all of the participants in person. Some are clients who participated in the past in person, but others have participated only online.

What happens in the group happens in real time, and it can feel even more immediate on the screen than in person. In person, the leader has some control over the group's environment; with virtual therapy, however, group members are in their own homes and are largely responsible for their environments. Also, confidentiality may have a different meaning for older adults than for young people: Some older people may be more distrustful of being watched on video. Caregivers or other family members may be in the home. They might be groomed in an acceptable manner for the home but not for an outside environment. Or they may not be comfortable making their homes visible. As one group member, who chose not to be seen, said: "We want to be heard. Isn't that what we all need?"

Although the groups I am facilitating online have been successful, and appreciated by their members, I think it is important to share an example of a group whose problems might more easily have been remedied in person, but caused the demise of the group online.

Before the pandemic, I was running a women's group affectionately called "Peace of Mind," for women suffering from anxiety, composed of six women from diverse backgrounds. When we moved to teletherapy, some of the women chose to take a leave of absence, saying they would come back when we could meet in person again, not anticipating the pandemic situation would last as long as it has. Only two of the women continued meeting to support one another through several crises. Only one of the two, whom I will call Gloria, wanted to be seen, and because she originally had gotten to know the other group member, Lina, in person, she did not object to Lina's participation with audio only. Lina had spoken openly about her cluttered home, and this was her reason for turning off the video.

The women decided to write something together about their life experiences shared in this intimate group, and asked me to join them. Gloria had suggested a three-woman show, and insisted that I be the narrator. In the end, we decided to write whatever came to us as long as it related to the group, and we would decide later how to put it together. Lina said our writing project was "like a patchwork quilt," it would be creative and might be a show, or it might be something else.

Gloria wrote a short piece describing her first time in the group in person, and the transition to teletherapy:

> No need to pause at the door. I knew where it was. My show of confidence was definitely not required for what greeted me; an empty room. I chose a neutrally placed chair and waited. That was the beginning. Many steps from the breakdown of 2018. Into group therapy, my first group therapy, unknown group therapy?
>
> The rest blends together. The patchwork of women shuffled in each week until the virus shut us down. So, a few months in our meetings it all evaporated. Poof! Pandemic! This is not the Middle Ages, yet everything closes. I ran seventy-seven miles north as a real refugee.[9]
>
> The first hundred days felt like a very long semi-joyful snow day. The novelty of the shifting sands quickly wore off. I returned to the city in anticipation of returning to the beauty of work. The group morphed down into two with the assistance of technology. Now I "Zoom" the meeting. That's the Morse Code version of how I got here.

Lina shared about the process of writing, and said: "One of the reasons I enjoy writing is because I get to change things, whereas in my real life it's not so easy to change things."

But after a few months of this deep connection, even though they were not physically present, they succumbed to a virtual "cabin fever." With the seeming endlessness of the pandemic and mounting frustration with only each other with whom to vent, they got on each other's nerves Seemingly out of the blue, Lina lit into Gloria, telling her that she was fed up with Gloria's trying to give her useless suggestions. Gloria tried not to lose her temper, but tensions were rising. I thought I had helped lower the temperature by the end of the session, but Lina called me after the session, to tell me she was leaving the group. To her credit, she attended the next session, as she said she didn't want to "just slink away." Had we been meeting in person, I might have been able to help the two women stay calm, address underlying frustrations causing misconceptions, and resolve their differences, particularly given that they had been so supportive of one another before this happened. Perhaps Lina would still have decided to leave, but trying to resolve this kind of conflict with teletherapy, especially when one of the clients did not want to be seen on the screen, was much more difficult.

CONCLUSION: SOME CAVEATS

Telehealth poses not only challenges but also possibilities for social workers. Teletherapy requires a different kind of concentration than that of in-person sessions. When we sit with a client in person, we can look away briefly to reflect on what the client is saying, but in telehealth, looking away from the screen may be interpreted as being distracted. Teletherapy sessions tend to have more interruptions, including technological difficulties, other phones ringing, people or pets coming into the room, or noises coming in from outside. Silences on the screen, or on the phone, may be more uncomfortable for both client and therapist.

Confidentiality online may mean something very different to young people than to older adults, as young people are used to sharing screens. One of my group members brought up her concerns about confidentiality when another group member joined the session while traveling on a train. Even though the client on the train was wearing headphones, the other client felt as though her sense of confidentiality was being compromised. If a client lives in a small space, an aide or family member may be in the room with the client, impinging on their sense of privacy. These issues are pertinent to teletherapy and should be addressed at the beginning of online treatment.

For telehealth to succeed with older adults, we need to ensure safety and confidentiality. We need to help older adults become more comfortable with technology and ensure that they have access to appropriate devices. Marva V. Foster and Kristen A. Sethares reviewed the literature on facilitation and barriers to telehealth and reported that because many older adults who avail themselves of telehealth have experienced physical and cognitive changes, the developers of new technology should involve end users, including both clients and caregivers, in the development of new devices.[10]

We need to be more creative in the ways in which we practice in the future and to take a proactive stance to ensure that telehealth continues to be covered by insurance. As Jacob C. Warren and K. Bryant Smalley have written, telehealth is not a panacea: it is offering "a critical avenue" for sustaining and expanding behavioral health services.[11] Teletherapy can bring help to many older adults who otherwise would not be able to receive our services.

NOTES

1. Jacob C. Warren and K. Bryant Smalley, "Using Telehealth to Meet Mental Health Needs During the COVID-19 Crisis," *Commonwealth Fund* (blog), June 18, 2020, https://www.commonwealthfund.org/blog/2020/using-telehealth-meet -mental-health-needs-during-covid-19-crisis.
2. Noah Y. Kim, "How the 1989 Pandemic Frayed Social Bonds," *The Atlantic*, March 31, 2020.
3. Ipsit V. Vahia, Dilip V. Jeste, and Charles F. Reynolds III, "Older Adults and the Mental Health Effects of COVID-19," *JAMA* 324, no. 22 (2020): 2253–54, https://doi.org/10.1001/jama.2020.21753.
4. Centers for Disease Control and Prevention, "Risk for COVID-19 Infection, Hospitalization, and Death by Race/Ethnicity," April 23, 2021, https://stacks.cdc .gov/view/cdc/105453.
5. Liat Ayalon et al., "Aging in Times of the COVID-19 Pandemic: Avoiding Ageism and Fostering Intergenerational Solidarity," *Journals of Gerontology: Series B* 76, no. 2 (2020): e49–e52, https://doi.org/10.1093/geronb/gbaa051.
6. Amy Novotney, "The Risks of Social Isolation," American Psychological Association, May 2019, https://www.apa.org/monitor/2019/05/ce-corner-isolation.
7. Candice Luo et al., "A Comparison of Electronically-Delivered and Face to Face Cognitive Behavioural Therapies in Depressive Disorders: A Systematic Review," *Lancet* 24, no. 100442 (2020), https://doi.org/10.1016/j.eclinm.2020 .100442.
8. Melanie Donahue, "Benefits of Using Telehealth for Senior Counseling," Blue Moon Senior Counseling, September 1, 2020, https://bluemoonsenior counseling.com/benefits-of-using-telehealth-for-senior-counseling/.
9. When the pandemic shutdown began, Gloria left the city to spend the first few months at the country home of some friends.
10. Marva V. Foster and Kristen A. Sethares, "Facilitators and Barriers to the Adoption of Telehealth in Older Adults," *Computers, Informatics, and Nursing* 32, no. 11 (2014): 523–33, https://doi.org/10.1097/cin.0000000000000105
11. Warren and Smalley, "Using Telehealth to Meet Mental Health Needs."

17

WEAVING LIFE WISDOM FROM EASTERN AND WESTERN NARRATIVE PRACTICES

IN THIS CONCLUDING CHAPTER, we invite our readers to join us in reflection, celebration, and anticipation of the transformative potential that narrative practice holds. Reflecting on the journey of writing this book on narrative practice with older adults, we are struck by the profound power and significance of life-story narratives shaped by diverse family and social identities. Throughout these chapters, we have discussed the intricate art of storytelling, witnessing how individuals skillfully learn to weave together the threads of their distinct identities and experiences, discovering deeper beauty, heroism, and hope within themselves. As we contemplated the importance of life-story narratives in our lives and professions as social workers, we found ourselves independently and serendipitously drawn back to our beginnings. It became clear to us that the act of reconstructing our daily thoughts to uncover the narrative points that imbue courage in both ourselves and others has established a lasting internal framework of hope. This narrative practice of reauthoring the stories of individuals and ourselves has breathed life into our professional journeys, resulting in a continuous cycle of reauthoring our lives.

In this chapter, we first summarize our perspective on narrative practice within the contexts of Eastern and Western cultures, recognizing the rich tapestry of influences that shape the ways in which older people remember, tell, and retell their life stories. Although Eastern and Western cultures are different, it is extremely important for narrative therapy (NT) practitioners to engage in reflective practice to reduce cultural stereotypes and ethnocentrism. An example of this is at the University of Melbourne and the Dulwich Centre, where every year, more than one hundred participants come from different countries to learn about NT in Australia, a country with a high degree of multiculturalism. The Dulwich Centre also has rich experience in accommodating practitioners from diverse cultural backgrounds. In the United States, NT practitioners also have to work with people from diverse sociocultural backgrounds. Therefore, instead of just highlighting the uniqueness of diverse cultural contexts, (i.e., individualism versus collectivism), it is extremely important for NT trainers to bear in mind the significance of enhancing the practitioners' cultural awareness and sensitivity, which can be informed by cultural theories. Second, we discuss the impact of the global crisis (i.e., COVID-19) on older adults and their autobiographical memory. We think that this will be important for all people, especially older populations, because their life-story narratives may be forever affected by COVID-19 pandemic. We will close the chapter with a discussion of the implications of NT practice for social work education.

Before we delve into these discussions, we want to pose three questions that will serve as a guiding framework for our reflection on the lessons and wisdom learned from our narrative practice experiences in the Eastern and Western cultural contexts. The first question we ask is: *Where were we?* As we take stock of the progress made thus far, we will evaluate the current state of NT practices across cultures. The second question that arises is: *Where are we now?* Our journey in writing this book took place during the challenging times of the COVID-19 pandemic, which has had a profound impact on our world and the way we engage with older people and provide services. We take a moment to reflect on these changes, acknowledging the shifts in the needs of the elderly and the adaptations we have made in our practice. Finally, we ask the question: *Where do we go from here?* As we envision the future trajectory of NT practice with older adults, we reflect on how our experiences and insights can shape social work education and practice, fostering a more inclusive and culturally sensitive approach to NT practice. By envisioning the path ahead, we aspire to further the global exploration, collaboration, and innovation in the realm of narrative practice.

WHERE WERE WE?

THE UNIQUENESS OF NARRATIVE THERAPY PRACTICE

NT diverges from conventional therapeutic approaches in several key ways.[1] First, narrative practice places significant emphasis on the *stories or narratives* that individuals construct about their lives, and how these narratives shape their emotional and behavioral responses. This contrasts with other therapeutic approaches that may prioritize emotions, behaviors, or thoughts. Second, narrative practice incorporates the concept of *externalization*, which involves separating the problem from the person. By perceiving individuals as distinct from their problems, this approach creates a space for rediscovering a sense of agency and empowerment, freeing individuals from being defined solely by their problems. In contrast, other therapeutic approaches may consider the problem as an intrinsic part of the individual.

Third, narrative practice adopts a *collaborative* approach, fostering a partnership between the therapist and the individual. The therapist supports the individual in exploring their narratives and facilitates the creation of new, more positive stories through a deliberate understanding of the self. Unlike more directive or prescriptive therapeutic approaches, the therapist does not impose their own perspective or solutions but rather assists the individual in uncovering their own strengths and resources within their narratives.

Finally, narrative practice is grounded in the *social constructionist* perspective, which posits that individuals shape their realities through their interpretations of the world around them. Consequently, the stories people tell about themselves and their experiences are not necessarily objective or factual but rather are influenced by cultural, social, and historical contexts. Overall, narrative practice distinguishes itself from other therapeutic approaches through its focus on narrative, externalization of problems, collaborative nature, and social constructionist viewpoint.

INSIGHT GAINED FROM NARRATIVE PRACTICE
BETWEEN EASTERN AND WESTERN CULTURES

This strengths-based approach is aligned with gerontological social work principles in both Eastern and Western cultures. When applying NT to older adults from diverse cultural backgrounds, such as Eastern and Western cultures, it is crucial to consider the cultural context, their respective use of language within the context, and its influence on an individual's self-worth and identity.[2] The subsequent insight sheds light on notable similarities and differences that should be taken into account when implementing NT practice within Eastern and Western cultures and possibly cultures of other kinds. This initial attempt to explore the use of NT in the two places with different cultures may provide a point of reference for future comparative analysis of NT practices beyond the Eastern-Western cultural boundary.

First, in terms of similarities, both Eastern and Western cultures recognize the significance of an individual's personal narrative in shaping their sense of self and meaning in life. NT encourages individuals to delve into and reflect on their life experiences, examining how these experiences have affected their beliefs, values, expectations, and behaviors. Second, in both Eastern and Western cultures, older adults are often esteemed for their life experiences and wisdom. NT practice values the insight and perspectives of older adults, encouraging them to share their stories and reflect upon their life experiences. Third, both Eastern and Western NT practitioners emphasize the process of meaning-making, wherein individuals create deep meaning for today by reauthoring meaning from their past life experiences. This concept is universally relevant and applicable to people from all cultural backgrounds.

In terms of differences, Eastern and Western cultures share similar values and beliefs, but diverge significantly in terms of weight and priority of their values and beliefs, which subsequently shape how older adults perceive themselves and their life experiences. For instance, Eastern cultures tend to emphasize the importance of family and community, whereas Western cultures tend to prioritize individualism and autonomy. Consequently, NT needs to consider these cultural disparities when working with older adults. In Western cultures, the therapy primarily focuses on reauthoring an individual's self-worth and identity by exploring their distinct experiences, strengths, and values. In contrast, Eastern cultures often emphasize collectivism and group-based values, necessitating collaboration with family members and an exploration of the individual's role within the family, community, and social networks.

In terms of self-concept and identity, Western cultures tend to view the self as an independent and autonomous entity, placing substantial emphasis on personal identity. In this context, NT may help older adults in exploring their individual accomplishments and personal growth. Conversely, Eastern cultures often emphasize interdependent self-concepts, in which an individual's identity is closely intertwined with their relationships and social roles. NT practice in these cultures may involve exploring the person's contributions to their family and community as well as their connections with others. Above all, communication styles between Eastern and Western cultures are significant.

COMMUNICATION STYLE DIFFERENCES BETWEEN EASTERN AND WESTERN CULTURES

Cultural sensitivity and competence are paramount considerations for NT practitioners when working with older adults from diverse cultural backgrounds. It is imperative for social workers and other professionals to undergo comprehensive training and grasp the significance of cultural competence in the provision of NT. Recognizing and respecting cultural differences in communication styles is vital for establishing effective therapeutic relationships and fostering mutual understanding. Moreover, communication styles may exhibit variations between Eastern and Western cultures, with certain cultures placing greater emphasis on indirect communication and nonverbal cues. To effectively engage with older adults, NT practice may need to adapt to these differences in communication styles.[3]

When comparing the communication styles of older adults in Eastern and Western cultures within a NT context, several key differences come to light.[4] First, regarding emotional expression, older adults in Eastern cultures may display a tendency to require more time for expressing their emotions than their Western counterparts. This inclination stems from Eastern societies' emphasis on high-context cultures, emotional restraint, and the maintenance of harmony within social relationships, leading to a more reserved expression of emotions. Conversely, older adults in Western societies, with low-context cultures, may exhibit a greater willingness to openly express themselves and may require a shorter period of time to feel secure in sharing their emotions.[5]

Second, in terms of the sense of safety, perceptions of safety in therapy can diverge between Eastern and Western cultures. In Eastern cultures, older adults may necessitate additional time to establish trust and a sense of safety within the therapeutic relationship because of cultural factors, such as hierarchical structures and the potential stigma associated with therapy for older adults. In this context, older adults in Eastern cultures may experience feelings of shame or a desire to "save face" even in the presence of a therapist, which underscores the importance of creating an environment that cultivates trust and nonjudgment.

Third, norms of social hierarchy, higher power distance, and respect for professionals hold greater prominence in Eastern cultures. Hierarchical relationships are highly valued, with older adults placing significant importance on maintaining respect and deference toward authority figures, including therapists. The narrative professional is often viewed as an expert who has the necessary know-how, and older adults may find comfort in a structured and hierarchical therapeutic dynamic. In contrast, Western cultures tend to adopt a more egalitarian approach, in which older adults expect a collaborative and equal partnership with the narrative practitioner. Thinking about these cultural differences in this regard leads to an examination of ways that therapists position themselves with respect to their clients in the therapeutic process. For example, if a therapist holds a traditional practice framework (e.g., "me big, you small") in directing and reframing the stories of her or his clients, instead of helping clients to externalize the problem, and reauthor their preferred identity, then the therapist will be operating from a hierarchical approach, even if this is not the therapist's intent. A therapist's tendency toward this practice framework is often more likely to occur or even be encouraged when older adults have or demonstrate a sense of powerlessness in the therapeutic process, as when they are economically worse off in society or suffer from poorer health conditions, such as long-term illnesses.

Last, seeking psychological support is not the cultural norm in Eastern cultures, as many people, especially older adults, may be hesitant to disclose family secrets or personal struggles to a social work professional. Eastern cultures prioritize saving face and maintaining social harmony, leading older adults to be more cautious about revealing vulnerabilities or personal challenges. Social workers must create a secure, encouraging, empowering, and accepting environment in which older adults feel comfortable sharing their experiences without fear of embarrassment or losing face or compromising confidentiality regarding personal or family matters.

In short, the communication styles of older adults in Eastern and Western cultures exhibit differences concerning emotional expression, the time required to establish a sense of safety, the influence of hierarchy and respect, perceptions of receiving narrative services, and an emphasis on saving face. Social work professionals should be mindful of these cultural disparities and adapt their approach accordingly, fostering trust, respect, and cultural sensitivity to effectively engage with older adults. Applying NT to older adults from Eastern and Western cultures necessitates a nuanced understanding of cultural differences and the ability to tailor the narrative approach accordingly. By incorporating cultural sensitivity and competence, NT practice can be a powerful tool in assisting older adults from diverse backgrounds in reshaping their life narratives. Indeed, there are possibilities of case-therapist mix, where cultural differences affect the therapeutic relationship, and thus NT practitioners need to be well trained to enhance their cross-cultural awareness and skills to reduce communication barriers.

WHERE ARE WE NOW?

Since the inception of this project, we have seen dramatic changes in the world, but perhaps the most salient for our older adult clients has been the pandemic. COVID-19 altered many life narratives and changed the way many of us work. Adding to the pandemic, many of the geopolitical changes of the past few years have affected older persons' narratives. In this section, we address how the COVID-19 pandemic has changed narratives and storylines of older adults and families and discuss the subsequent challenges they face as well as the opportunities.

THE IMPACT OF COVID-19 PANDEMIC ON OLDER POPULATIONS

The COVID-19 pandemic, reminiscent of a world war in its global impact, unleashed an overwhelming wave of stress, fear, and uncertainty on older adults worldwide. The magnitude of this impact cannot be overstated. For many older individuals, the pandemic represents one of the most significant life events they have ever encountered, leaving an indelible mark on their life-story narratives. As we discussed in chapter 1, autobiographical memory, a vital component of older adult storytelling, plays a crucial role in shaping their narratives.[6] It encompasses a wide range of memories, including singular moments, recurring themes, and extended experiences, all interwoven into a coherent self-narrative. Older adults draw on this reservoir of memories to construct and evaluate their life stories, which are influenced by their unique sociocultural perspectives.[7] It is important to consider the impact of the global pandemic crisis on the autobiographical memory of older individuals when engaging in narrative work with them, which is also relevant to educating students in social work and other disciplines.

Social work students need to be aware that autobiographical memory may contain powerful and impactful visual symbols and images that are associated with the COVID-19 pandemic. This imagery may reverberate deeply within the narratives of older people within their specific contexts.

For instance, lockdowns, depicted as shuttered doors and boarded windows, evoke a palpable sense of confinement, seclusion, and the loss of freedom. They stand as reminders of the isolation experienced by older individuals, forcing them to retreat from the outside world and severing precious social connections that once brought joy and companionship. Masks, worn as a protective measure, serve as a constant visual reminder of the potential dangers lurking in every interaction. The sight of these face coverings reflects the shared responsibility to safeguard oneself and others, but it also carries a weight of anxiety and caution. Masks blur the smiles and expressions that once conveyed warmth and empathy, replacing them with a sense of anonymity and the constant awareness of a pervasive threat.

Testing and retesting, the scenes of waiting and queuing outside testing booths, manifest the arduous and repetitive nature of pandemic life. These images signify the tireless efforts undertaken by older adults to ensure their safety and the safety of those around them. The hours spent in lines and the anticipation of results symbolize a collective yearning for reassurance, peace of mind, and a respite from the cycle of uncertainty. Vaccinations, represented by the sight of syringes and healthcare professionals administering doses, embody a glimmer of hope amid the darkness. They symbolize the scientific triumphs achieved in the face of adversity, offering older adults a lifeline to regain a sense of security and normality. The image of a Band-Aid on an arm can act as a totem: a visual testimony to resilience, signaling a step toward healing and protection from the insidious grip of the virus.

In contrast, throughout the pandemic, older adults also were confronted with an array of conflicting opinions and controversies surrounding vaccinations. These contrasting views have contributed to an increased sense of fear, confusion, and frustration within their personal narratives. Additionally, the pandemic has brought about the heartbreaking loss of family members and close friends, which has become an integral part of older adults' stories during this time. Grief and mourning have permeated their narratives, leaving a lasting impact on their collective memory. Social workers and narrative practitioners need to recognize and validate these experiences, providing a supportive space for older adults to express their emotions and integrate these significant events into their life stories.

In terms of social isolation, nursing home glass-door visits, a painful sight etched in the minds of many, depict the cruel separation between older adults and their families. The image of hands pressed against a windowpane, the longing gaze of an older person yearning for physical contact, and the inherent loneliness of being confined within the walls of long-term care facilities represent the isolation endured by older adults and the profound impact this isolation had on their emotional well-being. Video call visits, a novel form of connection born out of necessity, materialize as grids of faces on screens. They symbolize the paradox of virtual togetherness—a digital lifeline that simultaneously highlights the absence of physical presence. These images serve as bittersweet reminders of the resilience and adaptability of older adults as they strive to maintain relationships and seek solace in the pixelated embrace of their loved ones.

Social isolation and loneliness, starkly visible in the empty streets, desolate parks, and solitary figures behind closed doors, signify the emotional toll exacted by the pandemic. Older adults, already vulnerable to social disconnection, have endured prolonged periods of solitude, leading to a deep sense of loneliness and detrimental effects on mental health and well-being. These images capture their yearning for human connection, the ache for shared laughter, and the profound longing to be held in an embrace. Sudden heartbreaking losses, depicted through photographs of memorial altars, obituaries, and candles flickering in the darkness, serve as a testament to the immense grief experienced by older adults and their communities. These images symbolize the countless lives forever altered, the stories prematurely extinguished, and the mourning process disrupted by the constraints of the pandemic. They carry the weight of unspoken good-byes, unfinished conversations, and the profound sense of collective sorrow.

Psychologically, death and dying, a heart-wrenching reality that has touched countless lives, are imprinted in the memories of older adults. The visual representation of empty hospital beds, grieving families, and the stark reminder of the fragility of life evoke profound sorrow and loss. Funeral and memorial services with limited attendance, dead bodies wrapped in personal protective equipment, and the absence of traditional mourning rituals further compound the emotional weight carried by older individuals as they grapple with the irreparable void left by loved ones.

As we reflect on the impact of these visual symbols and images on the life-story narratives of older adults, we bear witness to the indomitable spirit that emerges amid adversity. Through this anguish and loss, older individuals also find strength, resilience, and a renewed appreciation for the moments of joy and connections that endure. These images will forever remain etched in their autobiographical memories, serving as a poignant reminder of their lived experiences during this unprecedented chapter in human history.

THE IMPACT OF GEOPOLITICAL CHANGES ON OLDER POPULATIONS

In addition to the ongoing pandemic, the recent domestic and geopolitical changes also have significantly affected the narratives of older people. Some express concerns for the future generations, whereas others remain indifferent, knowing they won't be around to witness potential devastation. In particular, Hong Kong, my hometown, has undergone significant political transformations since the social movement in 2019 and the enactment of the National Security Law (NSL) in 2020.[8] The NSL has imposed restrictions on free speech and assembly, resulting in the dissolution of numerous civil society organizations and student groups within university campuses. These changes have had a profound impact on Hong Kong society, with a large number of prodemocracy protestors being arrested and held in custody since 2020 without bail pending trial. Additionally, tens of thousands of families, with or without young children, have chosen to leave the city and seek refuge in countries, such as the United Kingdom, Australia, United States, and Canada. Because of the challenges and difficulties associated with uprooting the extended family, many of these individuals have left behind their older parents in Hong Kong, who often preferred to stay behind, perhaps because of their strong sociocultural connectedness to living in Hong Kong. These older Chinese individuals in Hong Kong have already experienced historical trauma, many having been refugees from mainland China in the 1940s and 1950s. They fled their communities decades ago with their parents, and now their own adult children have left Hong Kong. It is challenging to comprehend the potential triggers the current political situation may have on their autobiographical memories and how they envision their late-life circumstances.

In the Western Hemisphere, the United States has witnessed its share of political conflicts between various political parties and ideologies. These conflicts and tensions permeate not only the national political landscape but also extend into the fabric of everyday life, affecting relationships within extended families, workplaces, friendship circles, and other contexts. Apart from the ongoing pandemic, there is a palpable sense that civil discord may worsen. Within families, discussions around political matters can become contentious, straining relationships that have endured for decades. The workplace, once a space for collaboration and camaraderie, can become a battleground of conflicting viewpoints and impassioned debates. Even social gatherings and community events may be tinged with a sense of unease as differing political and ideological beliefs clash.

In the context of narrative practice with older adults, it is essential to acknowledge and address the potential division that can arise within families because of different perceptions of race and ideological issues, particularly in the current political climate. The intergenerational divide stemming from contrasting beliefs and attitudes toward race can become a significant source of stress and tension. Older adults and younger generations may hold divergent perspectives influenced by their unique cohort, life experiences and social contexts. As narrative professionals, it is crucial to provide a safe and inclusive space that encourages open dialogue, empathy, and understanding. By facilitating respectful conversations that validate each individual's lived experiences and perspectives, NT can promote healing and foster intergenerational connections within families. Emphasizing the power of storytelling and the cocreation of new narratives, narrative practice can contribute to fostering communication, reconciliation, and positive change in the face of racial tensions, ultimately promoting the well-being and harmony of older adults and their families.

The experiences of older Americans during this politically charged time are shaped not only by their personal opinions and perspectives but also by their lived experiences and generational values. Many have witnessed and lived through previous periods of societal upheaval, and the echoes of those times resonate with the current political climate. Navigating these conflicts can evoke a wide range of emotions, including anxiety, frustration, disappointment, and even a sense of despair as they witness the division and polarization within their communities. As the United States grapples with its political landscape, older Americans face the challenge of reconciling their beliefs and desires for a better future with the stark realities of a nation divided. In this climate of uncertainty and potential political upheaval, it becomes increasingly important to recognize the diverse experiences and perspectives of older Americans. Creating spaces for dialogue, empathy, and respect can foster a sense of unity and narrow the gaps that exist between generations and differing ideologies.

In the future, we hope that other researchers in the field of aging and narrative practice could undertake comprehensive qualitative research studies focusing on this pandemic cohort of older adults in both Eastern and Western contexts. These studies hold immense potential in unearthing invaluable insight into coping strategies, resilience, and accumulated wisdom, while their recollections of these profound sociopolitical circumstances remain vivid and accessible. By meticulously documenting and analyzing their lived experiences and perspectives, we can learn indispensable lessons and leverage their invaluable reservoir of knowledge to inform evidence-based practices and policymaking in the face of potential future conflicts and uncertainties. These research endeavors aim to uncover deepseated resilience and adaptive mechanisms that can contribute to the development of effective interventions and foster greater societal cohesion across generations, transcending geographic and cultural boundaries.

CHANGING NARRATIVES AND STORYLINES OF OLDER ADULTS AND FAMILIES

At the micro level, the COVID-19 pandemic has altered daily individual life. Disruptions in daily routines, remote work, increased social isolation especially from youth, closed worship buildings, and uncertainty about the future have had a global impact. The impact on adults already struggling with these issues has been even more profound as most were completely quarantined from all others, including their caregivers and significant social supports. Despite the challenges for older adults, the pandemic has highlighted their resilience and adaptability. The majority of our clients have learned to use technology, enabling them to stay connected to loved ones, participate in remote social activities, and access medical care. Some have even become more engaged in using technology than they were before the pandemic. Perhaps a lifetime of needing to adapt has provided many older individuals with resilience in the face of adversity as well as mortality.

When we first began to work remotely, it seemed challenging and unfamiliar. In time, we began to realize that remote work with older adults offers new avenues for creativity and connection. The possibility of screen-sharing allows us to enrich remote sessions with resources that are both practical and visually interesting. This very book is the result of resilience and adaptation to technological opportunities. Many of our older clients liked and continue to like the convenience of remote work, as it allows them to stay in the comfort of their homes. Before the pandemic, we were making home visits to homebound older clients, but not all of those welcomed someone into their homes. Now, they can make visible only what they wish to show. One of our group members initially kept her living room hidden by a video background, but when she started to feel more at home in the group, she removed the screen to reveal her living space. For survivors of trauma, the screen can provide a sense of physical safety, which has enabled some of our clients to speak more openly about their experiences. Phone sessions allow for another kind of intimacy, one that is purely auditory, but just as compelling. In teletherapy, as in in-person sessions, the narrative remains the essence of communication.

In terms of mortality and morbidity, most of the older adults we worked with said that they are not afraid of death, but they do fear becoming dependent. The concern over losing one's cognitive capability appears greater than the fear of physical decline. Death may be welcomed as a peaceful end to a life well-lived or as the final exit from a lifetime of pain, disappointment, or regret. Beliefs about death are rooted in culture and personal experience. For some, religion and spirituality provide a framework for end-of-life narratives; for others, rituals and traditions may give comfort. In the West, death is broadly seen as a tragedy, a subject to be avoided. By helping our older adults talk about death, and by truly listening to their end-of-life narratives, we can support them in finding deep meaning in the lives they have lived. This is the healing power of life stories.

WHERE DO WE GO FROM HERE?

This book offers a wealth of rich findings that carry significant implications for social work research, education, practice, and policy. While recognizing the broader impact, as dedicated social work educators, in this section, we focus exclusively on the implications for social work education.

Narrative serves as an invaluable tool in social work education, fostering a sense of community and shedding light on diverse themes. At the beginning of each semester, we encourage students to share the stories behind their names, revealing elements of parental expectations, cultural traditions, religious beliefs, popular culture influences, educational and professional aspirations, and language dynamics. This practice extends to our work with older adults, opening doors to a world of rich experiences and a more holistic approach to treatment. Case-based learning, essentially rooted in storytelling, forms a foundational aspect of social work student training. In our teaching, we share life stories of older adults, discussing our interactions in helping them "rewrite" problematic narratives, and occasionally acknowledging our mistakes. Empathy development is a key goal of case-based learning, alongside acquiring social work knowledge and skills.

Utilizing narrative in social work education necessitates establishing a solid theoretical understanding of narrative structure. Exploring concepts like recognizing dominant narratives and considering sociocultural and historical contexts in the formation of personal narratives is pivotal for student learning, enabling them to grasp the roots of individuals' life stories. Through case examples, social work students discover how NT can assist older adults in transforming problematic narratives into life-affirming ones. Furthermore, students can deepen their understanding of narrative power by interviewing older individuals and sharing their interviews, reflecting on their own reactions, identifying themes, recognizing challenges faced by interviewees, and appreciating their resilience. Cultural considerations and awareness of power dynamics, trauma history, and social inequities in shaping personal narratives guide students in adapting NT techniques accordingly. NT aligns with various treatment approaches and embodies a social work strengths-based perspective. Students are also encouraged to reflect on their personal narratives, identifying biases and assumptions that may arise when listening to older adults' stories.

Given that this book explores NT in both Eastern and Western contexts, although much is similar, it is essential to acknowledge the different influences on the meaning and understanding of narrative. Lauren, having been born and raised in New York City, brings forth a perspective shaped by Western training. She has been influenced by concepts of linear storytelling, individualism, professional identity, importance of personal time, and personal growth, among many others. Ada and Esther, who were both born and raised in Hong Kong (later receiving graduate education in the United States and Canada), both draw from their experiences in the East. Their perspectives have been shaped by communal roles, Eastern and Western educational attainment, teacher-student relationships, the importance of keeping active at all times, and immigration, among many others.

These are broad generalizations, and both Eastern and Western narrative traditions encompass diversity and overlap.[9] Globalization has led to the hybridization of narrative approaches in various cultural contexts. Regardless of the East-West distinction, equipping social work students with NT knowledge and skills empowers them to become effective agents of change for themselves, in their own practices, and in the world. In this light, we hope that you will gain from reading our narrative journeys in the afterword.

NOTES

1. Diane R. Gehart, *Mastering Competencies in Family Therapy: A Practical Approach to Theory and Clinical Case Documentation* (Boston: Cengage Learning, 2017); Alice Morgan, *What Is Narrative Therapy? An Easy-to-Read Introduction* (Adelaide, SA: Dulwich Centre, 2000); and Pei-Shan Yang and Ada C. Mui, *Foundations of Gerontological Social Work Practice in Taiwan* (Taipei: YehYeh Book Gallery, 2022).
2. Sylvia Xiaohua Chen et al., "The Added Value of World Views Over Self-Views: Predicting Modest Behaviour in Eastern and Western Cultures," *British Journal of Social Psychology* 56, no. 4 (2017): 723–49, https://doi.org/10.1111/bjso.12196; Katherine Nelson and Robyn Fivush, "The Emergence of Autobiographical Memory: A Social Cultural Developmental Theory," *Psychological Review* 111, no. 2 (2004): 486–511, https://doi.org/10.1037/0033-295X.111.2.486; and Qi Wang, "The Emergence of Cultural Self-Constructs: Autobiographical Memory and Self-Description in European American and Chinese Children," *Developmental Psychology* 40, no. 1 (2004): 3–15, https://psycnet.apa.org/doi/10.1037/0012-1649.40.1.3.
3. Chen et al., "The Added Value of World Views Over Self-Views."
4. Ada C. Mui and Suk-Young Kang, "Acculturation Stress and Depression Among Asian immigrant Elders," *Social Work* 51, no. 3 (2006): 243–55, https://

doi.org/10.1093/sw/51.3.243; Ada C. Mui and Tazuko Shibusawa, *Asian American Elders in the Twenty-First Century: Key Indicators of Well-Being*" (New York: Columbia University Press, 2008); Ada C. Mui et al., *Gerontological Social Work: Theory and Practice*, 2nd ed. (Shanghai: Truth and Wisdom, 2017); and Yang and Mui, *Foundations of Gerontological Social Work*.
5. Chen et al., "The Added Value of World Views Over Self-Views."
6. Nelson and Fivush, "The Emergence of Autobiographical Memory."
7. Wang, "The Emergence of Cultural Self-Constructs."
8. Hingchau Lam, "The Ouster Clause in the Hong Kong National Security Law: Its Effectiveness in the Common Law and Its Implications for the Rule of Law," *Crime, Law, and Social Change* 76 (2021): 543–61, https://doi.org/10.1007/s10611-021-09979-6.
9. Mui and Kang, "Acculturation Stress and Depression"; and Mui and Shibusawa, *Asian American Elders*.

PERSONAL REFLECTIONS ON NARRATIVE PRACTICE, IDENTITIES, AND LIFE JOURNEY

ESTHER OI-WAH CHOW

Being the eldest daughter of a typical Hong Kong Chinese family in the 1950s, my parents expected me to join the workforce after graduating from high school, as I had (and fortunately still have) four younger siblings, two of whom are the preferred male gender. Given this, I was privileged to be given the opportunity to complete five years of high school education in an English secondary school. However, any resources for university education were dedicated to my male siblings. Unless I was able to get admitted into university with a scholarship, as the eldest daughter, I had to work full time to help out the family. Knowing the chances of getting admitted into the local universities was low, not to mention getting a scholarship, I thought I had no choice and so I just followed my parents' words, accepting it as my narrative destiny.

I dreamed of studying abroad; however, studying abroad appeared to be unlikely as it meant adding a financial burden to my parents and our family. Ever since I was in primary school, I was fascinated by my teachers, who came from Canada, and the idea of studying in a foreign country, learning a new language, exploring foreign ideas, and experiencing a different culture inspired me. Yet, my parents thought high school was sufficient for girls, and that I did not need to receive a university education.

I was determined to pursue my dream for myself, to start following my own narrative apart from my family's ideas, by applying for university admission to several universities when I was in form six (equivalent to grade twelve in Canada). After months of hard work and determination,

I received an acceptance letter to a four-year undergraduate program from a Canadian University in Montreal. I was over the moon with excitement and could not wait to start my new life. My parents, however, were not pleased. They believed that I was making a mistake by leaving my family to study abroad. Knowing it was against my parents' wishes, I begged my parents for their support, and I promised to work hard to complete my studies within three years. Acknowledging my strong desire and efforts, my parents finally relented, and I arrived in Montreal with a suitcase containing some winter clothes, a heart full of hope, and a determination to succeed.

At first, things were tough for me. I had to adjust to a new culture, navigate the university system, and work part time to support myself financially, with limited French language proficiency. I missed my family terribly, but I cherished such a precious opportunity, and knew that I had to stay strong and focused on my goals.

Over time, I began to thrive in my new environment, made new friends, excelled in my studies, and even found a job that allowed me to work flexible hours and still have time for my studies. I was grateful for being able to become self-reliant and emotionally interdependent through the support from my peers whom I met at the university, who also had to work to support themselves.

After three years at university, I had attained my young life's dream of graduating from the honors program in sociology with high marks and was then admitted to the graduate school in social work. I had gained an expanded narrative of invaluable life experience and developed a sense of agency that would help me to flourish both personally and professionally. I was also able to prove to my parents that I was capable of taking care of myself, setting high goals and achieving my dreams. I returned to Hong Kong with a new perspective on life, with deep appreciation for the sacrifices that my parents had made for me, and for my teachers and peers who trusted and supported me during different stages of my studies.

Looking back, I can see that despite having a clear vision for myself, my parents had firmly in place their expectations of me adopted from the sociocultural norms at that time. It took great efforts to alter their minds to believe in my ability to attain higher career goals. Through my professional practice as a social worker, I worked with different people who have been in various life situations that have limited their choices and aspirations. It has become my career to reflect from my own life and practice to find ways to empower others to overcome their hardships, to actualize their life goals based on their strengths, to reconstruct their narratives instead of just going through the professional motions.

After I studied and became fluent in narrative therapy (trained by Australian colleagues from Dulwich Centre), I was inspired by peers coming from different countries with the knowledge, skills, and attitude needed to work collaboratively with people who consulted the practitioners. With funding support from Hong Kong Jockey Club Charities Trust, I launched the first randomized clinical trial in systematically applying narrative therapy with stroke survivors and their caregivers in 2009. This research has continued and extended evidence-based practice with other older people living with different chronicities. I am energized to rediscover their core values and preferred identity to make sense of the difficult life experiences they had undergone, to testify to their beliefs, to make meaning from those challenges that align with their purpose in life, and to become more resilient to live with their preferred identity, beyond their diagnostic labels.

My own story is a testament of the power of self-reliance, courage, determination, and perseverance to discover alternatives to change my designated path. Despite facing obstacles and opposition from those closest to me, I had not given up, and I explored different ways to grow and challenge myself. Nevertheless, at times, I felt caught in challenging life situations, such as feeling alone, especially during the first year of university when I arrived in Canada, including a new environment, different culture, different education context, and different use of languages. Yet, I was grateful to connect with a group of university classmates who shared the same goals of supporting ourselves financially and excelling in studies. Through my positive character traits of reaching out, being curious to new things, and being genuine and receptive, I made new friends across cultures. We helped and encouraged each other through positive, negative, and challenging times, and I gained lifelong friendships and developed deeper listening and respect for others. We studied together, supported each other, and were willing to "walk the extra mile" to overcome challenges to reach excellence.

The message that my life narrative gives to me is that when we encounter life challenges, if we are able to deeply connect with peers and supporters, then we can make sense of the negotiation process from those challenges. It makes a difference when we can help ourselves and one another; validate our self-worth, values, and beliefs; and solidify our identities over the lifespan. In this modern society, we cannot take this for granted. NT provides a "means" for us to understand, recollect, and interpret, and author/reauthor our life experiences. I am privileged and truly grateful to have the opportunities to work with and learn from those who have consulted me. Connecting different sparkling moments provides possibilities to narrate respective storylines through which rich and diverse life experiences can be rediscovered, expressed, told, and remembered, while other events are slowly forgotten and ignored. This process affirms that through open dialectic communication, people can generate solutions that align with their positive core values, which then can be applied to overcome life's challenges and live gracefully.

LAUREN TAYLOR

When Ada Mui and I first began discussing the possibility of writing this book, she had already started collaborating with Esther Chow on this project. Esther had submitted a proposal for a book on narrative therapy in Hong Kong, but Ada felt the topic needed to be broadened with a wider reach. I proposed looking at narrative therapy in the East and in the West, and we were all in agreement that this was a relevant scope; the world has changed dramatically since that conversation. The following is a personal reflection on my own journey, as a New Yorker, during the writing of this book.

Some events mark our lives and our language with "before" and "after." When I began writing for this book, COVID-19 had not yet become that event. Even when it did begin, during the first couple of months of the pandemic, while I was living in New York, it still seemed a distant problem, until suddenly it wasn't. The week before I fell ill, only days before everything shut down in New York, I had visited an elderly client in her home. She had broken both her wrists in a fall and had asked me to hold her cup of water to her lips. She was coughing and complaining of having difficulty breathing, but her doctor was not particularly concerned. She had been hospitalized the month before with pneumonia, and her doctor felt that these were likely residual symptoms. I was healthy, and I wasn't worried about catching whatever she had, thinking daily life would not be changed by a cough. A day later, her situation became critical, and her aide called 911. She was rushed to the hospital. I went to visit her the day before she died. She was already in and out of consciousness. The next day, I awoke with a fever, and my own nightmare began.

It has been more than a few years since that time, and I feel lucky to be alive. It took me a couple of years to recover, and despite some lingering symptoms, I am fine. Before the pandemic, I had written two chapters of this book. After COVID-19, I was unable to write for a long time, but when I finally started again, I was happy that I could, even though initially it was rocky. I wrote the beginning of a chapter, and went to check a reference in one of my prepandemic chapters, only to discover that I had written almost the same thing all over again. Discouraged at first, I was determined to try again. Fortunately, I had not lost my capacity to write, and to my surprise, I found it has been enriched.

COVID-19 changed my work, as it has for many, many people. Video calls have allowed me to go back to work much sooner than I could have if I had to return to working in person. At first it felt strange to meet new clients on the screen, knowing I would likely never meet them in person; speaking with clients I already knew was easier. Some, however, wanted phone sessions. Although I had been concerned about how this would work, phone sessions proved to be surprisingly intimate. One day, a new client who could not manage the video call platform, as she was virtually blind, accidently pressed FaceTime on her phone. For a brief moment I saw her, but she did not want to continue with the video. In the beginning, running groups on video calls was a challenge, but I have mastered this, and the groups are one of the most rewarding parts of my work. I have returned to working in person part time, and I have had the opportunity to see some old and some new clients face to face, but the majority of my work remains remote.

How has life changed for my clients? One died of COVID-19 early in the pandemic. I have been working with his widow. She couldn't visit him in the hospital, and she described how the nurses held up his phone so he could speak to her on the screen. He died four days later. Another had COVID-19 and survived, but she is still plagued with episodes of overwhelming fatigue. Most of my clients have been vaccinated and boosted (another word that has come into common parlance), and at this point, many have had a milder form of COVID-19. What has changed for so many clients, however, is a rise in anxiety. The anxiety engendered by the pandemic has been compounded by the political situation in the United States, racism and antisemitism, gun violence, global warming, the war in Ukraine, and many other challenges. We are also all a few years older. Before the pandemic, I didn't worry as much about my own health and my own aging. Now I do. But I am also a better clinician, as I have continued to grow and learn, despite my own challenging situation. Narrative has played an important role in this growth. As I tell my story, and listen to the stories of others, I become part of a collective experience of both survival and loss. I have become more intimately acquainted with mortality.

A number of my clients are approaching ninety, and a few are already in their nineties. I know they will likely begin to decline more rapidly now, and I will lose them. This is part of working with older adults, and it will not be the first time I have lost clients. But these losses seem more poignant in the context of today's world, perhaps as I came so close to losing my own life. I am more cognizant of how little time we have on this earth, and so, I have become more discerning in how I choose to live. But most of all, I feel enormously grateful for all of the people in my life who have enriched my narrative, and the connections we share. Narrative is a means of keeping the memories alive, as I remember their stories, and they remember mine. As one of my clients said: "My whole life is now history."

ADA C. MUI

As I look back on the journey of writing this book on narrative practice with older adults, I am struck by the profound power and significance of life-story narratives shaped by diverse family and social identities. Throughout these chapters, we have delved into the ways in which older individuals tell and retell their stories, interweaving the threads of their unique identities and experiences.

On a personal level, I feel compelled to offer a more intimate perspective—a glimpse into my own experiences and the identities that have influenced my understanding of this work. Beyond the titles of professor, teacher, researcher, preacher's wife, and dementia caregiver, lies a tapestry of narratives that have become an integral part of who I am. These narratives have shaped my worldview and life goals, influenced my interactions with others, and guided me through the complexities of my identity.

My passion for studying and working with older adults stems from a deeply rooted sense of empathy and compassion, nurtured by my upbringing in a challenging environment. Reflecting on my early years, growing up in the depths of extreme poverty in Hong Kong, I cannot help but acknowledge the profound impact this has had on shaping the person I am today. Despite the immense challenges, I have come to appreciate how these experiences served as a crucible, forging my resilience and igniting an unflinching determination to effect positive change in the world.

One of my role models who left an indelible mark on my journey was my extraordinary American missionary teacher at the church in Hong Kong. With a doctorate in education and a persistent devotion to her faith, she dedicated an astounding four decades of her life to serving children, youth, older adults, and families in poverty-stricken areas of China and Hong Kong. Her love for Jesus Christ propelled her to provide both tangible and spiritual support to those who needed it most.

I can still vividly recall the transformative impact she had on me during my time in her Sunday school class. Her steadfast commitment to others and her embodiment of the biblical teachings of selflessness resonated deeply within me. She truly exemplified the teachings of the Bible, "it is more blessed to give than to receive," and she lived by the principle that "much is given, much is expected."

What struck me the most about her remarkable journey was the stark contrast between her privileged upbringing in the United States and her chosen path of service to the less fortunate in impoverished areas. Coming from an affluent family, she recognized her privilege as a calling, a divine invitation to use her advantages to uplift those in need. Her decision to dedicate her life to serving others was a testament to her character, compassion, and firm Christian faith.

Through her tireless efforts, she not only provided education and support to countless children and young people, but she also instilled in me a profound sense of purpose. Witnessing her selfless dedication and sacrificial love for others sparked a fire within me—a deep desire to follow in her footsteps and make a meaningful impact in the lives of young and older people.

Her example taught me that our privileges and blessings are not meant to be hoarded, but rather to be shared and used as instruments of positive change. She taught me that true fulfillment lies in the act of giving, in uplifting others, and in embodying the Christian teachings of love, justice, kindness, humility, empathy, and compassion.

As we write the final pages of this book, I am humbled to pay homage to my beloved teacher, who not only provided me with an invaluable Bible education but also imparted timeless wisdom that continues to guide me. Her influence has shaped my perspective on narrative practice with older adults, as it has taught me the importance of honoring their stories and creating spaces where their voices can be heard.

ACKNOWLEDGMENTS

In the spirit of my Sunday school teacher's profound selflessness and steadfast devotion, I wholeheartedly dedicate this book to her and to all the remarkable individuals who, like her, have dedicated their lives to making a lasting impact. Their tireless efforts and resolute commitment serve as beacons of inspiration for us all. Before I continue delving into the narrative of my life, I feel compelled to express my heartfelt gratitude and admiration for two exceptional gerontologists who have played instrumental roles in shaping my academic journey. Drs. Nancy Morrow-Howell and Denise Burnette have been invaluable mentors and dear friends, whose unwavering support and guidance have accompanied me throughout the years.

Nancy, my esteemed dissertation adviser at Washington University Brown School of Social Work, has been a strong pillar of wisdom and support throughout my academic career. Her influence on my scholarly pursuits spans four decades since our paths first crossed in 1984. She not only has been a teacher and mentor to me but also a true friend, consistently championing my work and offering invaluable insight and emotional support.

Denise, my academic twin sister, shares a unique bond with me that extends beyond the professional realm. We embarked on our journey as gerontologists together when we were both hired by Columbia University School of Social Work in 1990. We have faced countless challenges and shed tears together, but we have also celebrated milestones and grown older as colleagues and cherished friends. We have traversed the academic landscape side by side, supporting and encouraging one another, knowing that we are stronger together. Our shared commitment to uplifting the lives of older adults has forged a bond that time cannot diminish.

As I reflect on the invaluable contributions of Nancy and Denise, I am reminded of the importance of collaboration and solidarity in our academic endeavors. Their legacies, like those of my Sunday school teacher and countless others, serve as powerful reminders that the power of narrative is not limited to personal stories alone. It is a tool that can be wielded to ignite compassion, foster understanding, and spark transformative change.

With this book, we hope to inspire future generations of professionals in aging to embrace the profound potential of storytelling and narrative practice. May the legacies of these remarkable individuals continue to guide us, nurturing a collective commitment to compassion and empathy. Together, let us harness the power of narrative as we strive to create a world that honors and uplifts the voices of older adults, fostering a society where every story is valued and cherished.

Witnessing firsthand the daily struggles and hardships that plagued my family and community during my upbringing in Hong Kong, I lived in dilapidated conditions and became acutely aware of scarcity, constantly grappling with the uncertainty of tomorrow. Amid the adversity, however, a profound lesson took root in the very core of my being—the power of the human spirit to endure and overcome.

These early formative experiences have become the bedrock of my personal narrative, fueling my passion for improving the lives of older adults from diverse backgrounds. Through my work, I have drawn on a deep understanding of their struggles and triumphs that I gained from my own journey. It is this empathy and connection that allows me to engage with and empower those who have faced similar challenges.

I firmly believe that our experiences, no matter how difficult, have the potential to be transformed into catalysts for growth and transformation. They teach us empathy, resilience, and the transformative power of kindness and compassion. My humble beginnings have endowed me with an unshakeable belief in the potential of every individual and a profound conviction that, with the right support and opportunities, we can rise above adversity and build a more equitable and inclusive society.

As we bring these journeys through the excerpts of our lives to a close, the integration of narrative practice into my professional life has been a transformative experience—one that continues to unfold and evolve. As a professor, I have been privileged to witness the power of storytelling in the lives of my students as they connect with their narratives and the narratives of others. Through their stories, I am reminded of the importance of fostering an inclusive and compassionate environment, in which all identities are celebrated and honored.

Parallel to my academic pursuits, my role as a dementia caregiver has provided me with a deeply personal understanding of the challenges faced by individuals and families living with dementia. Through their stories, I have witnessed the preservation of identity, resilience in the face of memory loss, and the enduring human spirit that transcends cognitive decline. The practice of narrative therapy has allowed me to guide individuals with dementia in reclaiming aspects of their life stories, preserving fragments of their identities, and promoting a sense of continuity and dignity. This journey has shaped me not only as a caregiver but also as a human being, reinforcing the profound impact that our stories can have on our well-being and sense of self.

In the process of writing this book, my collaboration with Esther and Lauren has been a source of inspiration and personal growth. Their unique perspectives, representing the merging of Eastern and Western cultures, have enriched our collective understanding of narrative practice. Through our shared experiences, conversations, and narratives, we have deepened our appreciation for the transformative potential of this approach.

On behalf of our team, we are deeply grateful for Melissa Gorton, L.C.S.W., a devoted alumna of Columbia University School of Social Work, whose persistent support, meticulous editing, and belief in the power of narratives have been instrumental in shaping this book. Her guidance and encouragement have allowed our voices to merge seamlessly, amplifying the importance of narrative practice in the lives of older adults.

We are also profoundly grateful to our dedicated research assistants, Ethan Siu Leung Cheung, Elsa Lee, Tsai Wan Yu, Lisa Li Chaoyu, Hardev Singh, Ava Hao, and Tracy To, and to our critical readers, Irene Ip and Pan Sam Chap, whose tireless efforts were instrumental in completing this book. Their invaluable contributions have been indispensable, and we are deeply indebted to them for their unwavering support.

As we conclude this afterword, we invite readers to embark on their own journey of self-reflection and exploration. Embrace the power of storytelling, not only as a means of understanding others but also as a way to connect with your own personal narratives and identities. Our stories hold the key to empathy, compassion, and the realization that, at our core, we are all connected by the universal human experience. May this book serve as a catalyst for further exploration, dialogue, and growth in the realm of narrative practice. Together, let us celebrate the rich tapestry of identities, the power of life stories, and the transformative potential that lies within each and every one of us.

BIBLIOGRAPHY

Adams, Richard E., Joseph A. Boscarino, and Charles R. Figley. "Compassion Fatigue and Psychological Distress Among Social Workers: A Validation Study." *American Journal of Orthopsychiatry* 76, no. 1 (2006): 103–8. https://doi.org/10.1037/0002-9432.76.1.103.

Adshead, Gwen. "The Life Sentence: Using a Narrative Approach in Group Psychotherapy with Offenders." *Group Analysis* 44, no. 2 (2011): 175–95. https://doi.org/10.1177/0533316411400969.

Ardelt, Monika. "Disentangling the Relations Between Wisdom and Different Types of Well-Being in Old Age: Findings from a Short-Term Longitudinal Study." *Journal of Happiness Studies* 17, no. 5 (2016): 1963–84.

Arendt, Hannah. *Men in Dark Times*. New York: Harcourt, Brace, 1968.

Audet, Cristelle T., and Robin D. Everall. "Therapist Self-Disclosure and the Therapeutic Relationship: A Phenomenological Study from the Client Perspective." *British Journal of Guidance and Counselling* 38, no. 3 (2010): 327–42.

Augusta-Scott, Tod, and Juergen Dankwort. "Partner Abuse Group Intervention: Lessons from Education and Narrative Therapy Approaches." *Journal of Interpersonal Violence* 17, no. 7 (2002): 783–805. https://doi.org/10.1177/088626050201700706.

Ayalon, Liat, Alison Chasteen, Manfred Diehl, Becca R. Levy, Shevaun D. Neupert, Klaus Rothermund, Clemens Tesch-Romer, and Hans-Werner Wahl. "Aging in Times of the COVID-19 Pandemic: Avoiding Ageism and Fostering Intergenerational Solidarity." *Journals of Gerontology: Series B* 76, no. 2 (2020): e49–e52. https://doi.org/10.1093/geronb/gbaa051.

Baars, Jan. "*Critical* Turns of Aging, Narrative, and Time." *International Journal of Ageing and Later Life* 7, no. 2 (2012): 143–65. https://doi.org/10.3384/ijal.1652-8670.1272a7.

Bailey, Andrew W, and Keith C Russell. "Volunteer Tourism: Powerful Programs or Predisposed Participants?" *Journal of Hospitality and Tourism Management* 19, no. 1 (2012): 123–32.

Bannon, Sarah, Jonathan Greenberg, Ryan A. Mace, Joseph J Locascio, and Ana-Maria Vranceanu. "The Role of Social Isolation in Physical and Emotional Outcomes Among Patients with Chronic Pain." *General Hospital Psychiatry* 69 (2021): 50–54.

Barnett, Jeffrey E. "Psychotherapist Self-Disclosure: Ethical and Clinical Considerations." *Psychotherapy* 48, no. 4 (2011): 315–21. https://psycnet.apa.org/doi /10.1037/a0026056.

Basu-Zharku, Iulia O. "Effects of Collectivistic and Individualistic Cultures on Imagination Inflation in Eastern and Western Cultures." *Inquiries Journal* 3, no. 2 (2011). http://www.inquiriesjournal.com/articles/1679/effects-of-collectivistic-and -individualistic-cultures-on-imagination-inflation-in-eastern-and-western-cultures.

Baumgartner, Barbara, and Brian Dean Williams. "Becoming an Insider: Narrative Therapy Groups Alongside People Overcoming Homelessness." *Journal of Systemic Therapies* 33, no. 4 (2014): 1–14. https://doi.org/https://doi.org/10.1521/jsyt .2014.33.4.1.

Beck, Aaron T, Robert A Steer, and Gregory Brown. "Beck Depression Inventory–II." *Psychological Assessment* (1996).

Benjamin, Diane, and Lori Zook-Stanley. "An Invitation to People Struggling with Trauma and to the Practitioners Working with Them." *International Journal of Narrative Therapy and Community Work* 3 (2012): 62–68.

Berggren, Kalle. "Sticky Masculinity: Post-Structuralism, Phenomenology and Subjectivity in Critical Studies on Men." *Men and Masculinities* 17, no. 3 (2014): 231–52. https://doi.org/10.1177/1097184x14539510.

Besley, Athlone Christine. "Foucault and the Turn to Narrative Therapy." *British Journal of Guidance and Counselling* 30, no. 2 (2002/05/01 2002): 125–43. https://doi.org/10.1080/03069880220128010.

Bloom, Martin, Joel Fischer, and John G. Orme. *Evaluating Practice: Guidelines for the Accountable Professional.* 6th ed. Boston: Pearson, 2009.

Bluck, Susan. "Remember and Review of Forget and Let Go? Views from a Functional Approach to Autobiographical Memory." *International Journal of Reminiscence and Life Review* 4, no. 1 (2017): 3–7. http://143.95.253.101/~radfordojs /index.php/IJRLR.

Bondemark, Lars, and Sabine Ruf. "Randomized Controlled Trial: The Gold Standard or an Unobtainable Fallacy?" *European Journal of Orthodontics* 37, no. 5 (2015): 457–61. https://doi.org/10.1093/ejo/cjv046.

Bottomley, Jamison S., Seth Abrutyn, Melissa A. Smigelsky, and Robert A. Neimeyer. "Mental Health Symptomatology and Exposure to Non-Fatal Suicidal Behavior: Factors That Predict Vulnerability and Resilience Among College Students." *Archives of Suicide Research* 22, no. 4 (2018): 596–614. https://doi.org/10.1080 /13811118.2017.1387632.

Bowe, Mhairi, Debra Gray, Clifford Stevenson, Niamh McNamara, Juliet R. H. Wakefield, Blerina Kellezi, Iain Wilson, et al. " A Social Cure in the Community:

A Mixed-Method Exploration of the Role of Social Identity in the Experiences and Well-Being of Community Volunteers." *European Journal of Social Psychology* 50, no. 7 (2020): 1523–39. https://doi.org/10.1002/ejsp.2706.

Bransford, Cassandra L. "Reconciling Paternalism and Empowerment in Clinical Practice: An Intersubjective Perspective." *Social Work* 36, no. 1 (2011): 33–41. https://doi.org/10.1093/sw/56.1.33.

Bressers, H., and P. J. Klok. "Fundamentals for a Theory of Policy Instruments." *International Journal of Social Economics* 15, no. 3/4 (1988): 22–41.

Bruner, Edward M. *The Anthropology of Experience.* Urbana: University of Illinois Press, 1986.

Bruner, Jerome. "Narratives of Aging." *Journal of Aging Studies* 13, no. 1 (1999): 7–9.

Buekens, Filip. "A Truth-Minimalist Reading of Foucault." *Le foucaldien* 7 (2021). https://doi.org/10.16995/lefou.7989.

Burns, David. "When Helping Doesn't Help: Why Some Clients May Not Want to Change." Psychotherapy Networker. March/April 1, 2017. https://www.psycho-therapynetworker.org/article/when-helping-doesnt-help.

Burns, G. W. *Healing with Stories in Your Casebook Collection for Using Therapeutic Metaphors.* Hoboken, NJ: Wiley, 2007.

Butera-Prinzi, Franca, Nella Charles, and Karen Story. "Narrative Family Therapy and Group Work for Families Living with Acquired Brain Injury." *Australian and New Zealand Journal of Family Therapy* 35, no. 1 (2014): 81–99. https://doi.org/10.1002/anzf.1046.

Butler, Robert N. "The Life Review: An Interpretation of Reminiscence in the Aged." *Psychiatry* 26, no. 1 (1963): 65–76. https://doi.org/10.1080/00332747.1963.11023339.

Carducci, Bernardo J. "Expressions of the Self in Individualistic vs. Collective Cultures: A Cross-Cultural-Perspective Teaching Module." *Psychology Learning and Teaching* 11, no. 3 (2012): 413–417. https://doi.org/10.2304%2Fplat.2012.11.3.413.

Carey, Maggie, and Shona Russell. "Externalising: Commonly Asked Questions." *International Journal of Narrative Therapy and Community Work* 2002, no. 2 (2002): 76–84.

——. *Narrative Therapy: Responding to Your Questions.* Adelaide, SA Dulwich Centre, 2004.

Carr, Alan. "Michael White's Narrative Therapy." *Contemporary Family Therapy* 20, no. 4 (1998): 485–503.

Carr, Eloise CJ, Graham McCaffrey, and Mia Maris Ortiz. "The Suffering of Chronic Pain Patients on a Wait List: Are They Amenable to Narrative Therapy?" *Canadian Journal of Pain* 1, no. 1 (2017): 14–21.

Catt, Isaac E. "Gregory Bateson's 'New Science' in the Context of Communicology." *American Journal of Semiotics* 19, no. 1/4 (2016): 153–72. https://doi.org/https://doi.org/10.5840/ajs2003191/47.

Caws, Peter. "What Is Structuralism?" *Partisan Review* 35, no. 1 (1968).

Centers for Disease Control and Prevention. "Risk for COVID-19 Infection, Hospitalization, and Death by Race/Ethnicity." April 23, 2021. https://stacks.cdc.gov/view/cdc/105453.

Chen, Sylvia Xiaohua, Jacky C. K. Ng, Emma E. Buchtel, Yanjun Guan, Hong Deng, and Michael Harris Bond. "The Added Value of World Views Over Self-Views: Predicting Modest Behaviour in Eastern and Western Cultures." *British Journal of Social Psychology* 56, no. 4 (2017): 723–749. https://doi.org/10.1111/bjso.12196.

Cheung, Chi, Siu-Wai Choi, Stanley Wong, and Yvonne Lee. "Changes in Prevalence, Outcomes, and Help-Seeking Behavior of Chronic Pain in an Aging Population over the Last Decade." *Pain Practice* 17 (10/01 2016). https://doi.org/10.1111/papr.12496.

Cheung, Chi Wai, Siu Wai Choi, Stanley Sau Ching Wong, Yvonne Lee, and Michael Garnet Irwin. "Changes in Prevalence, Outcomes, and Help-Seeking Behavior of Chronic Pain in an Aging Population over the Last Decade." *Pain Practice* 17, no. 5 (2017): 643–54.

Chow, Esther Oi-Wah. *I Have a Story with Chronic Pain: Narrative Practice in Application* (「我和疼痛有個故事」敘事治療小組實踐): *A Report*. Hong Kong: Neighbourhood Advice-Action Council, 2018.

——. *Narrating Faith. Love. Hope: A Practical Manual on Narrative Therapy* (敍出信。愛。望: 敍事治療實務手冊). 2nd ed. Hong Kong: City University of Hong Kong, 2016.

——. "Narrative Group Intervention to Reconstruct Meaning of Life Among Stroke Survivors: A Randomized Clinical Trial Study." *Neuropsychiatry* 8, no. 4 (2018): 1216–26. https://doi.org/10.4172/Neuropsychiatry.1000450.

——. "Narrative Group Interventions to Rediscover Life Wisdom Among Hong Kong Chinese Older Adults: A Waitlist RCT Study." *Innovation in Aging* 2, Suppl. 1 (2018): 992. https://doi.org/10.1093/geroni/igy031.3666.

——. "Narrative Therapy an Evaluated Intervention to Improve Stroke Survivors' Social and Emotional Adaptation." *Clinical Rehabilitation* 29, no. 4 (2015): 315–26. https://doi.org/10.1177/0269215514544039.

——. "Rediscovery of Older Adults' Life Wisdom: Application of Narrative Therapy Using a Tree-of-Life Metaphor." *Innovation in Aging* 4, Suppl. 1 (2020): 835. https://doi.org/10.1093/geroni/igaa057.3059.

——. "Responding to Lives After Stroke: Narrative Therapy with Stroke Survivors and Caregivers." *International Journal of Reminiscence and Life Review*. 10th Biennial Conference, New Orleans, LA, 2013.

——. "Responding to Lives After Stroke: Stroke Survivors and Caregivers Going on Narrative Journeys." *International Journal of Narrative Therapy and Community Work* 4 (2013): 1.

Chow, Esther Oi-Wah, and Chau-Kiu Cheung. "Contribution of Wisdom to Chinese Elders' Well-Being." *Innovation in Aging* 1, Suppl. 1 (June 30, 2017): 605. https://doi.org/10.1093/geroni/igx004.2117.

Chow, Esther Oi-Wah, and Doris Yuen Hung Fok. "Recipe of Life: A Relational Narrative Approach in Therapy with Persons Living with Chronic Pain." *Research on Social Work Practice* 30, no. 3 (2020): 320–29. https://doi.org/10.1177/1049731519870867.

Chow, Esther Oi-Wah, and Sai-Fu Fung. "Narrative Group Intervention to Rediscover Life Wisdom Among Hong Kong Chinese Older Adults: A Single-Blind Randomized Waitlist-Controlled Trial." *Innovation in Aging* 5, no. 3 (2021): igab027. https://doi.org/10.1093/geroni/igab027.

Chow, Esther Oi Wah, and Andrew Yiu Tsang. *Low Applications of Interactive Pedagogical Learning Model in Promoting Intergenerational Communication to Enhance Teaching and Learning*. Hong Kong: City University of Hong Kong, 2021–2023.

Clacherty, Glynis. "The Suitcase Project: Working with Unaccompanied Child Refugees in New Ways." In *Healing and Change in the City of Gold*, 13–30. Cham: Springer International, 2014. http://dx.doi.org/10.1007/978-3-319-08768-9_2.

Clark, Ashley A. "Narrative Therapy Integration within Substance Abuse Groups." *Journal of Creativity in Mental Health* 9, no. 4 (2014): 511–22. https://doi.org/10.1080/15401383.2014.914457.

Clark, Gregory, Neil Cummins, Yu Hao, and Daniel Diaz Vidal. *The Son Also Rises: Surnames and the History of Social Mobility*. Princeton Economic History of the Western World. Princeton, NJ: Princeton University Press, 2014.

Clemans, Shantih E. "Understanding Vicarious Traumatization: Strategies for Social Workers." *Social Work Today* 4, no. 2 (2004):13.

Cole, Thomas R. *The Journey of Life: A Cultural History of Aging in America*. New York: Cambridge University Press, 1992.

Combs, Gene, and Jill Freedman. "Narrative, Poststructuralism, and Social Justice: Current Practices in Narrative Therapy." *Counseling Psychologist* 40, no. 7 (2012): 1033–60. https://doi.org/10.1177/0011000012460662.

Costa, Rachel V., and Kenneth I. Pakenham. "Associations Between Benefit Finding and Adjustment Outcomes in Thyroid Cancer." *Psycho-Oncology* 21, no. 7 (2012): 737–44.

Cowley, Geoffrey, and Karen Springen. "Rewriting Life Stories: Mind: Instead of Looking for Flaws in People's Psyches, 'Narrative Therapy' Works at Nurturing Their Forgotten Strengths." *Newsweek* 125, no. 16 (1995): 70–74.

Creswell, John Ward. *Qualitative Inquiry and Research Design: Choosing Among Five Approaches*. 3rd ed. Los Angeles: SAGE, 2013.

Danner, Christine C., Beatrice Bean E. Robinson, Meg I. Striepe, and Pang Foua Yang Rhodes. "Running from the Demon: Culturally Specific Group Therapy for Depressed Hmong Women in a Family Medicine Residency Clinic." *Women and Therapy* 30, no. 1–2 (2007): 151–76.

Dean Webster, Jeffrey. "Measuring the Character Strength of Wisdom." *International Journal of Aging and Human Development* 65, no. 2 (2007): 163–83. https://doi.org/10.2190/AG.65.2.d.

De Hennezel, Marie. "La vulnérabilité dans l'accompagnement de fin de vie." Lecture at the Fourth Conference on Aging, *La cause des aînés: Pour vivre autrement . . . et mieux*, Paris, June 13, 2010.

De Medeiros, Kate. *Narrative Gerontology in Research and Practice*. New York: Springer, 2013.

Denborough, David. *Collective Narrative Practice: Responding to Individuals, Groups, and Communities Who Have Experienced Trauma*. Adelaide, SA Dulwich Centre, 2008.

——. "Healing and Justice Together: Searching for Narrative Justice." *International Journal of Narrative Therapy and Community Work* no. 3 (2013): 13–17. https:// doi.org/10.3316/informit.697583733979367.

——. *Kite of Life: From Intergenerational Conflict to Intergenerational Alliance*. Adelaide, SA: Dulwich Centre, 2010.

——. "Stories from Robben Island: A Report from a Journey of Healing." *International Journal of Narrative Therapy and Community Work* 2004, no. 2 (2004): 1–10.

——. "The Team of Life with Young Men from Refugee Backgrounds." *International Journal of Narrative Therapy and Community Work* 2 (2012): 44–53. https://doi.org/10.3316/informit.627063623957215.

Deng, CuiYu, Qi Lu, Lili Yang, Rui Wu, Yi Liu, LiYa Li, Shixiang Cheng, et al. "Factors Associated with Stigma in Community-Dwelling Stroke Survivors in China: A Cross-Sectional Study." *Journal of the Neurological Sciences* 407 (2018): 1–6. https://doi.org/10.1016/j.jns.2019.116459.

DeQuincy, Christian. "Intersubjectivity: Exploring Consciousness From a Second Person Perspective." *Journal of Transpersonal Psychology* 32, no. 2 (2001): 132–155.

Desai, Janhavi S. "Intergenerational Conflict Within Asian American Families: The Role of Acculturation, Ethnic Identity, Individualism, and Collectivism." *Dissertation Abstracts International* 67, (2006): 7369. https://www.worldcat.org /title/intergenerational-conflict-within-asian-american-families-the-role-of -acculturation-ethnic-identity-individualism-and-collectivism/oclc/437348983.

Dickson, Janelle. "The 'Mighty Oak': Using The Tree of Life Methodology as a Gateway to the Other Maps of Narrative Practice." *International Journal of Narrative Therapy and Community Work* 4 (2009): 9–23.

Doan, Robert E. "Narrative Therapy, Postmodernism, Social Constructionism, and Constructivism: Discussion and Distinctions." *Transactional Analysis Journal* 27, no. 2 (1997): 128–133. https://doi.org/10.1177/036215379702700208.

Donahue, Melanie. "Benefits of Using Telehealth for Senior Counseling." Blue Moon Senior Counseling. September 1, 2020. https://bluemoonseniorcounseling.com/benefits-of-using-telehealth-for-senior-counseling/.

Dover, Tessa L., Jeffrey M. Hunger, and Brenda Major. "Health Consequences of Prejudice and Discrimination." In *The Wiley Encyclopedia of Health Psychology*, vol. 2, ed. Lee Cohen, 231–38. Chichester, UK: Wiley, 2020.

Driscoll, Janette J., and Anthony A. Hughes. "Sexuality of Aging Adults: A Case Study Using Narrative Therapy." *Contemporary Family Therapy* 44 (2021): 373–80. https://doi.org/10.1007/s10591-021-09589-3.

Dunn, Robert G. "Self, Identity, and Difference: Mead and the Poststructuralists." *Sociological Quarterly* 38, no. 4 (1997): 687–705. https://doi.org/10.1111/j.1533-8525.1997.tb00760.x.

Erikson, Erik H. *Identity and the Life Cycle*. New York: Norton, 1980.

Faircloth, Christopher, et al., "Disrupted Bodies: Experiencing the Newly Limited Body in Stroke," *Symbolic Interaction* 27, no. 1 (2004).

Ferrazzi, Keith, and Tahl Raz. *Never Eat Alone, Expanded and Updated: And Other Secrets to Success, One Relationship at a Time*. New York: Crown, 2014.

Figley, Charles R. "Compassion Fatigue: Psychotherapists' Chronic Lack of Self Care." *Journal of Clinical Psychology* 58, no. 11 (2002): 1433–41. https://doi.org/10.1002/jclp.10090.

Fivush, Robyn, Jordan A. Booker, and Matthew E. Graci. "Ongoing Narrative Meaning-Making Within Events and Across the Life Span." *Imagination, Cognition and Personality* 37, no. 2 (2017): 127–152. https://doi.org/10.1177/0276236617733824.

Flood, Meredith, and Kenneth D. Phillips. "Creativity in Older Adults: A Plethora of Possibilities." *Issues in Mental Health Nursing* 28, no. 4 (2007): 389–411. https://doi.org/10.1080/01612840701252956.

Fond, Guillaume, Katlyn Nemani, Damien Etchecopar-Etchart, Anderson Loundou, Donald C. Goff, Seung Won Lee, Christophe Lancon, et al. "Association Between Mental Health Disorders and Mortality Among Patients with Covid-19 in 7 Countries: A Systematic Review and Meta-Analysis." *JAMA Psychiatry* 78, no. 11 (2021): 1208. https://doi.org/10.1001/jamapsychiatry.2021.2274.

Fond, Guillaume, Vanessa Pauly, Audrey Duba, Sebastien Salas, Marie Viprey, Karine Baumstarck, Veronica Orleans, et al. "End of Life Breast Cancer Care in Women with Severe Mental Illnesses." *Scientific Reports* 11, no. 1 (2021): 10167. https://doi.org/10.1038/s41598-021-89726-y.

Fort, Christin J. "Intersectionality, Intersubjectivity and Integration: A Two Person Therapy." *Journal of Psychology and Theology* 46, no. 2 (2018): 116–21. https://doi.org/10.1177/009164711876..7987.

Foster, Marva V., and Kristen A. Sethares. "Facilitators and Barriers to the Adoption of Telehealth in Older Adults." *Computers, Informatics, and Nursing* 32, no. 11 (2014): 523–33. https://doi.org/10.1097/cin.0000000000000105.

Foucault, Michel. The History of Sexuality. New York: Vintage Books, 1980.

——. "The Subject and Power." *Critical Inquiry* 8, no. 4 (1982): 777–95. http://www.jstor.org/stable/1343197.

——. "Just Listening: Narrative and Deep Illness." *Family Systems and Health* 16, no. 3 (1998): 197–212. https://doi.org/10.1037/h0089849.

——. *Letting Stories Breathe: A Socio-Narratology*. Chicago: University of Chicago Press, 2010.

Fredman, Glenda. "Weaving Net-Works of Hope with Families, Practitioners and Communities: Inspiration from Systemic and Narrative Approaches." *International Journal of Narrative Therapy and Community Work* 1 (2014): 34–44.

Freud, Sigmund. "Analysis Terminable and Interminable." *International Journal of Psycho-Analysis* 18 (1937): 373–405.

Fung, Helene H. "Aging in Culture." *Gerontologist* 53, no. 3 (2013): 369–377. https://doi.org/10.1093/geront/gnt024.

Fung, Sai-fu, Esther Oi-Wah Chow, and Chau-Kiu Cheung. "Development and Validation of a Brief Self-Assessed Wisdom Scale." *BMC Geriatrics* 20, no. 1 (2020): 1–8.

Gabbard, Glen O., Judith S. Beck, and Jeremy Holmes. *Oxford Textbook of Psychotherapy.* New York: Oxford University Press, 2005.

Gardner-Elahi, Catherine, and Sannam Zamiri. "Collective Narrative Practice in Forensic Mental Health." *Journal of Forensic Practice* 17, no. 3 (2015): 204–218. https://doi.org/10.1108/JFP-10-2014-0034.

Gardner, Paula J., and Jennifer M. Poole. "One Story at a Time: Narrative Therapy, Older Adults, and Addictions." *Journal of Applied Gerontology* 28, no. 5 (2009): 600–620. https://doi.org/10.1177/0733464808330822.

Gehart, Diane R. *Mastering Competencies in Family Therapy: A Practical Approach to Theory and Clinical Case Documentation.* Boston: Cengage Learning, 2017.

Gergen, K. J. "Psychological Science in a Postmodern Context." *American Psychologist* 56, no. 10 (2001): 803–13. https://doi.org/10.1037//0003-066x.56.10.803.

Han, Jessica Jungsook, Michelle D. Leichtman, and Qi Wang. "Autobiographical Memory in Korean, Chinese, and American Children." *Developmental Psychology* 34, no. 4 (1998): 701. https://doi.org/10.1037/0012-1649.34.4.701.

Hardy, Barbara. "Narrative as a Primary Act of Mind." In *The Cool Web: The Patterns of Children's Reading,* ed. Margaret Meek, Aiden Warlow, and Griselda Barton, 13. London: Bodley Head, 1977.

Hare-Mustin, Rachel T. "Discourses in the Mirrored Room: A Postmodern Analysis of Therapy." *Family Process* 33, no. 1 (1994): 19–35. https://doi.org/10.1111/j.1545-5300.1994.00019.x.

Hariton, Eduardo, and Joseph J. Locascio. "Randomised Controlled Trials—The Gold Standard for Effectiveness Research: Study Design: Randomised Controlled Trials." *BJOG: An International Journal of Obstetrics and Gynaecology* 125, no. 13 (2018): 1716. https://doi.org/10.1111/1471-0528.15199.

Haselhurst, Jessica, Kate Moss, Stewart Rust, James Oliver, Rhian Hughes, Catherine McGrath, Daniel Reed, Lucy Ferguson, and Joanne Murray. "A Narrative-Informed Evaluation of Tree of Life for Parents of Children with Physical Health Conditions." *Clinical Child Psychology and Psychiatry* 26, no. 1 (2021): 51–63.

Haug, Frigga. "Feminist Writing: Working with Women's Experience." *Feminist Review* 42, no. 1 (1992): 16–32. https://doi.org/10.1057/fr.1992.45.

Health Resources and Services Administration. Telehealth.NHS.gov. Accessed September 2, 2023. https://www.hhs.gov/coronavirus/telehealth/index.html.

Hedtke, Lorraine. "The Origami of Remembering." *International Journal of Narrative Therapy and Community Work* 4 (2003): 58–63. https://search.informit.org /doi/abs/10.3316/INFORMIT.661383982613964.

Helms, Janet E. *Black and White Racial Identity: Theory, Research, and Practice.* Westport, CT: Greenwood, 1990.

Herman, Judith L. *Trauma and Recovery: The Aftermath of Violence—From Domestic Abuse to Political Terror.* New York: Basic, 1992.

Hignett, Sue, and Hilary McDermott. "Qualitative Methodology for Ergonomics." In *Evaluation of Human Work*, ed. R. John Wilson and Sarah Sharples, 119–38. Boca Raton, FL: CRC, 2015.

Hong, Ying-yi, Grace Ip, Chi-yue Chiu, Michael W. Morris, and Tanya Menon. "Cultural Identity and Dynamic Construction of the Self: Collective Duties and Individual Rights in Chinese and American Cultures." Special issue, *Social Cognition* 19, no. 3 (2001): 251–268. https://doi.org/10.1521/soco.19.3.251.21473.

Hooyman, Nancy R., and H. Asuman Kiyak. *Social Gerontology: A Multidisciplinary Perspective.* Boston, MA: Pearson Education, 2018.

Hung, Suet Lin. "Collective Narrative Practice with Rape Victims in the Chinese Society of Hong Kong." *International Journal of Narrative Therapy and Community Work* 1 (2011): 14–31. https://doi.org/10.3316/informit.870589297245238.

Ipsit V. Vahia, Dilip V. Jeste, and Charles F. Reynolds III. "Older Adults and the Mental Health Effects of COVID-19." *JAMA* 324, no. 22 (2020): 2253–4. https:// doi.org/10.1001/jama.2020.21753.

Jacobs, Suzan F. M. "Collective Narrative Practice with Unaccompanied Refugee Minors: 'The Tree of Life' as a Response to Hardship." *Clinical Child Psychology and Psychiatry* 23, no. 2 (2018): 279–93. https://doi.org/10.1177/1359104517744246.

James, Ella L., Alex Lau-Zhu, Ian A. Clark, Renée M. Visser, Muriel A. Hagenaars, and Emily A. Holmes. "The Trauma Film Paradigm as an Experimental Psychopathology Model of Psychological Trauma: Intrusive Memories and Beyond." *Clinical Psychology Review* 47, (2016): 106–42. https://doi.org/10.1016/j.cpr.2016 .04.010.

Jetten, Jolanda, et al. Introduction to *The Social Cure: Identity, Health and Well-Being*, ed. Jolanda Jetten, Catherine Haslam, and Alexander, S. Haslam. London: Psychology Press, 2011. https://doi.org/10.4324/9780203813195.

Johnson, Judith. "Awakening to Hope Through Narrative Practices." *International Journal of Narrative Therapy and Community Work* 1 (2018): 49–56. https://search .informit.org/doi/abs/10.3316/informit.477108620072932.

Jones, Anne C. "Transforming the Story: Narrative Applications to a Stepmother Support Group." *Families in Society* 85, no. 1 (2004): 129–38. https://doi.org/10.1606 /1044-3894.242.

Josselson, Ruthellen. "Narrative Research and the Challenge of Accumulating Knowledge." *Narrative Inquiry* 16, no. 1 (2006): 3–10.

Kaptchuk, Ted J. "The Double-Blind, Randomized, Placebo-Controlled Trial: Gold Standard or Golden Calf?" *Journal of Clinical Epidemiology* 54, no. 6 (2001): 541–49. https://doi.org/10.1016/S0895-4356(00)00347-4.

Kim, Bryan S. K., Clara E. Hill, Charles J. Gelso, Melissa K. Goates, Penelope A. Asay, and James M. Harbin. "Counselor Self-Disclosure, East Asian Client Adherence to Asian Cultural Values, and Counseling Process." *Journal of Counseling Psychology* 50, no. 3 (2003): 324–32. https://psycnet.apa.org/doi/10.1037/0022-0167.50.3.324.

Kiser, L., and V. Ostrom. "Three Worlds of Action. A Metatheoretical Synthesis of Institutional Approaches." In *Strategies of Political Inquiry*, ed. E. Ostrom. Beverly Hills: Sage, 1985.

Kohrt, Brandon A, James L Griffith, and Vikram Patel. "Chronic Pain and Mental Health: Integrated Solutions for Global Problems." *Pain* 159, Suppl. 1 (2018): S85.

Korte, J., E. T. Bohlmeijer, P. Cappeliez, F. Smit, and G. J. Westerhof. "Life Review Therapy for Older Adults with Moderate Depressive Symptomatology: A Pragmatic Randomized Controlled Trial." *Psychological Medicine* 42, no. 6 (2012): 1163–73. https://doi.org/10.1017/S0033291711002042.

Kronsted, Christian. "The Self and Dance Movement Therapy: A Narrative Approach." *Phenomenology and the Cognitive Sciences* 19, no. 1 (2020): 47–58. https://doi.org/10.1007/s11097-018-9602-y.

Kropf, Nancy P., and Cindy Tandy. "Narrative Therapy with Older Clients: The Use of a "Meaning-Making" Approach." *Clinical Gerontologist* 18, no. 4 (1998): 3–16. https://doi.org/10.1300/J018v18n04_02.

Kurman, Jenny. "Self-Enhancement: Is It Restricted to Individualistic Cultures?" *Personality and Social Psychology Bulletin* 27, no. 12 (2001): 1705–1716. https://doi.org/10.1177%2F01461672012712013.

Lakshman, M., L. Sinha, M. Biswas, M. Charles, and N. K. Arora. "Quantitative Vs Qualitative Research Methods." *Indian Journal of Pediatrics* 67, no. 5 (2000): 369–77. https://doi.org/10.1007/BF02820690.

Lam, Hingchau. "The Ouster Clause in the Hong Kong National Security Law: Its Effectiveness in the Common Law and Its Implications for the Rule of Law." *Crime, Law, and Social Change* 76(2021): 543–61. https://doi.org/10.1007/s10611-021-09979-6.

Lamers, S. M. A., Ernst T. Bohlmeijer, Jojanneke Korte, and Gerben J. Westerhof. "The Efficacy of Life-Review as Online-Guided Self-Help for Adults: A Randomized Trial." *Journals of Gerontology, Series B: Psychological Sciences and Social Sciences* 70, no. 1 (2015): 24–34. https://doi.org/10.1093/geronb/gbu030.

Lee, Ho-Jin, Eun Joo Choi, Francis Sahngun Nahm, In Young Yoon, and Pyung Bok Lee. "Prevalence of Unrecognized Depression in Patients with Chronic Pain

Without a History of Psychiatric Diseases." *Korean Journal of Pain* 31, no. 2 (2018): 116–24.

Legowski, Teresa, and Keith Brownlee. "Working with Metaphor in Narrative Therapy." *Journal of Family Psychotherapy* 12, no. 1 (2001): 19–28. https://doi.org /10.1300/J085v12n01_02.

Lesher, Emerson L, and Jeffrey S Berryhill. "Validation of the Geriatric Depression Scale-Short Form Among Inpatients." *Journal of clinical psychology* 50, no. 2 (1994): 256–60.

Lesley, Grant. "Bringing Together Women Like You and Me: Collective Narrative Practice with Women and Trauma." *International Journal of Narrative Therapy and Community Work* 1 (2022): 1–8. https://doi.org/10.3316/informit.429037128627631.

Linder, S. H., and B. G. Peters. "The Study of Policy Instruments: Four Schools of Thought." In *Public Policy Instruments: Evaluating the Tools of Public Administration*, ed. B. G. Peters and F. K. M. Van Nispen. Cheltenham: Edward Elgar. 1998.

Lit, Siu Wai. "Dialectics and Transformations in Liminality: The Use of Narrative Therapy Groups with Terminal Cancer Patients in Hong Kong." *China Journal of Social Work* 8, no. 2 (2015): 122–35. https://doi.org/10.1080/17525098.2015 .1039171.

Looyeh, Majid Yoosefi, Khosrow Kamali, Amin Ghasemi, and Phuangphet Tonawanik. "Treating Social Phobia in Children Through Group Narrative Therapy." *Arts in Psychotherapy* 41, no. 1 (2014): 16–20. https://doi.org/10.1016/j.aip.2013.11.005.

Looyeh, Majid Yoosefi, Khosrow Kamali, and Roya Shafieian. "An Exploratory Study of the Effectiveness of Group Narrative Therapy on the School Behavior of Girls with Attention-Deficit/Hyperactivity Symptoms." *Archives of Psychiatric Nursing* 26, no. 5 (2012): 404–10. https://doi.org/10.1016/j.apnu.2012.01.001.

Lowenthal, Del. "Countertransference, Phenomenology and Research: Was Freud Right?" *European Journal of Psychotherapy and Counselling* 20, no. 4 (2018): 365–372. https://doi.org/10.1080/13642537.2018.1534676.

Lu, Qi, Dongrui Wang, Li Fu, Xue Wang, LiYa Li, Lihong Jiang, Cuiyu Deng, and Yue Zhao. "The Effect of Stigma on Social Participation in Community-Dwelling Chinese Patients with Stroke Sequelae: A Cross-Sectional Study." *Clinical Rehabilitation* 36, no. 3 (2022): 407–414. https://doi.org/10.1177/02692155211050558.

Luo, Candice, Nitika Sanger, Nikhita Singhal, Kaitlin Pattrick, Leta Shams, Hamnah Shams, Peter Hoang, et al. "A Comparison of Electronically-Delivered and Face to Face Cognitive Behavioural Therapies in Depressive Disorders: A Systematic Review." *Lancet* 24, no. 100442 (2020). https://doi.org/10.1016/j.eclinm.2020.100442.

Lustbader, Wendy. "Thoughts on the Meaning of Frailty." *Generations* 23, no. 4 (1999–2000): 21–24. https://www.jstor.org/stable/44877540.

Lutz, Wolfgang, and Clara E. Hill. "Quantitative and Qualitative Methods for Psychotherapy Research: Introduction to Special Section." *Psychotherapy Research* 19, no. 4–5 (2009): 369–73. https://doi.org/10.1080/10503300902948053.

Lyotard, Jean-François. *The Postmodern Condition: A Report on Knowledge*. Trans. Geoff Bennington, Brian Massumi, and Fredric Jameson. Vol. 10, *Theory and History of Literature*. 12th ed. Minneapolis: University of Minnesota Press, 1984.

Madigan, Ruth, and Moira Munro. "'House Beautiful': Style and Consumption in the Home." *Sociology* 30, no. 1 (1996): 41–57. https://doi.org/10.1177/0038038596030001004.

Madigan, Stephen. "Anticipating Hope Within Conversational Domains of Despair." *Hope and Despair* (2008): 104–12.

——. "Narrative Therapy-Informed Relational Interviewing—Emotionally Preparing Conflicted Couple Relationships for Possible Re-Unification, Separation, Mediation, and Family Courtrooms." *Fokus på familien* 45, no. 2 (2017): 138–58. https://doi.org/10.18261/issn.0807-7487-2017-02-05.

Madigan, Stephen Patrick. "The Application of Michel Foucault's Philosophy in the Problem Externalizing Discourse of Michael White." *Journal of Family Therapy* 14, no. 3 (1992): 265–79. https://doi.org/10.1046/j..1992.00458.x.

Marc-Antoine Crocq, and Louis Crocq. "From Shell Shock and War Neurosis to Posttraumatic Stress Disorder: A History of Psychotraumatology." *Dialogues in Clinical Neuroscience* 2, no.1 (2000): 47–55. https://doi.org/10.31887/DCNS.2000.2.1/macrocq.

Markus, Hazel R., and Shinobu Kitayama. "Culture and the Self: Implications for Cognition, Emotion, and Motivation." *Psychological Review* 98, no. 2 (1991): 224–253. https://doi.org/10.1037/0033-295X.98.2.224.

Marsten, David, David Epston, and Laurie Markham. *Narrative Therapy in Wonderland: Connecting with Children's Imaginative Know-How*. New York: Norton, 2016.

Maslow, Abraham Harold. *Motivation and Personality*. Prabhat Prakashan, 1981.

Mather, R. "Hegel, Dostoyevsky and Carl Rogers: Between Humanism and Spirit." *History of the Human Sciences* 21, no. 1 (2008): 33–48. https://doi.org/10.1177/0952695107086151.

Matt, Susan J. "Current Emotion Research in History: Or, Doing History from the Inside Out." *Emotion Review* 3, no. 1 (2011): 117–24. https://doi.org/10.1177/1754073910384416.

May, Todd. *Friendship in an Age of Economics: Resisting the Forces of Neoliberalism*. Lanham, Md: Lexington Books, 2012.

——. *A Fragile Life: Accepting Our Vulnerability*. Chicago: University of Chicago Press, 2017. https://doi:10.7208/9780226440019.

McLean, Kate C., and Marc A. Fournier. "The Content and Processes of Autobiographical Reasoning in Narrative Identity." *Journal of Research in Personality* 42, no. 3 (2008): 527–545. https://doi.org/10.1016/j.jrp.2007.08.003.

McLeod, John. "Psychotherapy, Culture and Storytelling: How They Fit Together." In *Narrative and Psychotherapy*. London: SAGE, 1997.

Merton, Robert. "The Self-Fulfilling Prophecy." *Antioch Review* 8, no. 2 (1948): 193–210. https://doi.org/10.2307/4609267.

Miley, Karla Krogsrud, Michael O'Melia, and Brenda DuBois. *Generalist Social Work Practice: An Empowering Approach.* 7th ed. Boston: Pearson, 2013.

Miller, Jean B. Introduction to *How Connections Heal: Stories from Relational-Cultural Therapy,* ed. Maureen Walker and Wendy B. Rosen. New York: Guildford, 2004.

Miller, Michael L. "Dynamic Systems and the Therapeutic Action of the Analyst: II. Clinical Application and Illustrations." *Psychoanalytic Psychology* 21, no. 1 (2004): 54–69. https://doi.org/10.1037/0736-9735.21.1.54.

Minuchin, Salvador. "My Many Voices." In *The Evolution of Psychotherapy,* ed. Jeffery K Zeig. New York: Routledge, 1987.

Moreira, André, Ana Cristina Moreira, and José Carlos Rocha. "Randomized Controlled Trial: Cognitive-Narrative Therapy for IPV Victims." *Journal of Interpersonal Violence* 37, no. 5–6 (2022): NP2998–NP3014. https://doi.org/10.1177/0886260520943719.

Morgan, Alice. *What Is Narrative Therapy? An Easy-to-Read Introduction.* Adelaide, SA: Dulwich Centre, 2000.Morrissey, Charles T. "Public Historians and Oral History: Problems of Concept and Methodology." *Public Historian* 2, no. 2 (1980): 22–29.

Morrow-Howell, Nancy, and Ada C. Mui. "Productive Engagement of Older Adults: International Research, Practice, and Policy Introduction." *Ageing International* 38, no. 1 (2013): 1–3. https://doi.org/10.1007/s12126-012-9175-y.

Mörtl, Kathrin, and Omar Carlo Gioacchino Gelo. "Qualitative Methods in Psychotherapy Process Research." In *Psychotherapy Research: Foundations, Process, and Outcome,* ed. Omar C. G. Gelo, Aldred Pritz, and Bernd Rieken, 381–428. Vienna: Springer Vienna, 2014.

Mui, Ada C., and Suk-Young Kang. "Acculturation Stress and Depression Among Asian Immigrant Elders." *Social Work* 51, no. 3 (2006): 243–55. https://doi.org/10.1093/sw/51.3.243.

Mui, Ada C., Terry Lum, and Iris Chi. *Gerontological Social Work: Theory and Practice.* 2nd ed. Shanghai: Truth and Wisdom, 2017.

Mui, Ada C., and Tazuko Shibusawa. *Asian American Elders in the Twenty-First Century: Key Indicators of Well-Being.* New York: Columbia University Press, 2008.

Mullen, Mary K. and Soonhyung Yi. "The Cultural Context of Talk About the Past: Implications for the Development of Autobiographical Memory." *Cognitive Development* 10, no. 3 (1995): 407–419. https://doi.org/10.1016/0885-2014(95)90004-7.

Muruthi, Bertranna, Megan McCoy, Jessica Chou, and Andrea Farnham. "Sexual Scripts and Narrative Therapy with Older Couples." *American Journal of Family Therapy* 46, no. 1 (2018): 81–95. https://doi.org/10.1080/01926187.2018.1428129.

Myerhoff, Barbara. "Life History Among the Elderly: Performance, Visibility, and Re-Membering." In *Remembered Lives: The Work of Ritual, Storytelling, and Growing Older*, ed. Barbara G. Myerhoff, Deena Metzger, Jay Ruby, and Viginia Tufte, 231–49. Ann Arbor: University of Michigan Press, 1992.

Natterson, Idell. "Turning Points and Intersubjectivity." *Clinical Social Work Journal* 21, no. 1 (1993): 45–56. https://doi.org/10.1007/BF00754911.

Ncube, Ncazelo. "The Tree of Life Project: Using Narrative Ideas in Work with Vulnerable Children in Southern Africa." *International Journal of Narrative Therapy and Community Work* 1 (2006): 3–16. https://doi.org/https://search.informit.org /doi/10.3316/informit.197106237773394.

Nelson, Katherine, and Robyn Fivush. "The Emergence of Autobiographical Memory: A Social Cultural Developmental Theory." *Psychological Review* 111, no. 2 (2004): 486–511. https://doi.org/10.1037/0033-295X.111.2.486.

Niedzwiedz, Claire L., Lee Knifton, Kathryn A. Robb, Srinivasa Vittal Katikireddi, and Daniel J. Smith. "Depression and Anxiety Among People Living with and Beyond Cancer: A Growing Clinical and Research Priority." *BMC Cancer* 19, no. 1 (2019): 943. https://doi.org/10.1186/s12885-019-6181-4.

Novotney, Amy. "The Risks of Social Isolation." American Psychological Association. May 2019. https://www.apa.org/monitor/2019/05/ce-corner-isolation.

Pargament, Kenneth I., James W. Lomax, Jocelyn S. McGee, and Qijuan Fang. "Sacred Moments in Psychotherapy From the Perspective of Mental Health Providers and Clients: Prevalence, Predictors, and consequences." *Spirituality in Clinical Practice* 1, no. 4 (2014): 248–262. https://doi.org/10.1037 /scp0000043.

Peters, B. G., and F. K. M. Van Nispen, eds. *Public Policy Instruments: Evaluating the Tools of Public Administration*. Cheltenham: Edward Elgar. 1988.

Phillips, Laurel. "A Narrative Therapy Approach to Dealing with Chronic Pain." *International Journal of Narrative Therapy and Community Work* no. 1 (2017): 21–30. https://doi.org/10.3316/informit.768720305988235.

Pia, Emily. "Narrative Therapy and Peacebuilding." *Journal of Intervention and Statebuilding* 7, no. 4 (2013): 476–91. https://doi.org/10.1080/17502977.2012 .727538.

Polard, José. "Home: écouter un sujet âgé dans son environnement." Lecture at the Fourth Conference on Aging, *La cause des aînés: Pour vivre autrement . . . et mieux*, Paris, 12 June 2010.

Portelli, Alessandro. "What Makes Oral History Different?" In *The Death of Luigi Trastulli and Other Stories: Form and Meaning in Oral History*, 42–54. Albany: State University of New York Press, 1991.

Portnoy, Sara, Isabella Girling, and Glenda Fredman. "Supporting Young People Living with Cancer to Tell Their Stories in Ways That Make Them Stronger: The Beads of Life Approach." *Clinical Child Psychology and Psychiatry* 21, no. 2 (2016): 255–67. https://doi.org/10.1177/1359104515586467.

Polkinghorne, Donald E. "Narrative Therapy and Postmodernism." In *The Handbook of Narrative and Psychotherapy: Practice, Theory and Research*, ed. Lynne E. Angus and John McLeod. Thousand Oaks, CA: Sage, 2004).

Radloff, LS. "Center for Epidemiologic Studies Depression Scale (CES-D)." (2012).

Rajaei, Afarin, Andrew S. Brimhall, Jakob F. Jensen, Abby J. Schwartz, and Essie Talina Torres. "Striving to Thrive: A Qualitative Study on Fostering a Relational Perspective through Narrative Therapy in Couples Facing Cancer." *American Journal of Family Therapy* 49, no. 4 (2021): 392–408. https://doi.org/10.1080/01926187.2020.1820402.

Randall, William. "Storied Worlds: Acquiring a Narrative Perspective on Aging, Identity, and Everyday Life." In *Narrative Gerontology: Theory, Research, and Practice*, ed. Gary M. Kenyon, Philip G. Clark, and Brian De Vries, 41. New York: Springer, 2001.

Randall, William L., and Gary M. Kenyon. "Time, Story, and Wisdom: Emerging Themes in Narrative Gerontology." *Canadian Journal on Aging (La Revue canadienne du vieillissement)* 23, no. 4 (2004): 333–46.

Rathore, Jaivir S, Lara E Jehi, Youran Fan, Sima I Patel, Nancy Foldvary-Schaefer, Maya J Ramirez, Robyn M Busch, Nancy A Obuchowski, and George E Tesar. "Validation of the Patient Health Questionnaire-9 (Phq-9) for Depression Screening in Adults with Epilepsy." *Epilepsy and Behavior* 37 (2014): 215–20.

Remen, Rachel N. *My Grandfather's Blessings: Stories of Strength, Refuge, and Belonging.* New York: Riverhead, 2001.

Rickard, Wendy. "Oral History—'More Dangerous than Therapy'? Interviewees' Reflections on Recording Traumatic or Taboo Issues." *Oral History* 26, no. 2 (1998).

Ritivoi, Andreea Deciu. *Yesterday's Self: Nostalgia and the Immigrant Identity.* Lanham, MD: Rowman and Littlefield, 2002.

Rivers, Ben. "Narrative Power: Playback Theatre as Cultural Resistance in Occupied Palestine." *Research in Drama Education* 20, no. 2 (2015): 155–172. https://doi.org/10.1080/13569783.2015.1022144.

Rodríguez Vega, B., C. Bayón Pérez, A. PalaoTarrero, and A. Fernández Liria. "Mindfulness-based narrative therapy for depression in cancer patients." *Clinical Psychological Psychotherapy* 21, no. 5 (2014): 411–19. https://doi.org/10.1002/cpp.1847.

Romanelli, Assael. "Deep Listening to the Heart of the Story." *Psychology Today*, September 3, 2021. https://www.psychologytoday.com/us/blog/the-other-side-relationships/202109/deep-listening-the-heart-the-story.

Rood, Bobbi. "A Time to Talk: Re-Membering Conversations with Elders." *International Journal of Narrative Therapy and Community Work* no. 1 (2009): 18–28.

Roughan, William H., Adrián I. Campos, Luis M. García-Marín, Gabriel Cuéllar-Partida, Michelle K. Lupton, Ian B. Hickie, Sarah E. Medland, et al. "Comorbid Chronic Pain and Depression: Shared Risk Factors and Differential Antidepressant Effectiveness." *Frontiers in Psychiatry* 12 (2021): 643609.

Rubin, Allen, and Earl R. Babbie. *Research Methods for Social Work*. Empowerment Series. Ninth edition. ed. Boston, MA: Cengage Learning, 2017.

Russell, Shona, and Maggie Carey. "Re-Membering: Responding to Commonly Ask Questions." *International Journal of Narrative Therapy and Community Work* 3 (2002): 23–31.

Rusu, Marinela. "The Process of Self-Realization" from the Humanist Psychology Perspective." *Psychology* 10, no. 8 (2019): 1095–115. https://doi.org/10.4236/psych .2019.108071.

Ruth Grossman, Dean. "A Narrative Approach to Groups." *Clinical Social Work Journal* 26, no. 1 (1998): 23–37.

Saakvitne, Karen W., and Laurie A. Pearlman. *Transforming the Pain: A Workbook on Vicarious Traumatization*. London: Norton, 1996.

Saarelainen, Suvi-Maria K. "Life Tree Drawings as a Methodological Approach in Young Adults' Life Stories During Cancer Remission." *Narrative Works* 5, no. 1 (2015): 68–91. https://journals.lib.unb.ca/index.php/NW/article/view/23785.

Samuel, Raphael. "Myth and History: A First Reading." *Oral History* 16, no. 1 (1988).

Sarfo, Fred Stephen, Michelle Nichols, Suparna Qanungo, Abeba Teklehaimanot, Arti Singh, Nathaniel Mensah, Raelle Saulson, et al. "Stroke-Related Stigma Among West Africans: Patterns and Predictors." *Journal of the Neurological Sciences* 375 (2016): 270–274. https://doi.org/10.1016/j.jns.2017.02.018.

Schiff, Brian. "The Function of Narrative: Toward a Narrative Psychology of Meaning." *Narrative Matters* 2, no. 1 (2012): 33–47. https://id.erudit.org/iderudit/nw2 _1art03.

Schriver, Joe M. *Human Behavior and the Social Environment: Shifting Paradigms in Essential Knowledge for Social Work Practice*. Connecting Core Competencies Series. 5th ed. Boston: Allyn and Bacon, 2011.

Semmler, Pamela L., and Carmen B. Williams. "Narrative Therapy: A Storied Context for Multicultural Counseling." *Journal of Multicultural Counseling and Development* 28, no 1 (2000): 51–62. https://doi.org/10.1002/j.2161-1912.2000 .tb00227.x.

Shakeri, Jalal, Seyed Mojtaba Ahmadi, Fateme Maleki, Mohammad Reza Hesami, Arash Parsa Moghadam, Akram Ahmadzade, Maryam Shirzadi, and Adele Elahi. "Effectiveness of Group Narrative Therapy on Depression, Quality of Life, and Anxiety in People with Amphetamine Addiction: A Randomized Clinical Trial." *Iranian Journal of Medical Sciences* 45, no. 2 (2020): 91–99. https://doi.org /10.30476/ijms.2019.45829.

Shakespeare, William. *All's Well that Ends Well*. 1623.

Shorten, Allison, and Joanna Smith. "Mixed Methods Research: Expanding the Evidence Base." *Evidence-Based Nursing* 20, no. 3 (2017): 74–75. https://doi.org /10.1136/eb-2017-102699.

Shulman, Lawrence. *Dynamics and Skills of Group Counseling*. Belmont, CA: Cengage Learning, 2010.

Siebold, Cathy. "What Do Patients Want? Personal Disclosure and the Intersubjective Perspective." *Clinical Social Work Journal* 39, (2011): 151–160. https://doi.org /10.1007/s10615-011-0338-1.

Sit, Regina W. S., S. W. Law, C. Y. Lam, and Martin C. S. Wong. "Management of Chronic Musculoskeletal Pain in Hong Kong." *Hong Kong Medical Journal (Xianggang yi xue za zhi)* 28, no. 3 (2022): 201–3.

Skillman, Gemma Dolorosa. "Intergenerational Conflict Within the Family Context: A Comparative Analysis of Collectivism and Individualism Within Vietnamese, Filipino, and Caucasian Families." PhD diss., Syracuse University, ProQuest Dissertations Publishing, 1999.

Sliep, Yvonne. "A Narrative Theatre Approach to Working with Communities Affected by Trauma, Conflict and War." *International Journal of Narrative Therapy and Community Work* 2005, no. 2 (2005): 47–52.

Smigelsky, Melissa A., and Robert A. Neimeyer. "Performative Retelling: Healing Community Stories of Loss through Playback Theatre." *Death Studies* 42, no. 1 (2018): 26–34. https://doi.org/10.1080/07481187.2017.1370414.

Smith, R. G. "Structuralism/Structuralist Geography." In *International Encyclopedia of Human Geography*, ed. Rob Kitchin and Nigel Thrift, 30–38. Oxford: Elsevier, 2009. https://doi.org/10.1016/B978-008044910-4.00748-3.

Spence, Donald P. *Narrative Truth and Historical Truth: Meaning and Interpretation in* Psychoanalysis. New York: Norton, 1982, 182.

Stahnke, Brittany, and Morgan E. Cooley. "End-of-Life Case Study: The Use of Narrative Therapy on a Holocaust Survivor with Lifelong Depression." *Journal of Contemporary Psychotherapy* 52 (2022): 191–98. https://doi.org/https://doi.org /10.1007/s10879-022-09532-z.

Staudacher, Carol. *A Time to Grieve: Meditations for Healing After the Death of a Loved One.* London: Souvenir, 1995.

Stefana, Alberto. *History of Countertransference. From Freud to the British Object Relations School.* London: Routledge, 2017.

Stern, Dafna. "Narrative Therapy at any Age." *International Journal of Narrative Therapy and Community Work* 1 (2011): 57–64.

Stern, Dafna, and Caroline Serrure. "Making a Meaning-Full Life at Montefiore." *International Journal of Narrative Therapy and Community Work* 3 (2014): 21–30.

Stiles, Deborah A., Esa Alaraudanjoki, Lisa R. Wilkinson, Keary L. Ritchie, and Kelly Ann Brown. "Researching the Effectiveness of Tree of Life: An Imbeleko Approach to Counseling Refugee Youth." *Journal of Child and Adolescent Trauma* 14, no. 1 (2021): 123–39.

Stiver, Irene P. "The Meaning of Care: Reframing Treatment Models." Wellesley Centers for Women. 1985. http://www.wcwonline.org/pdf/previews/preview_20sc .pdf.

Stompór, M., T. Grodzicki, T. Stompór, J. Wordliczek, M. Dubiel, and I. Kurowska. "Prevalence of Chronic Pain, Particularly with Neuropathic Component, and Its

Effect on Overall Functioning of Elderly Patients." *Medical Science Monitor* 25 (2019): 2695–701. https://doi.org/10.12659/msm.911260.

Strömbäck, Jesper. "Four Phases of Mediatization: An Analysis of the Mediatization of Politics." *International Journal of Press/Politics* 13, no. 3 (July 2008): 228–46. https://doi.org/10.1177/1940161208319097.

Sue, Derald W., and David Sue. *Counseling the Culturally Different: Theory and Practice.* 2nd ed. Washington, DC: Wiley, 1990.

Summerfield, Penny. *Reconstructing Women's Lives: Discourse and Subjectivity In Oral Histories of the Second World War.* Manchester: Manchester University Press, 1998.

Sun, Liying, Xueli Liu, Xiaoling Weng, Haiyan Deng, Qian Li, Jingpeng Liu, and Xiaorong Luan. "Narrative Therapy to Relieve Stigma in Oral Cancer Patients: A Randomized Controlled Trial." *International Journal of Nursing Practice* (2021): e12926. https://doi.org/10.1111/ijn.12926.

Szabo, Jozsef, Szilvia Toth, and Annamaria Karamanne Pakai. "Narrative Group Therapy for Alcohol Dependent Patients." *International Journal of Mental Health and Addiction* 12, no. 4 (2014): 470–476. https://doi.org/10.1007/s11469 -014-9478-1.

Tan, Meizi. "Recipes for Life: A Collective Narrative Methodology for Responding to Gender Violence." *International Journal of Narrative Therapy and Community Work* no. 2 (2017): 1–12.

Taylor, Lauren. "Resilience: Elder in East Harlem." In *Say It Forward: A Guide to Social Justice Storytelling,* ed. Cliff Mayotte and Claire Kiefer. Chicago: Hay-market, 2019.

——. "Sharing a Narrative Meal." In *Narrative in Social Work Practice: The Power and Possibility of Story,* ed. Ann Burack-Weiss, Lynn Sara Lawrence, and Lynne Bamat Mijangos. New York: Columbia University Press, 2017.

Theron, H., and D. Bruwer. "More About Mental Health in the Community." *CME* 24, no. 8 (2008): 449–50.

Toseland, Ronald W, and Robert F Rivas. *An Introduction to Group Work Practice.* Boston: Pearson/Allyn and Bacon, 2009.

Trevarthen, Colwyn. "The Foundations of Intersubjectivity." In *The Social Foundations of Language and Thought,* ed. David R. Olson, 216–42. New York: Norton, 1980.

Triandis, Harry C. "The Self and Social Behavior in Differing Cultural Contexts." *Psychological Review* 96, no. 3 (1989): 506–520. https://doi.org/10.1037/0033 -295X.96.3.506.

Trudinger, Mark. "Remembering Joan: Re-Membering Practices as Eulogies and Memorials." *International Journal of Narrative Therapy and Community Work* no. 1 (2009): 29–38.

Updike, John. *More Matter: Essays and Criticism.* New York: Random House, 1999.

U.S. Census Bureau. "America Counts: Stories Behind the Numbers." Accessed April 14, 2022. https://www.census.gov/library/stories.html.

Van Dijck, José, and David Nieborg. "Wikinomics and Its Discontents: A Critical Analysis of Web 2.0 Business Manifestos." *New Media and Society* 11, no. 5 (July 21, 2009): 855–74. https://doi.org/10.1177/1461444809105356.

Van Wyk, Rene. "Narrative House: A Metaphor for Narrative Therapy: Tribute to Michael White." 2008.

Walker, Maureen, and Wendy Rosen. *How Connections Heal: Stories from Relational Cultural Therapy.* New York: Guilford, 2004.

Walther, Sarah, and Hugh Fox. "Narrative Therapy and Outsider Witness Practice: Teachers as a Community of Acknowledgement." *Educational and Child Psychology* 29, no. 2 (2012): 8–17.

Wamsley, G. L., and H. B. Milward. "Policy Subsystems, Networks and the Tools of Public Management." In *Policy Implementation in Federal and Unitary Systems: Questions of Analysis and Design,* ed. K. I. Hanf and Th. A. J. Toonen. Dordrecht: Nijhoff, 1985.

Wang, Qi. "Culture Effects on Adults' Earliest Childhood Recollection and Self-Description: Implications for the Relation Between Memory and the Self." *Journal of Personality and Social Psychology* 81, no. 2 (2001): 220–33. https://doi.org/10.1037/0022-3514.81.2.220.

——. "The Emergence of Cultural Self-Constructs: Autobiographical Memory and Self-Description in European American and Chinese Children." *Developmental Psychology* 40, no. 1 (2004): 3–15. https://psycnet.apa.org/doi/10.1037/0012-1649.40.1.3.

Wang, Qi, Michelle D. Leichtman, and Katharine I. Davies. "Sharing Memories and Telling Stories: American and Chinese Mothers and their 3-Year-Olds." *Memory* 8, no. 3 (2000): 159–77. https://doi.org/10.1080/096582100387588.

Wang, QuanQiu, Rong Xu, and Nora D. Volkow. "Increased Risk of COVID-19 Infection and Mortality in People with Mental Disorders: Analysis from Electronic Health Records in the United States." *World Psychiatry* 20, no. 1 (2021): 124–30. https://doi.org/10.1002/wps.20806.

Wang, Yun-He, Jin-Qiao Li, Ju-Fang Shi, Jian-Yu Que, Jia-Jia Liu, Julia M. Lappin, Janni Leung, et al. "Depression and Anxiety in Relation to Cancer Incidence and Mortality: A Systematic Review and Meta-analysis of Cohort Studies." *Molecular Psychiatry* 25, no. 7 (2020): 1487–99. https://doi.org/10.1038/s41380-019-0595-x.

Warren, Jacob C., and K. Bryant Smalley. "Using Telehealth to Meet Mental Health Needs During the COVID-19 Crisis." *Commonwealth Fund* (blog), June 18, 2020. https://www.commonwealthfund.org/blog/2020/using-telehealth-meet-mental-health-needs-during-covid-19-crisis.

Webster, Jeffrey Dean. "An Exploratory Analysis of a Self-Assessed Wisdom Scale." *Journal of Adult Development* 10, no. 1 (2003): 13–22. https://doi.org/10.1023/A:1020782619051.

——. "Is It Time to Reminisce About the Future?" *International Journal of Reminiscence and Life Review* 1, no. 1 (2013): 51–4.

——. "Measuring the Character Strength of Wisdom." *International Journal of Aging and Human Development* 65, no. 2 (2007). https://doi.org/10.2190/AG.65.2.d.

Weick, Ann, Charles Rapp, Patrick W. Sullivan, and Walter Kisthardt. "A Strengths Perspective for Social Work Practice." *Social Work* 34, no. 4 (1989): 350–354. https://www.jstor.org/stable/23715838.

Weingarten, Kathy. "The Small and the Ordinary: The Daily Practice of a Postmodern Narrative Therapy." *Family Process* 37, no. 1 (1998): 3–15. https://doi.org/10.1111/j.1545-5300.1998.00003.x.

Westerhof, Gerben J, Ernst Bohlmeijer, and Jeffrey Dean Webster. "Reminiscence and Mental Health: A Review of Recent Progress in Theory, Research and Interventions." *Ageing and Society* 30, no. 4 (2010): 697–721. https://doi.org/10.1017/S0144686X09990328.

White, Michael. "Children, Trauma and Subordinate Storyline Development." Research Article. *International Journal of Narrative Therapy and Community Work* 2005, no. 3/4 (2005): 10–22. https://doi/10.3316/informit.244657580424321.

——. "Definitional Ceremony and Outsider-Witness Responses." Michael White Workshop Notes, 2005, Retrieved from https://www.dulwichcentre.com.au/michael-white-workshop-notes.pdf.

——. "The Externalizing of the Problem and the Re-Authoring of Lives and Relationships." *Dulwich Centre Newsletter* (Summer 1989).

——. "Family Therapy and Schizophrenia: Addressing the 'In-the-Corner' Lifestyle." *Dulwich Centre Newsletter* 1 (1987): 14–21.

——. "Journey Metaphors." *International Journal of Narrative Therapy and Community Work* 2002, no. 4 (2002): 12–18. https://search.informit.org/doi/10.3316/informit.662334264148132

——. *Map of Narrative Therapy.* Adelaide, SA Dulwich Centre, 2007.

——. *Maps of Narrative Practice.* New York: Norton, 2007.

——. "Working with People Who Are Suffering the Consequences of Multiple Trauma: A Narrative Perspective." *International Journal of Narrative Therapy and Community Work* 1 (2004): 44–75.

White, Michael, and David Epston. *Narrative Means to Therapeutic Ends.* New York: Norton, 1990.

Wood, Natale Rudland. "Recipes for Life." *International Journal of Narrative Therapy and Community Work* 2 (2012): 34–43.

World Health Organization. "Active Ageing: A Policy Framework." World Health Organization. April 2002. https://apps.who.int/iris/handle/10665/67215.

Yamagishi, Toshio, Hirofumi Hashimoto, Karen S. Cook, Toko Kiyonari, Mizuho Shinada, Nobuhiro Mifune, Keigo Inukai, Haruto Takagishi, Yutaka Horita, and Yang Li. "Modesty in Self-Presentation: A Comparison Between the USA and Japan." *Asian Journal of Social Psychology* 15, no. 1 (2012): 60–68. https://doi.org/10.1111/j.1467-839X.2011.01362.x.

Yang, Pei-Shan, and Ada C. Mui. *Foundations of Gerontological Social Work Practice in Taiwan.* Taipei: YehYeh Book Gallery, 2022.

Yeganeh Farzand, Seyedhadi, Kianoush Zahrakar, and Farshad Mohsenzadeh. "The Effectiveness of Narrative Therapy on Reducing the Fear of Intimacy in Couples." *Practice in Clinical Psychology* (2019): 117–24. https://doi.org/10.32598 /jpcp.7.2.117.

Yotis, L., C. Theocharopoulos, C. Fragiadaki, and D. Begioglou. "Using Playback Theatre to Address the Stigma of Mental Disorders." *Arts in Psychotherapy* 55 (2017): 80–84. https://doi.org/10.1016/j.aip.2017.04.009.

Yow, Valerie. "What Can Oral Historians Learn from Psychotherapists?" *Oral History* 46, no. 1 (2018). https://www.jstor.org/stable/44993454.

Yu, S. F., Doris, Sheung-Tak Cheng, Esther Oi-Wah Chow, Timothy Kwok, and Brendan McCormack. "Effects of Strength-Based Intervention on Health Outcomes of Family Caregivers of Persons with Dementia: A Study Protocol." *Journal of Advanced Nursing* 76, no. 10 (2020): 2737–2746. https://doi.org/10.1111 /jan.14470.

Zhou, De-Hui Ruth, Yu-Lung Marcus Chiu, Tak-Lam William Lo, Wai-Fan Alison Lo, Siu-Sing Wong, Chi Hoi Tom Leung, Chui-Kam Yu, Yuk Sing Geoffrey Chang, and Kwok-Leung Luk. "An Unexpected Visitor and a Sword Play: A Randomized Controlled Trial of Collective Narrative Therapy Groups for Primary Carers of People with Schizophrenia." *Journal of Mental Health* (2020): 1–12. https://doi.org/10.1080/09638237.2020.1793123.

Zimmerman, Jeffrey L., and Victoria C. Dickerson. *If Problems Talked: Narrative Therapy in Action.* New York: Guilford, 1996.

SOCIAL MEDIA

Support Community (@_were_all_mental). Instagram Photos and Videos. September 14, 2023. https://www.instagram.com/_were_all_mental/.

"This Weeks Mental Meetup Topic Is Anxiety." Support Community (@_were_all _mental). Instagram Photos and Videos. August 28, 2023. https://www.instagram .com/p/Cwd3I5LtBsQ/?utm_source=ig_web_copy_link&igshid=MzRlODBi NWFlZA==.

青春頌 | 青少年癌症 · 認識 · 同行 · 改變 (@youthcancerhk). Instagram Photos and Videos. (什麼是睪丸癌？). May 20, 2023. https://www.instagram.com/p /Csd9uICBxhW/?img_index=1.

青春頌 | 青少年癌症 · 認識 · 同行 · 改變 (@youthcancerhk). Instagram Photos and Videos. September 14, 2023. https://www.instagram.com/youthcancerhk/.

拿破輪劇團 (@narrative_playback_theatre). Instagram Photos and Videos. September 14, 2023. https://www.instagram.com/narrative_playback_theatre/.

INDEX

Page numbers in *italics* refer to figures or tables.

and, 68, 218–21; meaning and,
21, 55, 223–24; negative, 33–34,
114–15, 180, 217; society in conflict
with, 46; of therapist, 142, 153–54,
278–81
life review, 21–22, 107; oral history
compared to, 109–16; reminiscence
compared to, 80, 83
life stations, in Train-of-Life, 194–95
life story, 6, 15, 46–47, 169, *170*; beliefs
and, 182–83; change and, 153–60,
246, 265–67; COVID-19 and,
263; gerontology and, 21–22, 107;
narrative construction in, 7; problem-
saturated identities and, 55, 188–90;
reauthoring of, 63–65, 72–76
life wisdom, 35, 212, 224, 239;
narrative practice and, 258–60, 267;
rediscovery of, 173–76
linguistics, memory and, 8–9, 15
listeners, 108; group practice and,
102–5; oral history and, 109–10,
115, 117; outsider witness as, 72,
173; therapist as, 53, 99–101, 107,
109–10, 120–21, 154–55; trauma
and, 120–21, 125
loneliness, 33, 100, 246, 264–65; as
challenges, 274–75
Lorde, Audrey, 104
loss, 46, 104, 123; resilience and, 127–28,
265, 277–78
Lowenthal, Del, 94
Lucy, narrative of, 104
Lustbader, Wendy, 105

Mao Zedong, 13
Margaret, narrative of, 139–42
marginalized people, 47, 52–53, 214,
226, 235, 239; aging and, 217;
COVID-19 and, 247–48; preferred
identity and, 168, 230–31
Marion, narrative of, 113–15
marriage, 114, 127–28, 143–44, 165–
66, 250; abuse in, 100–101, 248–49;
caregivers and, 189, 247, 252; death
and, 23–25, 175; stroke and, 57,
208–9, 221. *See also* couples

Mary, narrative of, 99–101
Maslow, Abraham, 46–47
Matt, Susan, 117
Mauriac, François, 108
McLeod, John, 79–80, 89
meaning, vii, 3–4, 195, 216, 231;
abilities and, 23–25, 202–4; aging
and, 12; artifacts and, 147–49;
death and, 268; grief and, 104;
interpretation and, 45, 47–48,
51–52; intersubjectivity and, 91; of
life, 47–48, 206–7; life experiences
and, 21, 55, 223–24; memory and,
8; personhood and, 124; reauthoring
and, 260; reconstruction of,
21–27, 82, 201–6; society and, 55;
storytelling and, 47–48, 108–9;
support and, 45
media visibility, 237–38
memory, 108, 130; collective, 7–10,
264; community and, 156; food
and, 129, 181–82; linguistics
and, 8–9, 15; meaning and, 8; in
psychotherapy, 81–83; specific,
7–10; trauma and, 13, 81
mental health, 176, 180; isolation and,
247–48; RCTs and, 35; recovery
and, 89–90, 128; society and, 55;
stigma and, 27, 33. *See also* anxiety;
depression
metaphor: culture and, 181–82;
problem-saturated identity and,
33–34, 218–19, 231; stigma and, 34;
wisdom and, 168, 172
metaphoric frameworks: coconstruction
and, 195, 201; future and, 194–95,
204–5, 208; group practice and,
33–34, 167; in Hong Kong, 231–33;
preferred identity and, 174, 183–88,
201–4, 210; Recipe-of-Life, 34, 179–
90, *184, 186–87*, 232; ToL, 33–34,
165–77, *170–73*, 231–32; Train-of-
Life, 34, 193–210, *195–97*, 232–33
Mike, narrative of, 155
Miller, Jean Baker, 94–95, 130
Millie, narrative of, 159
Minuchin, Salvador, 110

Esther Oi-Wah Chow, MSW, RSW, MNTCW, PhD, is an esteemed social work professor and gerontologist in health and aging at the Department of Social Work of Hong Kong Shue Yan University (HKU). She is also a leading therapist, and her scholarship has created an impact on rethinking and shaping the knowledge of aging through narrative practice with older people who are confronted with late-life transitions to reconstruct meaning and purpose. In recognitions of her contributions to the field of gerontological social work, she has received numerous prestigious awards, including Fellow of Hong Kong Academy of Social Work (2023), Fellow of Gerontological Society of America (2015), Excellence in Knowledge Transfer Award by City University of Hong Kong (2021 and 2013), a Research Fellow of Sau Po Centre on Aging, HKU (2009), and a CADENZA fellow by Hong Kong Jockey Club (HKJC) (2008).

Lauren Taylor, MA, MS, LCSW, is a psychiatric social worker and oral historian, a senior lecturer at the Columbia University School of Social Work (CUSSW), and a graduate of Columbia's Oral History Master of Arts program. She has been on staff for many years at the Service Program for Older People (SPOP), a mental health clinic for older adults. She gives seminars and workshops on a wide variety of mental health issues related to the aging process, with a focus on the therapeutic use of narrative. She has made two educational films: about sexuality and aging in 2002, with CUSSW, and in 2005 a dialogue between young social work students and older women about the challenges facing women across the lifespan. As an oral historian, she has conducted dozens of life-history interviews with older adults, both in the United States and abroad, and is studying the subjective experience of aging through the medium of narrative in a cross-cultural context.

Ada C. Mui, MSW, PhD, is a world-renowned professor of social work at Columbia University, specializing in research and practice in productive aging, family caregiving, mental health, and dementia in the United States and Asia. A distinguished scholar, colleague, and researcher in cross-cultural gerontology, she has received numerous prestigious awards, including the Fulbright Specialist Scholarship and the Busse Research Award from the Pan-American Congress on Gerontology as well as the Outstanding Mentorship Award from the Gerontological Society of America.

GPSR Authorized Representative: Easy Access System Europe, Mustamäe tee
50, 10621 Tallinn, Estonia, gpsr.requests@easproject.com

www.ingramcontent.com/pod-product-compliance
Lightning Source LLC
Chambersburg PA
CBHW022137020426
42334CB00015B/937